Endocrine Pathophysiology

Endocrine Pathophysiology

Catherine B. Niewoehner, M.D.

Associate Professor of Medicine
University of Minnesota School of Medicine
Staff Physician, Endocrinology/Metabolism Section
Veterans Administration Medical Center
Minneapolis, Minnesota

Fence Creek
Publishing

Madison,
Connecticut

Typesetter: Pagesetters, Brattleboro, VT
Printer: Port City Press, Baltimore, MD
Illustrations by Visible Productions, Fort Collins, CO
Distributors:

United States and Canada
Blackwell Science, Inc.
Commerce Place
350 Main Street
Malden, MA 02148
Telephone orders: 800-215-1000 or 781-388-8250
Fax orders: 781-388-8270

Australia
Blackwell Science, PTY LTD.
54 University Street
Carlton, Victoria 3053
Telephone orders: 61-39-347-0300
Fax orders: 61-39-347-5001

Outside North America and Australia
Blackwell Science, LTD.
c/o Marston Book Service, LTD.
P.O. Box 269
Abingdon Oxon, OX 14 4XN England
Telephone orders: 44-1-235-465500
Fax orders: 44-1-235-465555

2 3 4 5 6 7 8 9 10

TABLE OF CONTENTS

CONTRIBUTORS

John P. Bantle, M.D.
Professor of Medicine
Division of Endocrinology and Diabetes
University of Minnesota School of Medicine
Minneapolis, Minnesota

Charles J. Billington, M.D.
Associate Professor of Medicine
University of Minnesota School of Medicine
Director, Special Diagnostic and Treatment Unit
Veterans Affairs Medical Center
Minneapolis, Minnesota

Erica A. Eugster, M.D.
Clinical Assistant Professor of Pediatrics
Indiana University School of Medicine
Department of Pediatrics
Riley Hospital
Indianapolis, Indiana

Susan L. Freeman, M.D.
Assistant Professor of Medicine
University of Minnesota School of Medicine
Minneapolis, Minnesota
Chief, Section of Endocrinology and
    Vice-President of Medical Affairs
Regions Hospital
St. Paul, Minnesota

Angeliki Georgopoulos, M.D.
Associate Professor of Medicine
University of Minnesota School of Medicine
Medial Director, Women Veterans Program
Veterans Affairs Medical Center
Minneapolis, Minnesota

J. Michael Gonzales-Campoy, M.D., Ph.D.
Clinical Assistant Professor of Medicine
University of Minnesota School of Medicine
Minneapolis, Minnesota

David M. Kendall, M.D.
Clinical Assistant Professor of Medicine
University of Minnesota School of Medicine
Park Nicollet Clinic and International Diabetes Center
Minneapolis, Minnesota

Virginia R. Lupo, M.D.
Assistant Professor of Medicine
University of Minnesota School of Medicine
Director, Maternal-Fetal Medicine
Department of Obstetrics and Gynecology
Hennepin County Medical Center
Minneapolis, Minnesota

Cary N. Mariash, M.D.
Professor of Medicine, Cell Biology, and Neuroanatomy
Interim Director, Division of Endocrinology and Diabetes
University of Minnesota School of Medicine
Minneapolis, Minnesota

Antoinette M. Moran, M.D.
Assistant Professor of Pediatrics
Department of Pediatrics
University of Minnesota School of Medicine
Minneapolis, Minnesota

Jack H. Oppenheimer, M.D.
Emeritus Professor of Medicine, Cell Biology, and Anatomy
Division of Endocrinology and Diabetes
University of Minnesota School of Medicine
Minneapolis, Minnesota

Elizabeth R. Seaquist, M.D.
Associate Professor of Medicine
Division of Endocrinology and Diabetes
University of Minnesota School of Medicine
Minneapolis, Minnesota

Joseph J. Sockalosky, M.D.
Assistant Professor of Pediatrics
University of Minnesota School of Medicine
Minneapolis, Minnesota
Director, Medical Education, Children's Health Care
St. Paul Children's Hospital
St. Paul, Minnesota

Christopher H. Sorli, M.D., Ph.D.
Assistant Professor of Medicine
Diabetes Division
University of Massachusetts School of Medicine
Worcester, Massachusetts

When preparing this book we have tried to keep in mind three major principles of medical practice: (1) the human body and its disorders are complex and wonderful; (2) we must ask the right questions in order to get answers; and (3) if we do not understand the underlying pathophysiology, we will not know the right questions to ask.

Endocrinology is about communication between tissues by chemical mediators. The field of endocrinology is expanding so rapidly that even endocrinologists become overwhelmed. We have tried to concentrate on basic principles of endocrine pathophysiology and to illustrate their significance with clinical problems. It seems more important to provide a framework within which students can begin to solve problems than to provide exhaustive detail. New approaches for treating endocrine disorders have been appearing quite rapidly. We have focused upon the pathophysiology underlying these approaches, rather than on the details of treatment, because these change constantly.

We have begun this book with a brief review of general concepts of hormone and receptor interaction that are introduced in the first year of medical school. Our discussion of specific areas of endocrinology begins with the pituitary gland, the "master gland," which, together with the hypothalamus, controls many target glands. This is followed by discussion of other classic glands of the endocrine system: the thyroid and adrenal glands and their disorders; the parathyroid glands and regulation of calcium homeostasis; and normal and abnormal hormonal regulation of blood glucose by the endocrine pancreas. Subsequent sections on lipid disorders and obesity emphasize control of fuel and energy metabolism. We conclude with the sections on the complex hormone regulation of male and female reproduction, growth, sexual development, puberty, pregnancy and lactation, which are affected by all of the hormone systems described previously.

Since endocrine disorders are very common, we hope that you will find the material relevant and exciting!

Catherine B. Niewoehner

ACKNOWLEDGMENTS

We are especially grateful to Jane Edwards at Fence Creek Publishing for her invaluable editing skills, her attention to details, and her patience. She has done her best to protect us from errors; those that remain are our responsibility. Matt Harris at Fence Creek Publishing provided the format for the book and has been a constant source of support. We would like to thank Claudia Durand for her secretarial assistance. The time and effort of the contributing authors also is appreciated.

To my students with thanks
To Elizabeth, Richard, and Christopher with pleasure
To Dennis Niewoehner with love

INTRODUCTION

Endocrine Pathophysiology is one of six titles in the *Pathophysiology Series* from Fence Creek Publishing. These books have been designed as course supplements and aids for board review for second- and third-year medical students who are studying the pathophysiology of individual organ systems. Each book in the series is an overview of a major organ system with an emphasis on pathophysiology. Diagnosis, treatment, and management of specific diseases are also covered at a level appropriate for preclinical study. Each chapter has one or more clinical cases integrated throughout the text; the resolution of these cases requires mastery of the pathophysiologic concepts presented in the chapter.

Each book in the *Pathophysiology Series* shares common features and formats. Difficult concepts are presented in a brief and focused format to provide a pedagogical aid that facilitates both knowledge acquisition and review. Extensive use of margin notes, figures, tables, and board-review questions illuminates the basic science principles of pathophysiology.

Given the long gestation period necessary to publish a book, it is often impossible for publishers to keep pace with the rapid changes and advances. However, the authors and the publisher recognize the need to have access to the most current information and are committed to keeping *Endocrine Pathophysiology* as up to date as possible between editions. As the field of endocrinology evolves, updates to this text may be posted on our web site periodically at http://www.fencecreek.com.

We hope that the student finds the format and the text material relevant, interesting, and challenging. The Fence Creek staff and the authors welcome your comments and suggestions for use in future editions.

Chapter 1

GENERAL CONCEPTS IN ENDOCRINOLOGY

Catherine B. Niewoehner, M.D.

■ CHAPTER OUTLINE

■ ENDOCRINOLOGY DEFINED

The endocrine system and the nervous system are the two major systems by which cells and tissues communicate. Originally endocrinology was defined as the study of glands that produce chemical mediators called *hormones*. Hormones are secreted directly (not via ducts) into the circulation and exert their effects by binding to receptors in or on target cells. It is now clear that virtually every tissue can produce substances that act like hormones and that hormones can act within the same cell (autocrine action), on neighboring cells (paracrine action), or on distal cells (endocrine action). The boundaries of endocrinology are somewhat arbitrary but include the following:

- Regulation of hormone synthesis and secretion
- Hormone-receptor interaction and how it results in specific biologic effects
- Interaction between endocrine organs and target tissues, including normal feedback loops, perturbed feedback loops, and use of feedback loops to monitor endocrine therapy
- Symptoms and signs of hormone excess or deficiency
- Regulation of energy metabolism, reproduction, and growth

■ HORMONE-RECEPTOR INTERACTIONS

HORMONE-RECEPTOR COMPLEX

Response to hormones requires:
Normal receptor protein structure
Receptor availability
Intact receptor signaling
Normal postreceptor events

Hormone receptors are proteins that bind hormones with high affinity and specificity. Each receptor usually binds only one kind of hormone efficiently. Cells respond only to certain hormones because they only have receptors for certain hormones. Each receptor has a domain that recognizes a specific hormone and a domain that generates a signal once the hormone is bound. Hormone-binding alters receptor conformation.

Receptors located in the cell membrane usually are present in excess of the amount needed for the maximum biologic response. Since hormones are present in low concentrations in the circulation, the maximum biologic response of cell surface receptors is determined by the hormone concentration. Nuclear receptors usually are present in low concentrations in the cell, and the number of receptors determines the extent of the biologic response.

Normal events at the postreceptor level are necessary for normal hormone action. Cells must also have a mechanism for release of bound hormone or destruction of the hormone-receptor complex to turn the action of a hormone off!

■ MAJOR CLASSES OF HORMONES

Hormones are divided into two main classes: *the peptide or glycoprotein hormones* and the *steroid and steroid-type hormones* (Table 1-1). The steroid-type hormones include thyroid hormones and 1,25-dihydroxyvitamin D. Although they are not true steroids in the structural sense, their mechanism of action places them in a class with steroid hormones.

Table 1-1
Peptide and Steroid Hormones

PEPTIDE HORMONES	DISTINGUISHING CHARACTERISTICS	STEROID AND STEROID-TYPE HORMONES	DISTINGUISHING CHARACTERISTICS
Hypothalamic hormones Corticotropin-releasing hormone (CRH) Growth hormone–releasing hormone (GHRH) Gonadotropin-releasing hormone (GnRH) Thyrotropin-releasing hormone (TRH)	Attach to receptors on cell surface Activation of G proteins and kinases Subsequent activation of second messengers Changes in cell calcium and phosphorylation state Changes in cell secretion and protein synthesis Water soluble Catabolized in gastrointestinal (GI) tract; poorly absorbed from skin Short half-life	**Steroid hormones: adrenal or gonadal hormones** Aldosterone Cortisol Dehydroepiandrosterone Progesterone Testosterone Dihydrotestosterone Estradiol	Enter cell cytoplasm and nucleus Interact with receptors in cytoplasm and nucleus Hormone-receptor complex interacts with DNA Changes in protein synthesis Fat soluble Absorbed from GI tract and skin Longer half-life if protein bound or stored in fat
Anterior pituitary hormones Adrenocorticotropic hormone (ACTH) Follicle-stimulating hormone (FSH) Growth hormone (GH) Thyroid-stimulating hormone (TSH) Prolactin (somatomammotropin)		**Steroid-type hormones** Triiodothyronine (T_3) Thyroxine (T_4) 1,25-Dihydroxyvitamin D [1,25(OH)$_2$ D]	
Posterior pituitary hormones Antidiuretic hormone (ADH) Oxytocin			
Pancreatic islet hormones Glucagon Insulin Somatostatin			
Calcium-regulating hormones Calcitonin Parathyroid hormone (PTH) Parathyroid hormone–related peptide (PTHrP)			
Additional peptide hormones Epinephrine Human chorionic gonadotropin (HCG) Human chorionic somatomammotropin (HCS) [human placental lactogen, HPL] Inhibin Insulin-like growth factor-1 (IGF-1) [somatomedin C]			

PEPTIDE AND PROTEIN HORMONES

Peptide hormone synthesis follows the typical sequence for protein synthesis: gene activation, transcription of DNA, formation of messenger RNA (mRNA), and translation of mRNA into protein. The initial, large preprohormone enters the endoplasmic reticulum. A signal sequence is cleaved; the remaining prohormone or hormone undergoes further modification, is packaged into vesicles, and delivered to the Golgi apparatus. Most of the hormone is stored in the gland in granules awaiting the appropriate stimulus for release. Sometimes peptide hormones are altered further while in the storage granules. For example, insulin is stored as a larger molecule, proinsulin, which is cleaved to insulin and another peptide at the time the insulin is released. Sugar molecules are added to some peptide hormones to form glycoproteins. Major peptide hormones are listed in Table 1-1.

Once released into the circulation, most peptide hormones travel unbound to carrier proteins. The unbound proteins are subject to attack by proteases, and therefore, they tend to have short half-lives. They cannot be given orally because they are hydrolyzed by acid in the stomach or peptidases in the intestine. Glycoprotein hormones are more stable and usually last longer in the circulation.

Peptide hormones are water soluble and cannot cross cell membranes easily. They bind to receptors on the cell surface. Binding of most peptide hormones to their receptors activates guanosine triphosphate (GTP)–binding proteins, which act as on/off switches. Binding of insulin activates tyrosine kinases. Coupling of peptide hormones (*first messengers*) to cell surface membrane receptors generates *second messengers*, which set off cascades of reactions, leading to changes in the phosphorylation state (Figures 1-1 and 1-2). For example, a combination of a peptide hormone with its receptor activates a GTP-binding protein. This results in increased or decreased adenyl cyclase activity, which, in turn, increases or decreases cyclic adenosine monophosphate (cAMP) formation. cAMP activates protein kinase A, which initiates a cascade of phosphorylation mediated by other kinases.

Alternatively, a combination of a peptide hormone with its receptor can activate a GTP-binding protein, which activates phospholipase C. This generates diacylglycerol, which activates protein kinase C. This, in turn, initiates a cascade of phosphorylation mediated by other kinases. Activation of phospholipase C also generates inositol triphosphate (IP_3), which increases cytosol calcium by increasing calcium release from intracellular membranes.

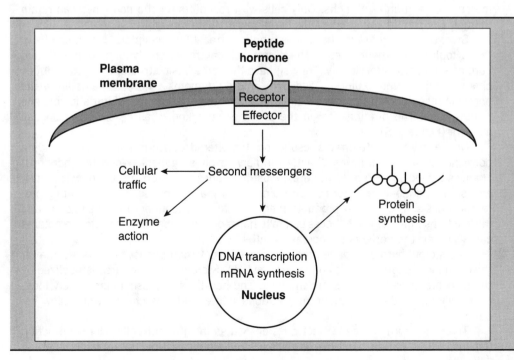

FIGURE 1-1
MECHANISM OF ACTION OF PEPTIDE HORMONES. Peptide hormones bind to receptors on the cell surface. Binding of hormones (first messengers) to their receptors changes the conformation of the receptors, which initiates reactions resulting in the formation of second messengers such as cyclic adenosine monophosphate (cAMP). Second messengers set off a reaction cascade, which results in changes in the phosphorylation state of cell components. This results in changes in cellular traffic, enzyme action, and protein synthesis.

FIGURE 1-2
PEPTIDE HORMONE RECEPTORS. Peptide hormone binding to its membrane receptor results in changes in receptor conformation, which are transmitted to the intracellular domain of the protein and initiate postreceptor events. The intracellular domains for receptors for hormones such as insulin and insulin-like growth factor-1 *(represented by the triangle)* have tyrosine kinase activity. Interaction of most peptide hormones *(represented by the rectangle)* with their membrane receptors (R) activates guanosine triphosphate–binding proteins (G). This results in increased concentrations of effectors (E) [also called second messengers] such as cyclic adenosine monophosphate (cAMP), inositol triphosphate (IP_3), or intracellular calcium (Ca^{2+}), which activate protein kinases.

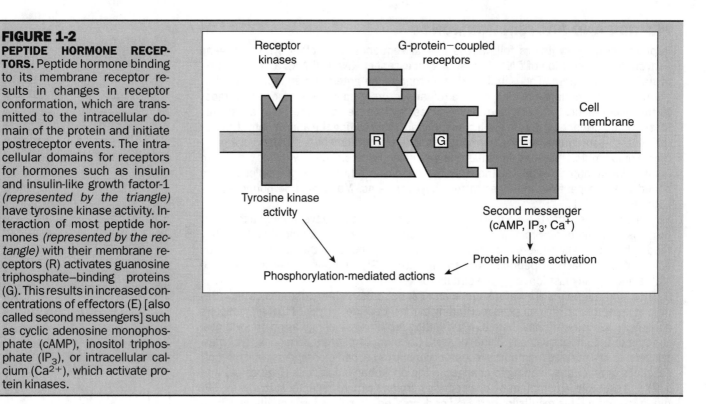

Changes in cell secretion and protein synthesis occur as a result of these changes in phosphorylation and intracellular Ca^{2+} concentration. These events can occur quickly and can be very transient.

STEROID AND STEROID-TYPE HORMONES

The basic steroid structure is derived from cholesterol. Steroid and steroid-type hormones are lipid soluble and must be carried in the circulation attached to carrier proteins such as sex hormone–binding globulin, thyroid hormone–binding globulin, and cortisol-binding globulin. They can be given orally. Since they are fat soluble, they can cross membranes and enter all cells. Only cells with receptors for the hormones can retain them. Major steroid and steroid-type hormones are listed in Table 1-1.

Steroid and steroid-type hormones bind to intracellular receptors, which can be in the cytoplasm or the nucleus. These intracellular receptors belong to the steroid hormone–receptor superfamily. They all have the same basic structure, which includes characteristic hormone-binding and DNA-binding domains. These domains allow the hormone-receptor complex to bind directly to DNA and alter the rate of initiation of gene transcription. The binding site on the target gene is known as a hormone response element (Figure 1-3).

Only a few hormone effects result from the altered transcription of genes binding hormone-receptor complexes directly (primary response genes). When this happens, changes can occur within 30 minutes. Most hormones act through secondary response genes. The hormone-receptor complex binds to primary response genes, initiating protein synthesis. The protein products then bind to the secondary response genes and initiate transcription. This process can take hours or days. Hormone-receptor complexes can also exert their effects by increasing mRNA stability.

The steroid hormone–generated cascade of events can persist for days, even after the hormone-receptor complex releases from DNA. Steroid hormones are metabolized by the cytochrome P-450 system in the liver. The half-lives in plasma can be very long, especially for synthetic hormone preparations with added side chains, which slow hepatic metabolism.

The same hormone can affect different genes in different cells. Hormone action depends on the presence of other gene regulatory proteins (transcription factors), which

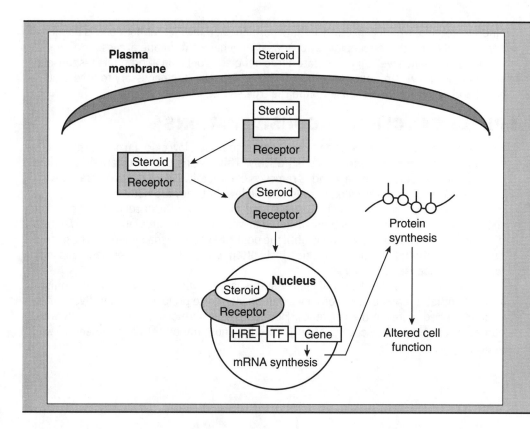

Plasma membrane

Steroid

Steroid / Receptor

Steroid / Receptor

Steroid / Receptor

Protein synthesis

Nucleus

Steroid / Receptor

HRE — TF — Gene

mRNA synthesis

Altered cell function

FIGURE 1-3
MECHANISM OF ACTION OF STEROID HORMONE. Steroid hormones bind to intracellular receptors in the cytoplasm or nucleus. The receptor changes conformation once the hormone-receptor complex has formed. The hormone-receptor complex enters the nucleus and binds directly to the DNA at the area of the gene known as the hormone response element (HRE). Binding results in activation of transcription factors (TFs), altered gene transcription, protein synthesis, and altered cell function.

can be specific to particular cells. Response to steroid and steroid-type hormones is abnormal if the receptor is defective or if there are mutations in the genes to which the hormone-receptor complexes bind.

▌ ADDITIONAL CONSIDERATIONS FOR HOMEOSTASIS

Hormones may have different actions at different times, depending on the presence of receptors and other modulators. One hormone may produce some effects in the fetus; different effects during childhood, puberty, or pregnancy; and other effects in adults, which change with age.

The endocrine system interacts with the nervous system, the immune system, and other systems. This is particularly evident in the interaction between the hypothalamus and the pituitary gland. As a result of this interplay, peptide hormones are secreted in pulsatile fashion, and normal pulse amplitude and duration are important for normal hormone action. There are also diurnal rhythms of hormone secretion and rhythms that are tied to the sleep–awake cycle.

In general, the system operates to maintain homeostasis. Excess hormone down-regulates the number of receptors. Decreased receptor availability diminishes tissue response to the excess hormone. Hormone depletion usually up-regulates receptors. Increased receptor availability increases the opportunity for tissue response.

Hormone secretion also is regulated by *feedback loops*. Hormones are secreted in response to a signal. The hormone acts on a target tissue to produce a response. When this response has returned the initial signal to normal, hormone secretion decreases.

Major Modulators of Hormone Secretion/Action
Age
Pregnancy
Nervous system
Immune system
Sleep–wake cycle
Feedback loops

▌ HORMONE EXCESS, HORMONE DEFICIENCY, AND HORMONE RESISTANCE

When control mechanisms fail, hormone excess and deficiency result in abnormal metabolism, growth, and reproduction. However, a high or low hormone level per se does not always represent the primary problem. A high hormone level can be an appropriate response to a persistent deficiency or represent an appropriate attempt by a gland to overcome hormone resistance (an abnormality at the receptor or postreceptor level in the target tissue). Some patients have polypeptide hormone receptors with abnormal GTP-binding proteins, which constantly initiate hormone action whether hormone is bound or not. Patients with these receptors appear as if they have a hormone excess.

A low hormone level might indicate a true deficiency or be an appropriate response to an abnormally low stimulus from a higher center. Usually it is necessary to assess both gland and target tissue response to find the true source of the problem.

■ PRACTICAL CLINICAL CONSIDERATIONS

Hormones are secreted in response to a specific signal (i.e., low calcium or high glucose), but some hormones are secreted constitutively. This means that circulating levels are usually undetectable unless a gland is removed completely. New sensitive assays reveal that in deficiency states hormone levels may be low, but they are not zero.

Since peptide hormones usually are stored in glands until needed, the signal for secretion often elicits an initial burst of stored hormone into the circulation, followed by a decrease in secretion of the hormone until the peptide synthetic machinery can be geared up. Hormone stimulation or suppression tests often are needed to assess gland capacity for normal response.

Hormone replacement for deficiency states is becoming more and more sophisticated. Synthetic replacement hormones can be altered to prolong their half-lives in the circulation and increase their potency. Hormones and hormone disorders usually were named at the time of discovery, often before the most important hormone action was known.

■ REVIEW QUESTIONS

Directions: For each of the following questions, choose the **one best** answer.

1. Several peptide hormone analogs are being considered for development. Based on hormone physiology, a hormone with prolonged action is most likely to be successful because

   (A) it needs to be taken orally only once a day
   (B) it is very tightly bound to its transport protein in plasma
   (C) it inactivates its receptor guanosine triphosphate (GTP)–binding protein
   (D) it is tightly bound to the hormone response element on DNA
   (E) it elicits a prolonged second messenger response

2. A large family is remarkable because many members have reduced responses to all of their steroid hormones. The problem in this family is most likely to be

   (A) decreased binding of hormone-receptor complexes to hormone response elements
   (B) decreased steroid hormone catabolism by the hepatic cytochrome P-450 system
   (C) decreased synthesis of a gene regulatory protein (transcription factor) in target tissue

Directions: The group of questions below consists of lettered choices followed by several numbered items. For each numbered item, select the appropriate lettered option with which it is most closely associated. Each lettered option may be used once, more than once, or not at all.

Questions 3–5

Gland X produces hormone A, which stimulates target tissue Y to produce hormone B. For each clinical situation described below, select the expected hormone level.

   (A) high A, high B
   (B) high A, low B
   (C) low A, high B
   (D) low A, low B

3. A patient has a congenital defect, causing gland X to function at a very low level.

4. A patient has a tumor, causing gland X to overproduce hormone A.

5. A patient is resistant to hormone A because of a receptor defect in target tissue Y.

▌ANSWERS AND EXPLANATIONS

1. The answer is E. Peptide hormones (first messengers) produce their effects by interacting with cell membrane receptors coupled to GTP-binding proteins. This generates second messengers such as cyclic adenosine monophosphate (cAMP) and intracellular calcium (Ca^{2+}), which activate kinases and alter cell phosphorylation. The more prolonged the second messenger response, the longer the effects of the hormone persist. Peptide hormones cannot be taken orally because they are digested by acid in the stomach and peptidases in the intestine. Most peptide hormones are not attached to binding proteins in plasma. Peptide hormones normally act through GTP-binding proteins and cannot exert their effects without them. Peptide hormones interact with receptors in the cell membrane. They do not enter the cytoplasm and nucleus and do not interact directly with DNA.

2. The answer is A. A defect that alters the binding of the superfamily of steroid hormone receptors to the response elements on DNA would confer a generalized defect in steroid hormone action. This would not be the result of decreased hormone catabolism, which would be likely to prolong hormone availability. Gene regulatory proteins allow steroid hormones to produce different actions in different cells because they are specific to particular cells. A defect in only one target tissue would not produce a generalized defect in steroid hormone action.

3–5. The answers are: 3-D, 4-A, 5-B. As a result of the congenital defect, gland X produces too little of hormone A. Without the stimulus of hormone A, target tissue Y cannot produce hormone B.

Overproduction of hormone A results in excessive stimulation of target organ Y, which then overproduces hormone B.

Tissue Y does not produce hormone B because it cannot respond to hormone A without receptors for A. The endocrine system is designed to maintain homeostasis. Therefore, lack of hormone B signals gland X to produce excess hormone A in an attempt to overcome the deficit.

▌REFERENCES

Chirgwin JM: Molecular biology for nonmolecular biologists. *Diabetes Care* 13:188–197, 1990.

Clark JH, Schrader WT, O'Malley BW: Mechanism of action of steroid hormones. In *Williams Textbook of Endocrinology*, 8th ed. Edited by Wilson JD, Foster DW. Philadelphia, PA: W. B. Saunders, 1992, pp 35–91.

Kahn CR, Smith RL, Chin WW: Mechanism of action of hormones that act at the cell surface. In *Williams Textbook of Endocrinology*, 8th ed. Edited by Wilson JD, Foster DW. Philadelphia, PA: W. B. Saunders, 1992, pp 91–104.

Lefkowitz RJ: G proteins in medicine. *N Engl J Med* 332:186–187, 1995.

Linder ME, Gilman AG: G proteins. *Sci Am* 267:56–61, 64–65, 1992.

Miller WL: Molecular biology of steroid hormone synthesis. *Endocrine Rev* 9:295–318, 1988.

Roth J, Le Roith D, Rosenzweig JL, et al: The evolutionary origins of hormones, neurotransmitters, and other chemical messengers. *N Engl J Med* 306:523–527, 1982.

Chapter 2
THE ANTERIOR PITUITARY

Susan L. Freeman, M.D.

■ CHAPTER OUTLINE

Case Study: *Introduction*	A 30-year-old man was referred to the endocrinology clinic because he had been impotent for 18 months. He had also complained of fatigue, weakness, and loss of libido. He used to shave daily but now only had to shave every other day. He had had intermittent headaches but no other illnesses or trauma. The only other change he noticed was that his shoe size had increased two sizes over the last 3 years. He could no longer remove his wedding ring, which previously had slipped off easily.

On physical examination, he was 6'2" and weighed 260 lbs. There was prominent frontal bossing (prominent supraorbital ridges) and a wide nose. There were no cranial nerve defects, and extraocular eye motion was intact. Peripheral vision was diminished bilaterally to confrontation. His tongue appeared to be of normal size; however, there were spaces between the teeth and dental malocclusion consistent with mandibular enlargement. The hands were enlarged and of a spade-like configuration. The thyroid gland was of normal size and consistency. The lungs were clear bilaterally, and the cardiovascular examination was unremarkable. The liver edge was palpable, but the abdomen was otherwise unremarkable. The testes were small and soft.

Laboratory studies revealed an elevated serum prolactin (PRL) level of 742 ng/mL (normal: 1–20 ng/mL). The growth hormone (GH) level was 7.5 ng/mL (normal: 0–5 ng/mL in men). The somatomedin-C (insulin-like growth factor-1 [IGF-1]) level was elevated at 324 ng/mL (normal: 51–115 ng/mL). The serum testosterone level was low at 92 ng/dL (normal: 300–1200 ng/dL in men). Luteinizing hormone (LH) and follicle-stimulating hormone (FSH) levels were also low. The remainder of the laboratory tests, including serum cortisol, thyroxine (T_4), and thyroid-stimulating hormone (TSH) levels, were all within normal limits. A fasting serum glucose level was 110 ng/dL (normal: 65–115 ng/dL). An oral glucose tolerance test was ordered, but the patient failed to keep the appointment.

■ INTRODUCTION TO THE PITUITARY GLAND

The anterior pituitary gland (adenohypophysis) is a central feature of the endocrine system. The word "pituitary" comes from the Greek *ptuo* (to spit) and the Latin *pituita* (mucus). It was thought that mucus produced by the brain was excreted through the nose by the pituitary gland. Today, of course, we know that the pituitary produces hormones, not mucus, and that its secretions are released into the bloodstream, not the nose. In fact, the pituitary is part of an elaborate hormonal system. It receives signals from the brain and hypothalamus and responds by sending pituitary hormones to target glands. The target glands produce hormones that provide negative feedback at the level of the hypothalamus and pituitary. It is the feedback mechanism that enables the pituitary to regulate the amount of hormone released into the bloodstream by the target glands. The pituitary's central role in this hormonal system and its ability to interpret and respond to a variety of signals has led to its designation as the "master gland."

ANATOMY

The pituitary gland is located at the base of the skull in a saddle-shaped cavity of the sphenoid bone called the sella turcica (Figure 2-1). This bony structure protects and surrounds the pituitary bilaterally and inferiorly. The dura, a dense layer of connective tissue, forms the roof of the sella (the diaphragm sella). An external layer of the dura continues into the sella to form its lining. As a result, the pituitary is extradural and is not normally in contact with cerebrospinal fluid (CSF). The pituitary stalk (or infundibular stalk) passes through a foramen in the dura, resulting in the appearance of the pituitary as a cherry on a stem. The anterior pituitary gland is called the adenohypophysis; the posterior pituitary gland is called

FIGURE 2-1

PITUITARY ANATOMY. The pituitary gland, which is connected to the hypothalamus by the pituitary stalk, lies within the sella turcica below the diaphragm sella. Posterior pituitary hormones are synthesized in hypothalamic nuclei and transported through the pituitary stalk to nerve terminals in the posterior pituitary. Anterior pituitary hormones are made within the anterior pituitary in response to hypothalamic-releasing hormones. Hypothalamic-releasing hormones are made in hypothalamic neurons and secreted into the hypothalamic-hypophyseal portal vessels, which carry them to the anterior pituitary. Note the location of the optic chiasm above the anterior pituitary.

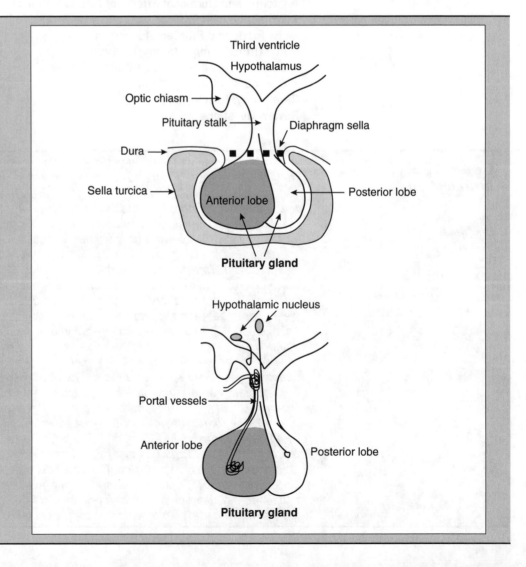

the neurohypophysis. The anterior lobe of the pituitary constitutes about 80% of the gland. It may double in size during pregnancy and shrinks in old age.

EMBRYOLOGY

The anterior pituitary is derived from Rathke's pouch, which is an ectodermal pouch of the primordial oral cavity. By 6 weeks gestation, the connection between Rathke's pouch and the oropharynx is totally obliterated, and the pouch establishes a direct connection with the downward extension of the hypothalamus, which gives rise to the pituitary stalk. The lumen of Rathke's pouch in humans is eventually obliterated by the developing pituitary gland. (Remnants of Rathke's pouch can persist as small cysts, which can give rise to tumors called craniopharyngiomas.) Secretory granules are seen in the developing pituitary at the end of the first trimester of pregnancy, and hormones can be measured as early as the seventh week of gestation. However, functional maturation of the pituitary axes is not fully developed until well into postnatal life.

Several cell types in the pituitary gland depend on a nuclear transcription factor, pit-1, for normal development. A deletion or mutation of the gene for this protein is associated with failure of these cell types to develop.

VASCULAR SUPPLY

The arterial blood supply of the pituitary gland originates from the internal carotid arteries via the superior, middle, and inferior hypophyseal arteries (see Figure 2-1). This network of vessels forms a unique portal circulation connecting the hypothalamus and the pituitary (see Figure 2-1). The branches of the superior hypophyseal arteries penetrate the stalk and form a network of vessels. All of these vessels drain into a series of long portal vessels, which transverse the pituitary stalk and terminate in a network of capillaries within the anterior lobe. It is through this portal venous system that hypothalamic hormones are delivered to the anterior pituitary gland.

CELL TYPES

The anterior pituitary is composed of a variety of cell types, which are responsible for synthesis, storage, and release of specific hormones. Most of these have been identified by immunohistochemical staining techniques using antisera for specific hormones and electron microscopy.

Somatotrophs produce growth hormone (GH). Lactotrophs produce prolactin (PRL). Corticotrophs produce adrenocorticotropic hormone (ACTH). Gonadotrophs produce luteinizing hormone (LH) and follicle-stimulating hormone (FSH), and thyrotrophs produce thyroid-stimulating hormone (TSH).

TSH, LH, and FSH are glycoprotein hormones composed of an α-subunit noncovalently linked to a β-subunit. The α-subunit is the same for all three hormones. It is the β-subunit that confers specificity of action. GH and PRL are composed of single chains of amino acids.

Anterior pituitary hormones are secreted in pulses. The pulsatile pattern of pituitary hormone release is essential for efficient and effective signaling of target tissues. Abnormalities in this pattern lead to target organ dysfunction.

▌HYPOTHALAMIC-PITUITARY REGULATION

Each pituitary hormone is regulated by one or more hormones synthesized and released by the hypothalamus. These hypothalamic hormones are transported into the pituitary via the hypothalamic-pituitary portal circulation. The hormones produced by the different pituitary cell types and the hypothalamic hormones that stimulate or inhibit their release are shown in Table 2-1.

The hypothalamic hormones bind to high-affinity cell membrane receptors on the appropriate pituitary cell types. The pituitary cells respond by secreting specific pituitary hormones that stimulate target glands. The target glands produce hormones that feed back to the hypothalamus and pituitary and regulate further release of pituitary hormones. This is called long-loop feedback (Figure 2-2). Feedback can be positive or negative and involves releasing factors and inhibitory factors. Short-loop feedback occurs when pituitary hormones feed back to the hypothalamus. If a target gland fails, there is a reduction in negative feedback, which leads to increased secretion of hypothalamic and

---

Two Different Tissues of the Pituitary Gland
Anterior pituitary (adenohypophysis) is derived from primitive oral cavity. Posterior pituitary (neurohypophysis) is an extension of the nervous system.

Anterior Pituitary Anatomy: Key Points
Well protected by bony sella
Highest blood flow of any tissue
Vascular (not physical) communication with hypothalamus
Hypothalamic hormones reach pituitary via portal venous system.

Anterior Pituitary

Cell Types	Percent
Somatotrophs	50%
Corticotrophs	15%
Lactotrophs	15%–20%
Gonadotrophs	10%
Thyrotrophs	5%

pituitary hormones. The pituitary is truly a "master gland" because it integrates signals from the brain and target organs and modifies its own hormone secretion to maintain a normal endocrine state.

Table 2-1
Hypothalamic-Pituitary-Target Organ Axes and Their Actions

Hypothalamic hormones	Growth hormone–releasing hormone and somatostatin (inhibitory)	Thyrotropin-releasing hormone	Corticotropin-releasing hormone	Gonadotropin-releasing hormone	Dopamine (inhibitory)
Pituitary cell type	Somatotroph	Thyrotroph	Corticotroph	Gonadotroph	Lactotroph
Pituitary hormones	Growth hormone	Thyroid-stimulating hormone	Adrencorticotropic hormone	Luteinizing hormone and follicle-stimulating hormone	Prolactin
Target organs	Liver, cartilage, and other tissues	Thyroid gland	Adrenal cortex	Ovaries and testes	Breast
Target organ hormones	Insulin-like growth factor-1 (somatomedin-C)	Thyroxine (T_4) and triiodo-thyronine (T_3)	Glucocorticoids (cortisol), mineralocorticoids, and androgens	Estrogen, progesterone, and testosterone	
Target organ hormones—major actions	Linear growth[a] and cell proliferation	Thermogenesis, growth,[a] and CNS maturation[a]	Stress response and sodium retention	Sexual maturation, menstrual cycle, gamete production, libido, and fertility	Milk production
Pituitary hyperfunction	Acromegaly and gigantism[a]	Hyperthyroidism (rare)	Hypercortisolism (Cushing's disease)		Galactorrhea, amenorrhea, infertility, and impotence
Pituitary hypofunction	Dwarfism[a]	Hypothyroidism	Adrenal insufficiency	Amenorrhea, infertility, decreased libido, and impotence	No lactation postpartum

Note. CNS = central nervous system.
[a] Seen only in children.

FIGURE 2-2
FEEDBACK LOOPS. Hypothalamic hormones stimulate anterior pituitary hormone release. Anterior pituitary hormones in turn stimulate target gland hormone release. Target gland hormones provide feedback to both the hypothalamus and the anterior pituitary. Anterior pituitary hormones also provide some feedback to the hypothalamus.

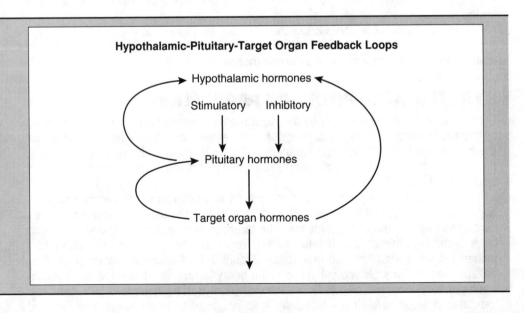

Hypothalamic-Pituitary-Target Organ Feedback Loops

Hypothalamic hormones

Stimulatory   Inhibitory

Pituitary hormones

Target organ hormones

HYPOTHALAMIC-PITUITARY AXES AND ASSOCIATED ANTERIOR PITUITARY HORMONES

HYPOTHALAMIC-PITUITARY-THYROID AXIS AND TSH

TSH is stored in secretory granules and released into the circulation in response to thyrotropin-releasing hormone (TRH), which is produced by the hypothalamus (Figure 2-3). When TRH is released, it interacts with a high-affinity membrane receptor on pituitary thyrotrophs and initiates a cascade of intracellular effects that lead to the synthesis and release of TSH. TRH has a direct effect on the transcription rates of both the TSH α- and β-subunit genes. TRH also is necessary for glycosylation of the subunits. Glycosylation is necessary for appropriate folding so that the tertiary structure of the peptides is stable.

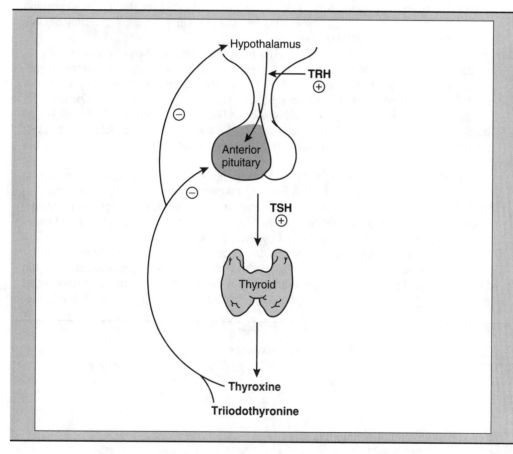

FIGURE 2-3
HYPOTHALAMIC-PITUITARY-THY-ROID AXIS. TRH = thyrotropin-releasing hormone; TSH = thyroid-stimulating hormone.

After TSH is released into the bloodstream, it binds to specific thyroid cell membrane receptors. This activates adenylate cyclase, which increases intracellular cyclic adenosine monophosphate (cAMP) levels and activates protein kinase A. This results in phosphorylation of proteins that regulate thyroid cells. These proteins increase the synthesis and release of thyroid hormones (thyroxine [T_4] and triiodothyronine [T_3]). TSH also increases the size and vascularity of the thyroid gland.

Once T_4 and T_3 are released into the bloodstream, they begin feedback inhibition of the production of TRH and TSH (see Figure 2-3). Within the pituitary gland, T_3 binds to specific nuclear receptors to form an activated T_3-receptor complex. This complex binds to specific nucleotide sequences on the TSH subunit gene and inhibits transcription. T_3 suppresses TSH levels within hours. Thyroid hormones also may decrease TRH stimulation of TSH secretion.

If the thyroid gland fails, T_4 and T_3 levels decrease, and TSH levels increase. If the thyroid is overactive, T_4 and T_3 levels increase, and TSH levels fall. Although T_3 and T_4 are the main regulators of TSH, several other hormones interact with the hypothalamic-pituitary-thyroid axis. Dopamine and glucocorticoids inhibit TSH secretion. The hypothalamic hormone somatostatin inhibits both TRH and TSH secretion.

HYPOTHALAMIC-PITUITARY-ADRENAL AXIS AND ACTH

ACTH is a 39–amino acid peptide, which is synthesized in pituitary corticotrophs as part of a much larger precursor molecule called pro-opiomelanocortin (POMC). ACTH release is accompanied by release of other peptide components of POMC. These include α-melanocyte–stimulating hormone (α-MSH) and corticotropin-like intermediate lobe peptide (CLIP), which are part of the ACTH molecule, and β-lipotropin (β-LPH), which contains the peptides β-melanocyte–stimulating hormone (β-MSH), γ-lipotropin (γ-LPH), and β-endorphin. The function of the other peptides is beyond the scope of this chapter. ACTH release is governed by the central nervous system (CNS) and hormonal mechanisms.

ACTH is secreted in a pulsatile manner, which is a reflection of its neural control. ACTH secretory bursts increase in frequency during sleep, resulting in a diurnal rhythm of hormone secretion. The highest levels of ACTH are present in the morning, about the time of normal awakening; levels gradually decrease through the day, reaching a trough around midnight. Reversal of the normal sleep–awake pattern results in a corresponding change in the diurnal pattern of ACTH secretion.

Corticotropin-releasing hormone (CRH) from the hypothalamus stimulates the production of ACTH. Psychologic stress and physical stresses like trauma, surgery, hypoglycemia, and fever also increase ACTH production. Some of these responses are mediated through interleukin-1, -2, and -6. Stress also increases the production of ACTH through catecholamines, serotonin, acetylcholine (ACh), or angiotensin II, depending on the type of stress present. Even exercise increases ACTH and β-endorphin levels in proportion to the intensity of exercise and the level of training. The more intense the exercise, the higher the levels.

ACTH acts on the adrenal gland through specific cell membrane receptors located in the adrenal cortex. The actions of ACTH are mediated through an adenylate cyclase mechanism resulting in synthesis and secretion of glucocorticoids (cortisol), mineralocorticoids (aldosterone), and adrenal androgens. ACTH also stimulates protein synthesis, which can lead to adrenocortical hypertrophy and hyperplasia.

The cortisol that is produced by the adrenal cortex feeds back negatively to inhibit both CRH and ACTH secretion within seconds or minutes and ACTH production within days (Figure 2-4). This is another example of a classic hypothalamic-pituitary-target gland feedback loop. If the adrenal glands fail, cortisol levels drop, and ACTH levels rise.

FIGURE 2-4
HYPOTHALAMIC-PITUITARY-ADRENAL AXIS. CRH = corticotropin-releasing hormone; ACTH = adrenocorticotropic hormone.

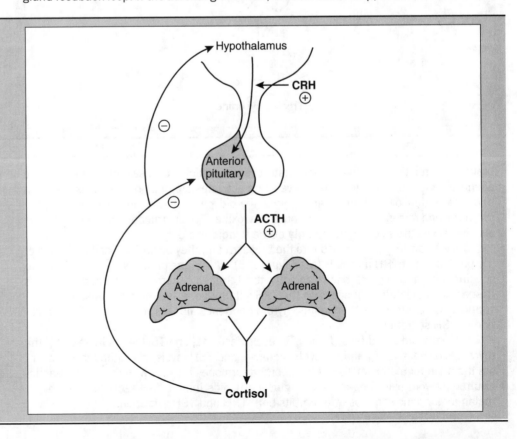

HYPOTHALAMIC-PITUITARY-GONADAL AXIS AND LH AND FSH

LH and FSH are the two anterior pituitary hormones that regulate gonadal function. Both hormones are released in response to the hypothalamic hormone gonadotropin-releasing hormone (GnRH). This hormone is also called luteinizing hormone–releasing hormone (LHRH).

There are several unique features of the hypothalamic-pituitary-gonadal axis. The first is that GnRH must be released in a pulsatile manner; the amplitude and frequency of the pulses determine the magnitude of the LH and FSH response. If GnRH is administered continuously, its receptors on pituitary cells are down-regulated, and LH and FSH release decreases.

Second, GnRH regulates the release of both LH and FSH, but the two hormones are secreted in different amounts at different times. There are variations in the sensitivity of LH and FSH to gonadal hormone feedback and also variations in sensitivity to the frequency and amplitude of GnRH pulses. If the GnRH pulse frequency increases, LH levels may rise more than FSH levels.

Third, LH and FSH have different functions in men and women. In men, LH binds to specific receptors on Leydig cells and stimulates the production of testosterone, which is essential for spermatogenesis, development of secondary sexual characteristics and sexual function, and maintenance of bone, mineral, and protein metabolism. FSH is essential for the normal function of Sertoli cells and spermatogenesis. Testosterone exerts negative feedback at the level of the pituitary and the hypothalamus (Figure 2-5). Gonadal failure results in increases in both LH and FSH.

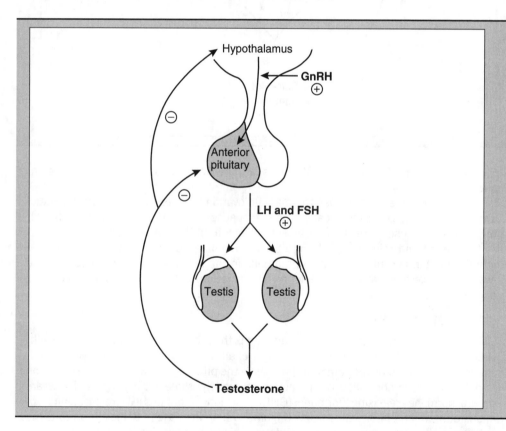

FIGURE 2-5
HYPOTHALAMIC-PITUITARY-TESTICULAR AXIS. In men, luteinizing hormone (LH) stimulates testosterone production in Leydig cells in the testes. Follicle-stimulating hormone (FSH) stimulates sperm formation in the seminiferous tubules. GnRH = gonadotropin-releasing hormone.

In women, the hypothalamic-pituitary-gonadal axis regulates the complex events of the menstrual cycle. GnRH from the hypothalamus stimulates pituitary gonadotrophs to release LH and FSH (Figure 2-6). FSH is critical for recruitment and maturation of a dominant ovarian follicle. As the follicle matures, the combined effects of LH and FSH stimulate the secretion of the ovarian hormone estradiol. This increase in estradiol inhibits FSH secretion by negative feedback, and plasma FSH levels fall. On the other hand, the LH pulse frequency increases, causing an increase in estradiol. The positive feedback of estradiol on the production of LH is a unique feature of the female gonadotropin axis. After ovulation, LH stimulates production of estradiol and progesterone by the ovary. These hormones exert negative feedback, causing GnRH pulses and LH and

FIGURE 2-6
HYPOTHALAMIC-PITUITARY-OVA-RIAN AXIS. In women, follicle-stimulating hormone (FSH) and luteinizing hormone (LH) regulate the events of the menstrual cycle. GnRH = gonadotropin-releasing hormone.

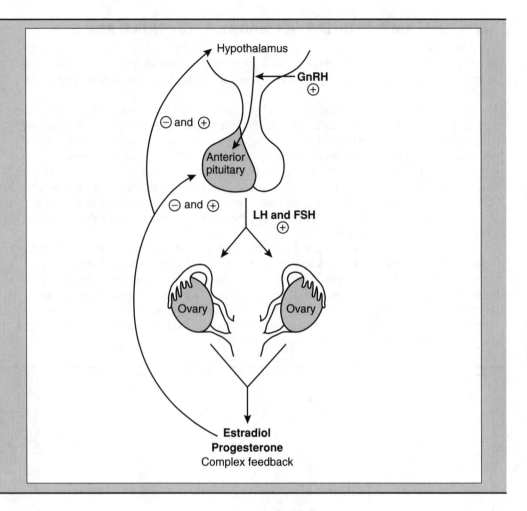

Unique Features of the Hypothalamic-Pituitary-Gonadal Axis

Normal action requires pulsatile GnRH and LH and FSH secretion.

GnRH regulates LH and FSH simultaneously but differently.

The axis is different in men and women.

In women, ovarian hormones provide both negative and positive feedback.

Effects of Growth Hormone

Increased

Linear growth

Bone thickness

Soft tissue growth

Nitrogen retention, amino acid uptake, and protein synthesis

Fatty acid release from adipose tissue

Insulin resistance and blood glucose

Decreased

Muscle glucose uptake

FSH levels to fall. When LH and FSH levels fall, the GnRH pulse frequency rises again, and the cycle repeats itself.

Menstrual cycles cease when there are no ovarian follicles left to produce estradiol and progesterone. This time is called the menopause. FSH and LH levels are high after menopause because there is no negative feedback from the ovarian hormones.

Secretion and release of LH and FSH are regulated by other peptides, including inhibin. Inhibin is synthesized by Sertoli cells in the testes and granulosa cells in the ovaries and exerts negative feedback on FSH secretion. Actions of inhibin are complex and are not well understood.

GROWTH HORMONE (GH)

GH is well named because its primary function is the promotion of normal linear growth. Growth hormone is a 191–amino acid single chain polypeptide, which is synthesized, stored, and secreted by the somatotroph cells in the pituitary. Growth hormone secretion is pulsatile and is controlled by the action of two hypothalamic hormones. These are growth hormone–releasing hormone (GHRH), which stimulates GH release, and somatostatin, which inhibits GH release (Figure 2-7). An increase in GH levels inhibits the action of GHRH and stimulates somatostatin. This is the short feedback loop.

The long feedback loop involves GH-induced production of insulin-like growth factor-1 (IGF-1), which is also called somatomedin-C. IGF-1 is produced and used locally by many tissues, but in the liver, IGF-1 is regulated by the action of GH on GH receptors. IGF-1 is secreted by the liver, exerts negative feedback on GH release, and stimulates somatostatin release. This creates the long feedback loop regulating GH production. Both GH and IGF-1 interact with different cell types to promote growth.

Physiologic factors also regulate GH secretion (Table 2-2). Sleep is associated with GH peaks. Growth hormone is secreted in response to exercise and physical stress. Insulin-induced hypoglycemia stimulates GH release 30–45 minutes after the blood

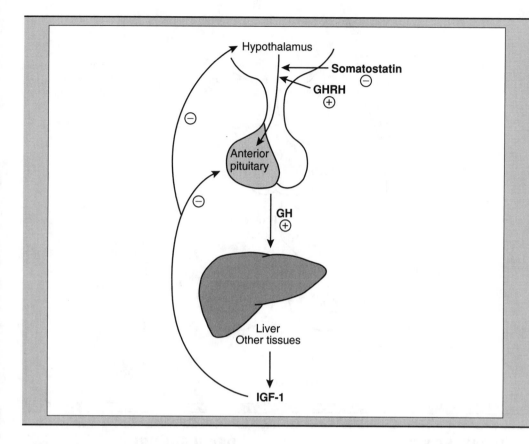

FIGURE 2-7
HYPOTHALAMIC-PITUITARY-GROWTH AXIS. Both somatostatin and growth hormone–releasing hormone (GHRH) from the hypothalamus regulate growth hormone (GH) secretion. Insulin-like growth factor-1 (IGF-1) is produced by the liver and released into the circulation. It also is produced locally in many tissues.

INCREASE GH	DECREASE GH
GH-releasing hormone (GHRH)	Somatostatin
Sleep	Hyperglycemia
Exercise	Hypothyroidism
Trauma	Glucocorticoids (decrease GH action)
Acute Illness	
Hypoglycemia	
Gonadal hormones (increase GH action)	

Table 2-2
Major Regulators of Growth Hormone (GH)

glucose level reaches its nadir. On the other hand, high blood glucose inhibits GH secretion. Low thyroid hormone levels are associated with low GH levels. Glucocorticoids (cortisol) inhibit somatic growth either by increasing somatostatin release or by causing damage to pituitary somatotrophs. Gonadal hormones play a role in the neuroregulation of GH secretion at the time of puberty.

Growth hormone is secreted in adults even after linear growth stops. In addition to its growth action on bone and soft tissues, GH also affects protein, carbohydrate, and fat metabolism.

PROLACTIN (PRL)

PRL is a 199–amino acid peptide made in the pituitary lactotrophs, which are also called mammotrophs. The regulation of PRL secretion is unique among pituitary hormones because PRL is secreted constitutively unless secretion is actively inhibited. Tonic inhibition of PRL is due to dopamine produced by neurons in the hypothalamus (Figure 2-8). Dopamine action at lactotroph receptors inhibits adenylate cyclase; this inhibits both PRL synthesis and secretion. Dopamine agonists suppress PRL secretion.

Because the hypothalamic action on PRL is inhibitory, disruption of the hypothalamus or the pituitary stalk can cause PRL levels to increase. Any dopamine antagonist increases PRL levels (e.g., phenothiazines, opiates, haloperidol). High levels of TRH in patients with hypothyroidism also increase PRL levels. When the hypothyroidism is treated, PRL levels return to normal. Other pathologic processes that increase PRL secretion are listed in Table 2-3.

The regulation of PRL secretion is unique among pituitary hormones because dopamine from the hypothalamus is required to keep PRL secretion suppressed.

FIGURE 2-8
HYPOTHALAMIC REGULATION OF PROLACIN (PRL) SECRETION. Hypothalamic dopamine inhibits pituitary PRL secretion. Suckling stimulates PRL synthesis via a neural reflex arc.

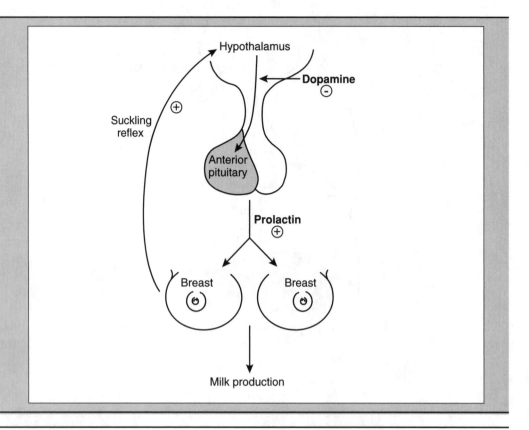

Table 2-3
Major Regulators of Prolactin (PRL) Secretion

INCREASE PRL	DECREASE PRL
Pregnancy (estrogen effect)	Dopamine antagonists
Suckling	
Nipple stimulation	
Chest wall trauma	
Sleep	
Exercise	
Hypothyroidism (high thyrotropin-releasing hormone)	
Pituitary stalk lesions	
Pituitary tumors	
Renal failure	
Liver failure	

PRL production is stimulated by high estrogen levels during pregnancy and by suckling in the postpartum period. The suckling effect is mediated by neural arcs. Pituitary lactotroph hyperplasia occurs during pregnancy and lactation.

The primary physiologic actions of PRL are preparation of the breasts for lactation and stimulation of milk production postpartum. During pregnancy, PRL is one of many hormones stimulating the development of the milk secretory apparatus. Lactation does not occur during pregnancy because of very high levels of estrogen and progesterone. After delivery, estrogen and progesterone levels drop, and high levels of PRL stimulated by suckling initiate lactation. Continued secretion of PRL is required if lactation is to be maintained.

PRL receptors have been found in other tissues. It is unclear what the physiologic action of PRL is at sites other than the breast. It also is not clear why men produce PRL.

Case Study:
Continued

At his initial visit, the patient had symptoms and signs of abnormal sexual function and abnormal growth of his hands, feet, nose, and jaw. The frontal bossing indicated enlargement of his frontal sinuses. His PRL level was high. GH and IGF-1 levels were also high, indicating a problem with GH regulation. His testosterone level was low. If his hypothalamic-pituitary-gonadal axis had been working normally, lack of negative feedback from testosterone should have stimulated the pituitary gland to produce high levels of FSH and LH. Since FSH and LH levels actually were low, the problem clearly was in the pituitary gland (or hypothalamus), not in the testes. The combination of abnormal PRL, GH, LH, and FSH levels and his history of headaches also strongly suggested a pituitary problem.

Six months after his first visit, the patient presented to his ophthalmologist for evaluation of vision problems. He had difficulty changing lanes when driving because of decreased peripheral vision. Formal visual field testing revealed bitemporal hemianopsia. The ophthalmologist obtained a magnetic resonance imaging (MRI) scan of the head, which showed a 3.3 × 4.3 × 3.0 cm enhancing intrasellar mass. The mass extended superiorly and impinged on the optic chiasm. It also extended into the cavernous sinuses bilaterally. It displaced both of the carotid siphons laterally. There was also some erosion of the floor of the sella. There were no calcifications or cystic areas in the mass.

Case Study:
Continued

ANATOMIC AND HORMONAL EFFECTS OF PITUITARY TUMORS

Pituitary tumors are seldom malignant and seldom metastasize. The problems they cause are related to (1) their space-occupying effects, (2) excessive hormone production, and (3) loss of function of the remaining gland.

Pituitary tumors that grow beyond the small, confined area of the sella turcica can impinge on or expand into surrounding structures (Figure 2-9) and produce significant signs and symptoms. A tumor that erodes the floor of the sella or extends into the sphenoid sinus may allow CSF to leak into the sphenoid sinus and into the nose, causing CSF rhinorrhea. Tumors extending laterally into either cavernous sinus can surround the carotid artery and produce unilateral defects in cranial nerves III, IV, $V_{1,2}$ (the ophthalmic and maxillary branches), and VI. The optic chiasm is located superiorly to the sella; in 80% of people, it is directly over the gland, separated from the pituitary only by the thin fold of dura called the diaphragm sella. The hallmark of chiasmal compression by a tumor expanding upward is the visual field defect called bitemporal hemianopsia (loss of peripheral vision). The eyes may not be affected equally, and other visual field defects, loss of visual acuity, and diplopia also are possible.

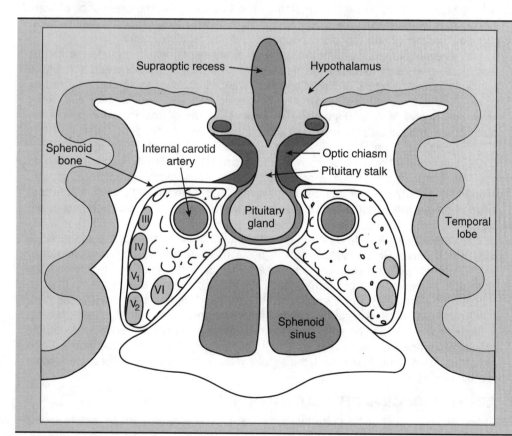

FIGURE 2-9
STRUCTURES SURROUNDING THE PITUITARY GLAND THAT ARE VULNERABLE TO EXPANDING PITUITARY TUMORS. (*Source:* Reprinted with permission from Lechan RM: Neuroendocrinology of pituitary hormone regulation. *Endocrinol Metab Clin North Am* 16:587, 1987.)

If a pituitary tumor is not producing a hormone, its space-occupying effects may be the first clues to its presence. A pituitary tumor should be considered in any patient who presents with headaches or visual changes. After the examination is complete, the presence of a pituitary tumor is best evaluated with an MRI scan. (MRI and computed tomography [CT] scans ordered for other reasons have resulted in the discovery of many pituitary tumors that might otherwise have gone undetected.) Tumors are loosely classified by size: a microadenoma is less than 10 mm in diameter; a macroadenoma is greater than 10 mm in diameter.

Hormone-secreting pituitary adenomas are thought to arise because of mutations occurring in the pituitary cells, not because of hypothalamic tumors overproducing releasing hormones. Almost all secreting pituitary tumors are monoclonal. Approximately 90% of pituitary tumors secrete *one or more* of the anterior pituitary hormones.

Pituitary Tumor Hormone Secretion	Percent of Tumors Diagnosed
Prolactin	60%
GH	20%
ACTH	10%
TSH, LH, and FSH	rare
Nonfunctional	10%

PROLACTINOMAS

The classic signs of a prolactinoma in a premenopausal woman are galactorrhea (leakage of milk from the breasts) and amenorrhea or infertility. Amenorrhea occurs because hyperprolactinemia suppresses pulsatile LH secretion and perhaps GnRH pulses as well. When the gonadotropin levels are suppressed, estrogen production is lower, and ovulation does not occur. The consequences are infertility and decreased libido and sexual function.

Men and postmenopausal women with prolactinomas frequently present because of symptoms created by the space-occupying effects of the tumor. Their tumors usually are larger than those in premenopausal women because premenopausal women with menstrual irregularities frequently seek medical attention sooner. Over 90% of men with prolactinomas have macroadenomas. Further evaluation often reveals impotence, loss of libido, and infertility.

The primary treatment for a prolactinoma is administration of a dopamine agonist such as bromocriptine. Transsphenoidal surgery may also be used, but a surgical cure for a prolactinoma is difficult to achieve. Radiotherapy can be used if all else fails.

GH-PRODUCING PITUITARY ADENOMAS

GH hypersecretion is often associated with hypersecretion of other pituitary hormones, particularly PRL.

GH-producing tumors cause the syndrome called acromegaly. The prevalence of acromegaly is 5–6 cases per 100,000 population, so even though it is the second most common disorder of pituitary overproduction, it is still relatively rare.

Acromegaly derives its name from the acral segments, which include the hands, feet, nose, chin, and forehead. Stimulation of growth of these bony and soft tissue segments is the hallmark of this disorder. Advanced acromegaly is characterized by spade-like hands, large feet, prognathism (prominent lower jaw), a large and fleshy nose, and frontal bossing (Figure 2-10). Progressive dental malocclusion occurs because of mandibular enlargement, and spaces form between the teeth. Often, a history of increasing hat, collar, shirt, glove, ring, and shoe size suggests the diagnosis. These changes occur insidiously over many years, so patients and family members often do not note them. In children, GH-producing tumors cause accelerated linear growth, resulting in gigantism. In adults, the epiphyseal plates have already closed, and further longitudinal growth is not possible. Additional symptoms and signs of acromegaly are listed in Table 2-4.

GH levels may fluctuate widely in an individual patient. This is not true of the IGF-1 level, which makes IGF-1 a more useful diagnostic measurement. Glucose suppression of GH is the best test for diagnosing acromegaly. Plasma GH is measured before and one hour after administration of oral glucose (75–100 g). In normal persons, but not in people with acromegaly, GH is suppressed to less than 2 ng/mL after this glucose load.

Treatments for acromegalic patients include surgery if the tumor is large, a long-acting somatostatin analog such as octreotide to suppress GH secretion, a dopamine agonist like bromocriptine (less effective with acromegaly than with prolactinomas), and radiation therapy. Suppression of GH may take years. A combination of these treatments is often necessary.

ACTH-PRODUCING PITUITARY TUMORS

Excess ACTH production by a pituitary tumor causes the adrenal gland to secrete excess glucocorticoids and androgens. The resulting syndrome is called Cushing's disease. Microadenomas account for 80%–90% of these tumors. The clinical manifestations of Cushing's disease reflect the biologic effects of adrenal corticosteroids (see Chapter 5).

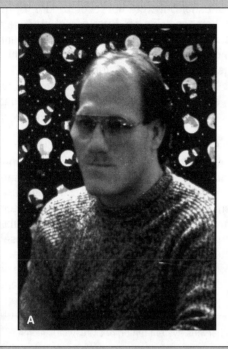
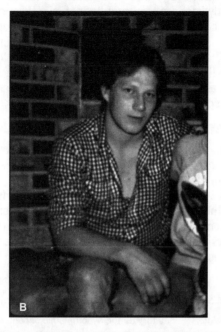

FIGURE 2-10
(A) A man with acromegaly. (B) The same man many years earlier. Note the coarsening of facial features, supraorbital prominence, and enlarged lower jaw in A as compared with the normal facial features in B.

Table 2-4
Symptoms and Signs of Acromegaly

Skeleton
Enlarged sinuses and prominent supraorbital ridges (frontal bossing)
Enlarged lower jaw (prognathism) and widely spaced teeth
Thickened bones (including the calvarium)
Large hands and feet

Connective tissue
Thickened synovium, resulting in painful joints
Large tongue and thickened tracheal cartilage, resulting in sleep apnea
Thickened vocal cords, resulting in a deeper voice
Thickened ligaments, resulting in carpal tunnel syndrome
Increased cartilage
Thick palms and soles

Muscles
Enlarged muscles with fiber atrophy, resulting in nerve entrapment, weakness, and fatigue

Viscera
Enlarged brain, lungs, liver, and kidneys
Increased heart size and hypertension, resulting in left ventricular hypertrophy, arrhythmias, cardiomyopathy, and congestive heart failure

Skin
Thickened with enlarged sweat glands and excess sebum production

Metabolism
Increased glucose production and increased insulin resistance, resulting in impaired glucose tolerance
Increased lipolysis
Increased protein synthesis
Increased tubular resorption of phosphate and increased urine calcium
Increased salt and water retention

These include central obesity, hypertension, purple abdominal striae, hirsutism, a round and plethoric face, easy bruising, glucose intolerance or diabetes, acne, and superficial fungal infections. Menstrual disorders, impotence, proximal muscle weakness, and back pain are also part of this disorder. Depression and other psychiatric disorders can be associated with Cushing's disease.

Cushing's disease occurs more frequently in women (female-to-male ratio 8:1). The symptoms are frequently insidious in onset. The diagnosis is established by determination of serum or urine cortisol levels and lack of suppression of cortisol levels with dexamethasone (see Chapter 5). Treatment for this disorder usually involves transsphenoidal surgery.

OTHER HORMONE-SECRETING PITUITARY TUMORS

Pituitary tumors that secrete excess TSH are very rare. They cause the classic symptoms of hyperthyroidism (see Chapter 4). Plasma levels of TSH and thyroid hormones are high. Treatment involves removing the thyroid gland or the pituitary tumor.

Gonadotropin-producing tumors are not unusual but were not recognized until recently because they secrete inefficiently and their secretion products do not produce a clinically recognizable syndrome. Gonadotroph tumors secrete intact gonadotropins and their subunits. The α-subunit, which is common to both LH and FSH, is frequently synthesized in excess of the β-subunit, so the synthesis of the β-subunit becomes the rate-limiting factor in the formation of intact hormones. As a result, gonadotroph adenomas are recognized only if they become large enough to produce symptoms related to the space-occupying effect of the tumor.

DISORDERS OF PITUITARY FAILURE

Failure of the pituitary gland is called hypopituitarism. Failure of individual cell types causes isolated hormonal deficiencies. Failure of the entire gland is called panhypopituitarism.

Specific disorders causing hypopituitarism are listed in Table 2-5. Pituitary tumors are the most common cause of hypopituitarism in adults. Impingement or compression of the anterior pituitary gland or the stalk by a large pituitary tumor can result in decreased functioning of the entire pituitary. Accidental head trauma is the leading cause of hypopituitarism seen at trauma centers.

Pathophysiology of Hypopituitarism
Primary pituitary disorder—loss of hormone secreting cells
Hypothalamic disorder—loss of releasing hormones
Extrinsic destruction of the hypothalamus, stalk, or pituitary gland

If hypopituitarism is due to damage to the hypothalamus, all pituitary hormones may be deficient except PRL, which normally is inhibited by dopamine from the hypothalamus.

Table 2-5
Major Causes of Pituitary Insufficiency

Invasion:	pituitary tumor, hypothalamic or central nervous system tumor, or craniopharyngioma
Injury:	head trauma
Infarction:	postpartum necrosis and pituitary apoplexy
Infiltration:	sarcoid and hemochromatosis
Infection:	tuberculosis
Iatrogenic:	pituitary surgery or radiation
Immune:	autoimmune hypophysitis
Idiopathic	

Postpartum pituitary necrosis, known as Sheehan's syndrome, occurs in women who experience massive blood loss, hypovolemic shock, or both during delivery. The pituitary gland enlarges during pregnancy, and hypotension or hemorrhage creates vasospasm in the hypophyseal vessels and ischemia. A hemorrhage that occurs in a preexisting pituitary adenoma is called pituitary apoplexy. Rapid expansion of the hemorrhage presents as severe headache, visual field defects, and acute hypopituitarism. This situation requires immediate surgery for decompression of the pituitary fossa.

The empty-sella syndrome also can be associated with hypopituitarism. An empty sella really is not empty. The pituitary gland is flattened against the wall of the sella by penetration or herniation of the subarachnoid space and CSF in the sella turcica. Primary empty-sella syndrome due to an incompetent diaphragm sella occurs predominantly in obese, multiparous, middle-aged women who are often hypertensive. One-third of these patients demonstrate some endocrine disturbance. Secondary empty-sella syndrome occurs in patients who have undergone pituitary surgery or radiotherapy for pituitary tumors.

Patients with pituitary failure usually are pale with fine skin and fine facial wrinkles. Symptoms and signs are due to the failure of the target organs to produce their hormones. A precipitous drop in ACTH causes a decrease in glucocorticoids, which can lead to hypotension and cardiovascular collapse. Because this is life-threatening, glucocorticoids are administered if this diagnosis is suspected, even before diagnostic testing is complete. Usually ACTH deficiency occurs gradually, causing chronic symptoms of glucocorticoid deficiency: weakness, lethargy, fatigue, nausea, arthralgias, myalgias, and vomiting (see Chapter 5). Chronic or partial ACTH deficiency may be exacerbated by an acute illness.

Hypopituitarism can also include TSH deficiency, which results in symptoms of hypothyroidism. These include fatigue, cold intolerance, constipation, dry skin, slow heart rate, and delayed drug metabolism. There is no goiter in the absence of TSH stimulation of the thyroid gland (see Chapter 4).

Hypopituitarism is treated by replacing target organ hormones, not pituitary hormones. Pituitary hormones must be given in pulsatile fashion. They have very short half-lives, and they cannot be given orally because they are destroyed in the gastrointestinal tract.

Deficiency of LH and FSH produces symptoms consistent with hypogonadism. Women develop amenorrhea and infertility. Men develop impotence and infertility. Both men and women experience loss of secondary sex characteristics and loss of libido. Whether GH deficiency causes significant increase in central fat mass, loss of lean body mass and weakness in adults is uncertain. Deficiency of PRL does not generally produce symptoms in adults except for the absence of lactation in the postpartum period.

Laboratory evaluation includes measurement of pituitary and target organ hormones (both should be low). Hypothalamic hormone concentrations in the peripheral circulation are too low to measure. Further evaluation (imaging, dynamic testing) depends upon the suspected cause of pituitary failure.

Case Study: Resolution

This patient had an enlarging pituitary adenoma producing PRL and GH. The space-occupying effects of his tumor caused his headaches, and extension of his tumor to the optic chiasm caused his bitemporal hemianopsia. The elevated GH levels resulted in typical symptoms and signs of acromegaly. The acromegaly was confirmed by a glucose suppression test. His GH level did not fall below 2 ng/mL in response to the glucose load.

His high PRL level suppressed LH pulses, which resulted in decreased testosterone production. In turn, his low testosterone levels resulted in decreased facial and body hair, decreased libido, and impotence. Destruction of FSH- and LH-producing cells by the tumor may also have contributed to his low testosterone level.

Although this patient's tumor was large, it did not compress and destroy the anterior pituitary completely. Adequate amounts of TSH and ACTH were being secreted to prevent hypothyroidism and adrenal insufficiency.

The patient underwent transsphenoidal surgery to remove the tumor. The bitemporal hemianopsia resolved immediately. Postoperatively the PRL level remained elevated, and he was placed on bromocriptine, which he continues to take. His GH and IGF-1 levels have returned to normal. He needs follow-up PRL and IGF-1 levels and glucose suppression tests to be sure that the tumor is adequately resected. These tumors often recur over time, since it is difficult to remove them completely. He might require additional therapy, such as treatment with a long-acting somatostatin analog in the future.

▌REVIEW QUESTIONS

Directions: For each of the following questions, choose the **one best** answer.

1. A 65-year-old woman is brought to the hospital 1 week after an automobile accident. For 2 months before the accident she complained of headaches. She had a psychiatric disorder, for which she was taking a phenothiazine, and a history of chronic renal failure. Physical examination revealed no signs of acromegaly or adrenal insufficiency, but she did have signs of a thyroid disorder. An magnetic resonance imaging (MRI) scan of the head and thyroid hormone, thyroid-stimulating hormone (TSH), luteinizing hormone (LH), follicle-stimulating hormone (FSH), and prolactin (PRL) levels were ordered. A high PRL level in this patient would most likely be due to

   (A) damage to the pituitary stalk during the accident
   (B) stimulation of dopamine secretion by the phenothiazine
   (C) a hypothalamic tumor producing gonadotropin-releasing hormone (GnRH)
   (D) a pituitary tumor producing TSH

2. A 60-year-old woman complains of cold intolerance, fatigue, constipation, and dry skin. Her physician suspects hypothyroidism and wonders whether it is due to a thyroid problem or a pituitary problem. If her laboratory tests show that she has hypothyroidism due to an abnormal thyroid gland, and her pituitary gland is functioning normally, which set of laboratory test results would she be most likely to have?

   (A) Low TSH, low thyroid hormones, and high FSH and LH
   (B) High TSH, low thyroid hormones, and high FSH and LH
   (C) Low TSH, low thyroid hormones, and low FSH and LH
   (D) High TSH, low thyroid hormones, and low FSH and LH

3. A 45-year-old man is referred to his physician by his dentist because of increasing malocclusion of his teeth and an enlarging lower jaw. He has been asked to bring old photographs with him. His features are coarser than in the past, and he has prominent supraorbital ridges, oily skin, very thick hands and feet, and a large tongue. His growth hormone (GH) level is 7 ng/mL after a glucose load. He is most likely to have

   (A) decreased lipolysis
   (B) decreased protein synthesis
   (C) decreased insulin action
   (D) decreased insulin-like growth factor-1 (IGF-1) levels
   (E) decreased gluconeogenesis

4. A 35-year-old man is undergoing an evaluation for impotence and infertility. His testicles are soft, and he has less body hair than he had in the past. He complains of fatigue. Testosterone, luteinizing hormone (LH), and follicle-stimulating hormone (FSH) levels are low. An MRI scan reveals a probable craniopharyngioma (tumor arising from primitive remnants of Rathke's pouch), which is quite large. If this tumor expands further, this patient is at risk for

   (A) impaired vision due to impingement on the optic chiasm
   (B) bilateral defects in cranial nerves IX, X, and XII
   (C) headaches due to shrinkage of the dura
   (D) excess cortisol production due to Cushing's disease
   (E) low prolactin (PRL) due to damage to the pituitary stalk

5. A 10-year-old child had radiation to the pituitary during treatment for a brain tumor 6 years ago. If radiation damage has caused loss of pituitary function, this child is most likely to experience which of the following?

   (A) Increased cortisol production in response to stress
   (B) Accelerated sexual maturation during puberty
   (C) Absence of the normal growth spurt during puberty
   (D) Development of hypothyroidism and a goiter (enlarged thyroid)

■ ANSWERS AND EXPLANATIONS

1. The answer is A. Dopamine produced by the hypothalamus normally inhibits PRL secretion. If the pituitary stalk was severed during the accident so that the portal circulation from the hypothalamus to the pituitary was interrupted, dopamine could not reach the pituitary gland. Phenothiazines cause hyperprolactinemia because they *inhibit* dopamine. High PRL levels inhibit GnRH pulses, but GnRH does not inhibit PRL secretion. Hypothyroidism is associated with high PRL. When thyroid hormone levels are low, absence of negative feedback causes the hypothalamus to increase thyrotropin-releasing hormone (TRH) production. High concentrations of TRH stimulate PRL production; normal TRH concentrations do not. A TSH-producing pituitary tumor would result in hyperthyroidism, and the high levels of thyroid hormones would suppress TRH.

This woman might have a large PRL-producing tumor. Since she is a postmenopausal, she would not have early warning signs of excess PRL production (amenorrhea, galactorrhea, infertility), which might have brought her to medical attention earlier. Her renal failure also could cause a high PRL level.

2. The answer is B. Absence of negative feedback due to low thyroid hormone levels should stimulate the pituitary to produce TSH. Since the patient is a postmenopausal woman, her ovaries do not produce enough estrogen and progesterone to suppress the hypothalamus and pituitary. FSH and LH levels are high in postmenopausal women.

3. The answer is C. The patient's GH level was not suppressed to less than 2 ng/mL after a glucose load. This is the gold standard for the diagnosis of acromegaly. Patients with acromegaly have increased lipolysis, increased hepatic glucose production (gluconeogenesis), and decreased insulin action (insulin resistance) due to their high GH levels. This combination can produce hyperglycemia and diabetes mellitus. GH stimulates protein synthesis, which is necessary for longitudinal growth in children and tissue proliferation in adults. IGF-1 should be increased by high GH.

4. The answer is A. The optic chiasm is located superiorly to the sella. In most people, it lies directly over the pituitary gland and is separated from the pituitary only by the thin fold of dura called the diaphragm sella. A large tumor can cause the pituitary gland to expand upward until it impinges on the optic chiasm. The major sign of such compression is bitemporal hemianopsia. The cranial nerves affected by pituitary or hypothalamic tumors are nerves III, IV, V and VI. Pituitary tumors cause headaches by stretching the dura, not shrinking it. Cushing's disease is due to adrenocorticotropic hormone (ACTH)-producing tumors, not craniopharyngiomas. If the pituitary stalk is damaged, dopamine from the hypothalamus cannot reach the pituitary to inhibit PRL secretion, and PRL secretion increases.

5. The answer is C. The 10-year-old child is at risk for panhypopituitarism. If this has developed, the cortisol response to stress would be decreased due to low adrenocorticotropic hormone (ACTH). Sexual maturation and the normal growth spurt during puberty would not occur because of low levels of luteinizing hormone, follicle-stimulating hormone, gonadal hormones, growth hormone, insulin-like growth factor-1, thyroid-stimulating hormone (TSH), and thyroid hormones. A goiter would not develop without TSH to stimulate growth of thyroid tissue.

■ REFERENCES

Abboud CF, Laws ER: Diagnoses of pituitary tumors. *Endocrinol Metab Clin* 17(2):241–280, 1988.

Casanueva F: Physiology of growth hormone secretion and action. *Endocrinol Metab Clin* 21(3):483–517, 1992.

Frohman LA: Therapeutic options in acromegaly. *J Clin Endocrinol Metab* 72:1175–1181, 1991.

Herman V, Fagin J, Gonsky R, et al: Clonal origins of pituitary tumors. *J Clin Endocrinol Metab* 71:1427–1433, 1990.

Lechan RM: Neuroendocrinology of pituitary hormone regulation. *Endocrinol Metab Clin* 16(3):475–501, 1987.

Mantozoros CS, Moses A: Whither recombitant human growth hormone? *Ann Intern Med* 125(11):932–934, 1996.

Melen O: Neuro-ophthalmologic features of pituitary tumors. *Endocrinol Metab Clin* 16(3):585–608, 1987.

Melmed S: Pituitary tumors secreting growth hormone and prolactin. *Ann Intern Med* 105:238–253, 1986.

Melmed S: Acromegaly. *N Engl J Med* 322:966–976, 1990.

Vance ML: Hypopituarism. *N Engl J Med* 330(23):1651–1662, 1994.

Chapter 3

THE POSTERIOR PITUITARY, ANTIDIURETIC HORMONE, AND OXYTOCIN

David M. Kendall, M.D.

■ CHAPTER OUTLINE

Case Study:
Introduction

A 36-year-old woman with mild mental retardation and a 5-year history of bipolar affective disorder was hospitalized on the inpatient psychiatry service. She had had several similar hospitalizations due to episodes of agitated depression, hallucinations, and mania. She failed to respond to multiple medications in the past and had stopped taking her psychotropic medication. Admission examination revealed a blood pressure of 110/68 mm Hg, a heart rate of 84 beats/min, regular respirations of 20 breaths/min, and temperature of 99.6°F. The neurologic examination was significant for intermittent tremor. She was minimally interactive with paranoid behavior.

During the first 3 days of hospitalization, the patient was described as "not eating well but drinking plenty of fluid." Serum sodium (Na$^+$) at that time measured 140 mEq/L (normal: 135–147 mEq/L); potassium (K$^+$), 3.7 mEq/L (normal: 3.5–5.0 mEq/L); blood urea nitrogen (BUN), 6 mg/dL (normal: 10–20 mg/dL); and creatinine, 0.8 mg/dL (normal: 0.8–1.4 mg/dL). On the sixth hospital day, she was still drinking large amounts of water. Nursing notes described "large amounts of clear urine voided." Because of her ongoing paranoid behavior, she was transferred to a closed psychiatric unit where free access to fluids was not allowed. On the ninth hospital day, the endocrinology service was asked to evaluate her excessive urination and thirst. Laboratory tests at that time revealed the following: serum Na$^+$, 155 mEq/L (normal: 137–145 mEq/L); K$^+$, 4.0 mEq/L; chloride (Cl$^-$), 115 mEq/L (normal: 95–105 mEq/L); bicarbonate (HCO$_3^-$), 25 mEq/L (normal: 22–28 mEq/L); BUN, 12 mg/dL (normal: 8–18 mg/dL); and creatinine, 0.8 mg/dL. Serum osmolality measured 312 mOsm/L (normal: 280–300 mOsm/L). Urine specific gravity was 1.005 units with a urine osmolality of 156 mOsm/L (both values at the low end of normal range). She had no glucose in her urine.

■ INTRODUCTION

Antidiuretic hormone is a nine–amino acid peptide synthesized in neurons of the hypothalamus. Its release is regulated by plasma osmolality and vascular volume.

The posterior pituitary gland is an extension of hypothalamic neurons, whose terminals lie closely opposed to the anterior pituitary gland. The major hormones secreted by the posterior pituitary—antidiuretic hormone (ADH) and oxytocin—are synthesized in specific hypothalamic nuclei (Figure 3-1). ADH plays a central role in the maintenance of water balance by inhibiting diuresis. In pharmacologic amounts, ADH raises vascular tone (blood pressure), so it is also known as arginine vasopressin (AVP). The term ADH will be used in this chapter.

FIGURE 3-1
SCHEMATIC REPRESENTATION OF THE HYPOTHALAMIC-POSTERIOR PITUITARY AXIS AND RELATED ANATOMIC STRUCTURES. Neuronal cell bodies within the paraventricular and supraoptic nuclei synthesize antidiuretic hormone (ADH) and oxytocin. These hormones are stored in the neuron terminals of the posterior pituitary gland.

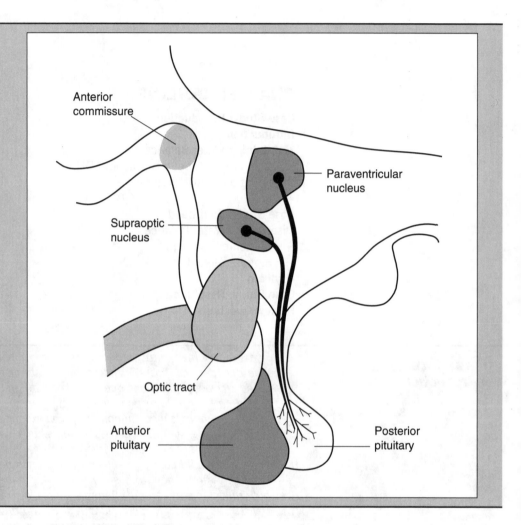

ADH is synthesized in the supraoptic and paraventricular nuclei of the hypothalamus and then transported along neuronal projections of these nuclei to the posterior pituitary gland. It is stored in the nerve terminals of the posterior pituitary until it is released in response to changes in plasma osmolality and intravascular volume. Separate cells within these same hypothalamic nuclei are thought to synthesize oxytocin, which also is transported to nerve terminals in the posterior pituitary for storage.

■ MAINTAINING WATER BALANCE

Water balance in humans depends on the complex interaction between water loss and water repletion. Total body water is maintained within a narrow range (defined by serum osmolality) through the balance of water ingestion and water loss in urine, feces, sweat, and water vapor. The water repletion reactions that maintain this balance are shown in Figure 3-2.

Water acquisition and water conservation are stimulated simultaneously by an increase in serum osmolality or by a decline in vascular volume. An increase in serum

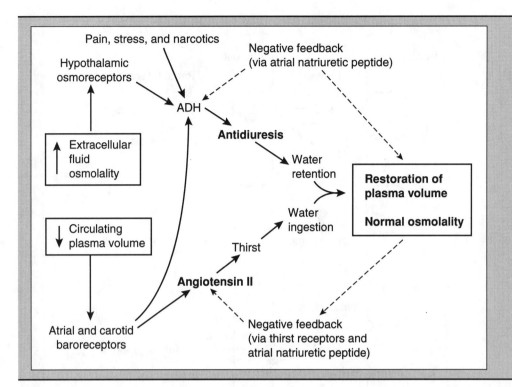

FIGURE 3-2
WATER REPLETION. The complex interaction between vascular volume and plasma osmolality is depicted. Note that antidiuretic hormone (ADH) release is dependent on both plasma volume and plasma solute. Negative feedback suppressing ADH release is provided by atrial natriuretic peptide.

osmolality is sensed within putative osmoreceptors located in the hypothalamus. This results in release of ADH, which causes antidiuresis. An increase in serum osmolality also increases thirst, which is regulated in an unknown fashion via release of angiotensin II. Changes in vascular volume are recognized by carotid and atrial baroreceptors. Stimulation of these osmo- and baroreceptors ultimately stimulates water conservation. This coordinated water repletion reduces extracellular fluid osmolality and increases circulating blood volume. Re-establishment of normal osmolality or vascular volume stimulates release of atrial natriuretic peptide (ANP) from the atrium, which provides negative feedback to inhibit further ADH release and angiotensin II production (see Figure 3-2).

Water balance in humans is primarily regulated by water ingestion (under the control of thirst) and water retention (under the control of ADH).

ACTION OF ANTIDIURETIC HORMONE (ADH)

ADH regulates water conservation at the level of the kidney by increasing the permeability of the renal collecting duct to water. In the absence of ADH, the renal collecting duct remains impermeable to water, and the dilute urine created in the distal nephron is excreted, resulting in free water loss. In the presence of ADH, water channels are translocated to the luminal cell membrane. This allows water to pass freely down its concentration gradient from the tubular lumen into the hypertonic renal interstitium. The urine becomes concentrated. The concentrating effect of ADH is critically dependent on the solute gradient across tubular cells, which is established in the renal medulla. A schematic representation of the effect of ADH on the collecting tubule is shown in Figure 3-3.

The mechanism by which ADH stimulates translocation of water channels involves interaction with its receptors in the collecting duct, which activates specific G proteins. This results in increased cellular adenylate cyclase activity. The increase in cellular cyclic adenine nucleotides creates downstream signals, which result in water channel translocation.

ADH is also a potent pressor agent (hence the alternate name AVP). However, plasma concentrations of ADH required to increase blood pressure are many times higher than normal physiologic concentrations. There is little evidence that ADH plays a significant role in maintaining normal blood pressure or causes hypertension in humans. Whether this pressor effect of ADH has a physiologic role in maintaining water balance is not known.

FIGURE 3-3
ANTIDIURETIC HORMONE (ADH) EFFECT ON RENAL COLLECTING TUBULE. In the absence of ADH, the collecting duct is impermeable to water. The dilute urine created in the distal nephron is excreted, resulting in free water loss. If ADH is present, water channels are transposed to the tubular cell membrane and water passes freely down its concentration gradient from the collecting tubule lumen into the hypertonic renal interstitium.

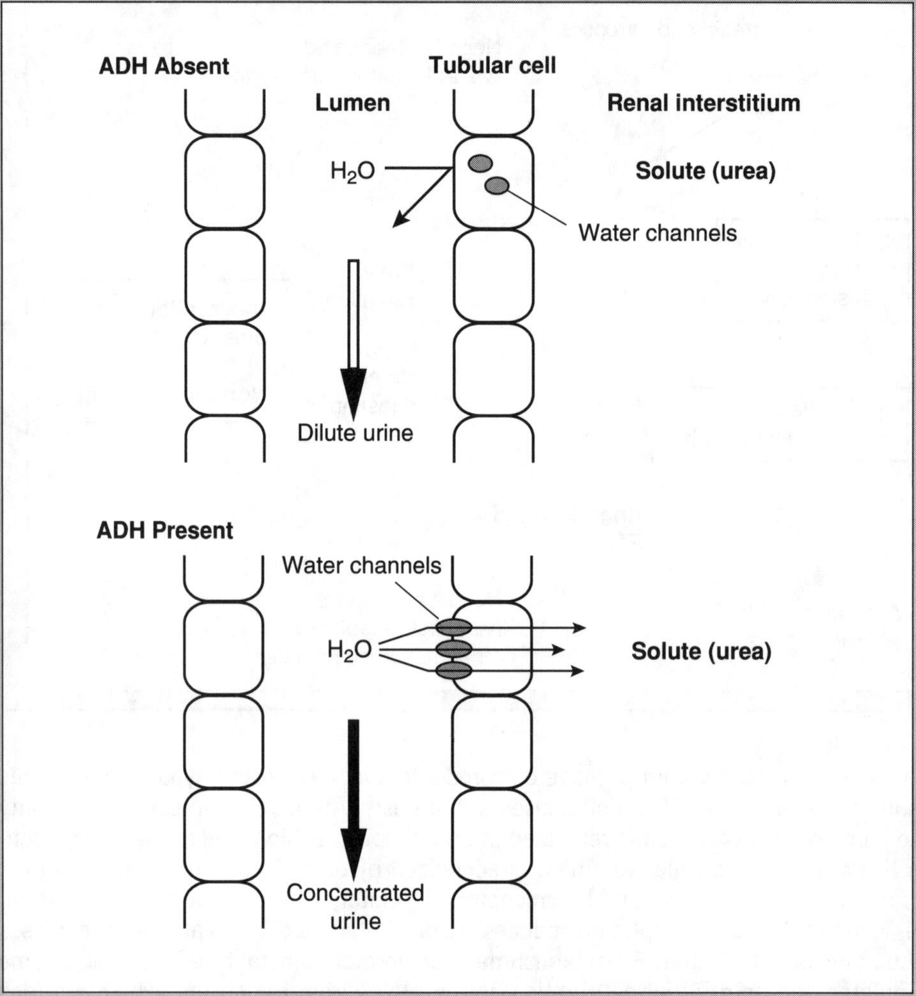

The **normal threshold** for ADH release *and* for stimulation of thirst is plasma osmolality greater than 285 mOsm/L.

REGULATION OF ADH RELEASE

ADH is released from the posterior pituitary in response to osmotic and nonosmotic stimuli. To maintain normal plasma osmolality between 275 and 300 mOsm/L, ADH secretion must respond to small changes in plasma solute concentration (Figure 3-4). As noted earlier, the osmotic stimulation of ADH release occurs through activation of putative osmoreceptors in the hypothalamus. The precise location and nature of these hypothalamic osmoreceptors are not clearly understood. As plasma osmolality rises, and water moves out of cells, the osmoreceptors become dehydrated, and ADH is released. This increase in osmolality requires an increase in *nonpermeable* solutes such as Na+ or glucose.

Nonosmotic stimulation of the posterior pituitary occurs predominantly through sensing of intravascular volume by baroreceptors in the atria and carotids. The relationship between blood volume, osmolality, and ADH release is such that a decrease in blood volume stimulates ADH release even if plasma osmolality is normal (or low). In dehydrated patients, low intravascular volume is a more important stimulus for water conservation than osmotic pressure.

THIRST

Regulation of the thirst response depends on many of the same factors as ADH release. Thirst is stimulated by a 2%–3% increase in plasma tonicity. Normal serum osmolality can be maintained even in the absence of ADH if enough water is ingested. The osmotic regulation of thirst occurs through osmoreceptors in the hypothalamus, which are

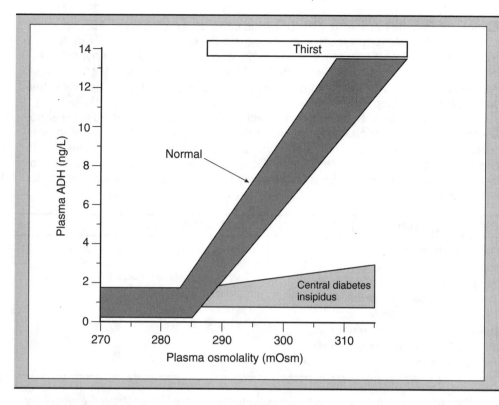

FIGURE 3-4
SCHEMATIC REPRESENTATION OF THE RELATIONSHIP OF PLASMA OSMOLALITY TO ANTIDIURETIC HORMONE (ADH) LEVEL IN NORMAL HUMANS (*DARK GRAY AREA*). Increased ADH release occurs at plasma osmolality above 285 mOsm/L. Individuals with central diabetes insipidus fail to increase ADH in response to plasma osmolality above 285 mOsm/L (*light gray area*). (*Source:* Reprinted with permission from Robertson GL: Vasopressin in osmotic regulation in man. *Ann Rev Med* 25:317, 1974.)

thought to be near the receptors that stimulate ADH release. Volume depletion detected by baroreceptors in the cardiac atria also regulates the water drinking response. Satiation of thirst occurs in response to many stimuli, including normalization of osmolality and esophageal stretch. These mechanisms control the ingested volume of liquids very accurately as osmolality approaches normal.

Case Study: *Continued*

The patient's increased urination and thirst and her high serum Na+ and plasma osmolality indicated a hypertonic state after she was deprived of free access to water. Her fluid restriction was lifted. Her serum Na+ fell to the normal range within 48 hours after she was allowed access to water. She continued to exhibit polydipsia and polyuria with a fluid intake of approximately 7–9 L/d. Review of her medical records revealed that she had been treated previously with lithium carbonate and that polydipsia and polyuria were noted at that time. A water deprivation test was ordered.

■ DISORDERS OF WATER BALANCE

Disorders of water balance can result in either hyper- or hypotonicity. Disorders related to the posterior pituitary are due to deficient or excessive secretion of ADH.

HYPERTONIC DISORDERS

Hypertonic disorders result from excess free water loss, inadequate free water intake, an impaired thirst mechanism, solute diuresis, defective ADH secretion, or defective ADH action. Major causes of hypertonic disorders are listed in Table 3-1. The ADH-related disorders result in two different forms of *diabetes insipidus*.

Table 3-1
Major Causes of Hypertonic Disorders

Excess free water loss	Inadequate free water intake
Central diabetes insipidus (DI)	Impaired thirst
Nephrogenic DI	Inadequate access to water
Sweating	**Solute diuresis**
Diarrhea	Hyperglycemia
Severe burns	Hypertonic intravenous infusion

Central (Neurogenic) Diabetes Insipidus
Decreased ADH secretion

Nephrogenic Diabetes Insipidus
Decreased ADH action

Etiology of Diabetes Insipidus (DI). DI is due either to a deficiency of ADH secretion from the posterior pituitary (central or neurogenic DI) or to renal insensitivity to ADH (nephrogenic DI). Water conservation in the distal collecting tubules cannot occur because ADH either is not present or is inactive. The dilute urine created in the proximal nephron is not concentrated as it passes through the renal parenchyma, and excess free water losses occur (see Figure 3-3).

The major causes of DI are outlined in Table 3-2. Conditions associated with central DI include trauma to the pituitary stalk and posterior pituitary destruction by a number of mechanisms. Transient DI after anterior pituitary surgery is common, perhaps due to edema temporarily affecting the pituitary stalk. Permanent DI is rare after anterior pituitary surgery; the risk is higher after surgery for a hypothalamic tumor. The risk for permanent DI depends on the extent of the damage to the pituitary stalk.

Table 3-2
Major Causes of Central and Nephrogenic Diabetes Insipidus (DI)

CENTRAL (NEUROGENIC) DI	NEPHROGENIC DI
Trauma to pituitary stalk	Toxins or drugs (demeclocycline, lithium, others)
Hypothalamic or pituitary surgery	
Tumors (infiltration)	Vascular (sickle cell disease)
Granulomatous disease (tuberculosis, sarcoid)	Infection (pyelonephritis)
Ischemia (postpartum hemorrhage)	Infiltration (amyloid)
Infection (viral encephalitis, meningitis)	Familial (X-linked)
Inflammation (autoimmune hypophysitis)	
Familial (autosomal dominant)	

Nephrogenic DI usually is due to chronic renal disease, which destroys the medullary concentrating gradient, or to drugs that inhibit ADH action, like demeclocycline and lithium. Nephrogenic DI also can be the result of rare congenital defects in the ADH receptor or postreceptor pathways.

The clinical picture of polyuria and thirst is the same regardless of the cause of DI. The symptoms were described eloquently by Quain in the *Dictionary of Medicine* published in 1883:

> Regarding the clinical history of polyuria, thirst and watery urine are the two prime symptoms, for there may be little wasting and the general health may be good. As long as drink is supplied in plenty, the condition of the patients is very tolerable, were it not for the broken sleep caused by the increased thirst and the desire to pass water. But any attempt to restrict the quantity of fluid gives rise to intense discomfort . . . the urine is inordinate in its quantity, and the specific gravity little above that of spring water . . . persistently at 1.001. If the drink is restricted, more will be passed than is consumed by the abstraction of water from the body.

Symptoms and Signs of Diabetes Insipidus
Excessive thirst
High fluid intake
High urine output
Plasma osmolality high or normal
Urine osmolality low

Urine volumes in excess of 6 L/24 hr can be generated. Maximal 24-hour urine volume is approximately 18 L, the total glomerular filtrate generated daily. The free water loss and increased osmolality stimulate profound thirst. If access to water is denied, hypertonicity worsens. However, if the thirst mechanism is intact, osmolality can be maintained within the normal range as long as water intake is equivalent to water loss.

Differential Diagnosis of DI. DI should be suspected whenever patients present with unexplained thirst, high fluid intake, large urine volumes, and dilute urine (urine osmolality less than plasma osmolality). The initial problem in differential diagnosis usually is distinguishing DI from psychogenic polydipsia (compulsive water drinking) or an abnormal thirst mechanism. Psychogenic water drinkers ingest large volumes of water, which dilutes plasma, suppresses ADH, and results in large volumes of dilute urine.

Evaluation of patients with suspected DI begins with laboratory tests of plasma and urine osmolality (Table 3-3). Psychogenic water drinkers should have decreased plasma osmolality, and patients with DI should have increased osmolality or normal osmolality if water intake is adequate. The next step in the evaluation is the water deprivation test. Patients are deprived of water in a controlled setting to avoid dangerous dehydration and surreptitious water ingestion. Urine osmolality will not increase in patients with either form of DI but should increase in patients with psychogenic polyuria.

	CENTRAL DI	NEPHROGENIC DI	PSYCHOGENIC WATER DRINKING
Plasma osmolality	Increased or normal	Increased or normal	Decreased
Urine osmolality	Decreased	Decreased	Decreased
Urine osmolality during water deprivation	No change	No change	Increased
Urine osmolality after dDAVP	Increased	No change	Increased
Plasma ADH	Low	Normal to high	Low

Note. dDAVP = D-desaminoarginine vasopressin; ADH = antidiuretic hormone.

Table 3-3
Laboratory Studies in Cases of Polyuria: Diabetes Insipidus (DI) versus Psychogenic Polydipsia

To differentiate central DI from nephrogenic DI, a plasma sample for ADH measurement is obtained at the end of the water deprivation period, and the patient is then given a bolus of subcutaneous aqueous vasopressin or D-desaminoarginine vasopressin (dDAVP or desmopressin). Urine osmolality is measured again. Patients with central or neurogenic DI have inappropriately low plasma ADH levels after water deprivation but are able to increase urine osmolality in response to the ADH injection. Patients with nephrogenic DI have high plasma ADH levels in response to water deprivation but are not able to increase urine osmolality after the ADH bolus.

Evaluation of Diabetes Insipidus
Plasma and urine osmolality
Water deprivation test
Plasma ADH levels

Treatment of DI. The treatment of DI depends on its cause. Free access to water is essential for all patients. Patients with central DI can be treated with vasopressin or one of its pharmacologic analogs such as dDAVP to diminish urine output and alleviate the need for chronic water drinking. Treatment of nephrogenic DI is more difficult because exogenous ADH cannot overcome renal insensitivity to the hormone. Maintaining adequate free water intake is the principal therapy.

HYPOTONIC DISORDERS

Disorders that result in decreased serum osmolality are common (Table 3-4). These disorders result from decreased water excretion in euvolemic states, hypovolemic states that result in preservation of plasma volume at the expense of decreased serum osmolality, or excess water ingestion. Urine osmolality is inappropriately concentrated considering the hypotonic plasma.

Decreased water excretion—euvolemic states
ADH excess due to syndrome of inappropriate ADH (SIADH)
  Pain and physical stress
  CNS infection, tumor, and trauma
  Ectopic tumors producing ADH
  Lung disease (tumor, tuberculosis, pneumonia)
Drug-induced ADH release
  (opiates, analgesics, others)

Decreased water excretion—hypovolemic states
  (decreased distal solute delivery)
  Congestive heart failure
  Cirrhosis
  Nephrotic syndrome
  Adrenal insufficiency
  Starvation

Excess water ingestion
  Psychogenic polydipsia

Table 3-4
Major Causes of Hypotonic Disorders

Note. ADH = antidiuretic hormone; CNS = central nervous system.

Syndromes of Decreased Water Excretion Due to Excess ADH. The most common hypotonic disorder is the syndrome of inappropriate ADH (SIADH). Patients with SIADH have *normal vascular volume* and inappropriate ADH release in the *absence* of any osmotic stimulus. In some of these patients, nonosmotic stimuli including pain, physical stress, and central nervous system disorders of various kinds stimulate ADH release despite normal plasma volume and osmolality. Some tumors secrete ectopic ADH. Lung cancers and other pulmonary diseases are particularly likely to be associated with SIADH, but the syndrome occurs with many other disorders as well. Inappropriate ADH can be caused by drugs, such as narcotic analgesics, beta agonists, barbiturates and nicotine, which stimulate or potentiate the effects of ADH.

Criteria for the Diagnosis of SIADH
Low plasma osmolality
Inappropriately high urine osmolality for plasma osmolality
Hyponatremia
Normal plasma volume
Normal renal and adrenal function

If ADH release and water ingestion continue unchecked, serum Na+ concentration and plasma osmolality continue to decrease. The treatment of choice is to limit free water intake. Water restriction to 1.0–1.5 L/d often is necessary to maintain normal serum osmolality. If this is unsuccessful, drugs such as demeclocycline or chlorpropamide that reduce the effect of ADH at the renal tubule can be used. Sodium chloride can be given cautiously to avoid heart failure if absolutely necessary.

Decreased Distal Solute Delivery Causing Increased ADH. Conditions that cause intravascular volume depletion and decreased solute delivery to the distal tubules result in excess ADH release. Examples are shown in Table 3-4.

Psychogenic Polydipsia. This pathologic condition, in which patients repeatedly ingest very large amounts of fluid, results in hypotonicity with suppressed ADH levels.

∎ OXYTOCIN

Oxytocin is the other major peptide hormone produced in hypothalamic nuclei and stored in the posterior pituitary. Oxytocin has two major physiologic actions in humans. It stimulates uterine contractions at the time of labor and delivery in response to distention of the reproductive tract, and it stimulates smooth muscle contraction in the breast during suckling, which results in milk let down. Suckling and distention of the reproductive tract stimulate oxytocin release through neural pathways.

Oxytocin has a minor role in the regulation of water homeostasis. Release is stimulated by increased plasma tonicity. In pharmacologic amounts, oxytocin potentiates water retention. Severe water intoxication can occur in women who receive high doses of oxytocin to promote uterine contractions during labor.

Case Study:
Resolution

A presumptive diagnosis of DI was made in this patient on the basis of her increased urination, thirst, high serum Na+, and plasma osmolality coupled with her dilute urine. She had no history of excessive sweating, diarrhea, or burns to cause excessive water loss and nothing to suggest a solute diuresis. Plasma and urine glucose were normal, and she had not been given a solute load. Her symptoms were compatible with psychogenic water drinking, but this results in hypotonicity (low plasma osmolality), not hypertonicity.

Her water deprivation test resulted in continuing urinary hypotonicity and significant free water loss, with urinary volumes up to 1 L/hr. Water deprivation was stopped after she had lost 3% of her body weight. She was given a bolus of dDAVP, but there was no increase in urine osmolality or reduction in urine volume. The diagnosis of nephrogenic DI was confirmed.

Her nephrogenic DI was thought to be related to the prior lithium carbonate therapy. Lithium carbonate is known to cause nephrogenic DI, and symptoms can persist for many years after the drug is discontinued. The treatment of nephrogenic DI can be difficult and definitely requires that patients have free access to water to replace their water loss. It is imperative to monitor their serum osmolality, serum Na+, and urinary water losses.

■ REVIEW QUESTIONS

Directions: For each of the following questions, choose the **one best** answer.

1. In the maintenance of normal water balance, a complex process that requires the integration of many signals, which of the following occurs?

    (A) Thirst is suppressed by hypovolemia and angiotensin II
    (B) ADH suppresses translocation of water channels to the surface of the collecting duct lumen
    (C) ADH stimulates water flow from the renal interstitium to the collecting duct lumen
    (D) Increased plasma osmolality and loss of plasma volume elicit ADH release

Questions 2 and 3

A 26-year-old woman developed polyuria 2 days after surgical removal of a large non–hormone-producing pituitary tumor. Now her urine volume is in excess of 6 L/d, and she is drinking large amounts of water.

2. What is the most likely cause of this woman's polyuria?

    (A) An impaired thirst mechanism due to surgical damage
    (B) Nephrogenic diabetes insipidus (DI)
    (C) Central DI
    (D) Syndrome of inappropriate ADH release (SIADH)
    (E) Excess intravenous fluid administration

3. Unfortunately, this patient's polyuria is permanent. Urine and plasma osmolality and a water deprivation test support the diagnosis. In light of this information, which of the following statements is likely to be true?

    (A) Her urine osmolality is higher than her plasma osmolality
    (B) Her water deprivation test shows no response to vasopressin
    (C) High plasma osmolality indicates psychogenic water drinking
    (D) A long-acting ADH agonist is the treatment of choice

4. A 64-year-old man was hospitalized 3 days ago for a laparotomy and cholecystectomy (gallbladder removal). He has had an uncomplicated postoperative course, although he has been given intravenous fluid (5% dextrose in 0.5% normal saline) and intravenous morphine for postoperative pain control. He has no complaints other than moderate pain due to his abdominal incision. Laboratory studies include Na$^+$ 127 mEq/L (normal: 137–145 mEq/L); K$^+$, 4.1 mEq/L (normal). Which of the following is the most likely explanation for this patient's hyponatremia?

    (A) Excessive water ingestion
    (B) Starvation with decreased solute delivery to the distal nephrons
    (C) Syndrome of inappropriate ADH release
    (D) Drug-induced suppression of ADH release

5. A 75-year-old man is evaluated for weight loss. An ADH level is measured as part of a research protocol. His ADH level is low. This would be expected in which of the following situations?

    (A) Ectopic ADH secretion by a tumor
    (B) Psychogenic water drinking
    (C) Nephrogenic diabetes insipidus (DI)
    (D) Hypovolemia due to dehydration

■ ANSWERS AND EXPLANATIONS

1. The answer is D. Osmoreceptors in the hypothalamus are exquisitely sensitive to cellular dehydration, which occurs when extracellular osmolality becomes greater than intracellular osmolality and water exits from cells. Baroreceptors are sensitive to volume depletion. Both stimuli elicit ADH release. Low osmolality suppresses ADH secretion. Thirst is stimulated by hypovolemia and angiotensin II. ADH increases translocation of water channels to the surface of the collecting duct lumen and stimulates water flow from the collecting duct lumen to the interstitium.

2. The answer is C. Transient DI following pituitary surgery occurs in up to 10% of cases. The patient's thirst mechanism is intact, as she is drinking large amounts of water. Recent pituitary surgery makes sudden onset of central DI much more likely than nephrogenic DI in this setting. SIADH and excess intravenous fluids do not cause thirst.

3. The answer is D. The patient has central DI. Since she cannot secrete ADH, she is unable to concentrate her urine, and urine osmolality is lower than plasma osmolality. Her kidneys should respond to exogenous ADH, which is given as part of the water deprivation test, and the treatment of choice is a long-acting ADH agonist. Psychogenic water drinking results in a hypotonic state, so plasma osmolality would be low.

4. The answer is C. The syndrome of inappropriate ADH is common in hospitalized postoperative patients. Continued infusion of hypotonic solution with concomitant ADH release from the posterior pituitary results in inappropriate free water retention. The ADH release is likely stimulated by physiologic stressors, including postoperative pain and the opiate analgesic. The test of choice would be measurement of urine osmolality. Urine osmolality should be inappropriately high (inappropriate concentration of urine in the setting of dilute plasma osmolality) in this patient. There is no evidence for any of the other choices.

5. The answer is B. Psychogenic water drinkers have hypotonic plasma and are volume replete, so ADH should be suppressed. In patients with nephrogenic DI, urine cannot be concentrated, and plasma osmolality rises. ADH is secreted in response to hypertonicity, but the renal collecting tubule cannot respond. Hypovolemia from any cause stimulates ADH secretion. ADH would be inappropriately high if the patient had an ectopic tumor secreting ADH, because secretion by ectopic tumors is not suppressed when normal osmolality and plasma volume have been achieved.

■ REFERENCES

Berl T, Anderson RJ, McDonald KM, et al: Clinical disorders of water metabolism. *Kidney Int* 10:117–132, 1976.

Blevins LS Jr, Wand GS: Diabetes insipidus. *Crit Care Med* 20:69–79, 1992.

Geele NG, Keil LC, Kravik SE: Inhibition of plasma vasopressin after drinking in dehydrated humans. *Am J Physiol* 247:R968–R971, 1984.

Goldsmith SR: Vasopressin as vasopressor. *Am J Med* 82:1213–1219, 1987.

Kovacs L, Robertson GL: Syndrome of inappropriate diuresis. *Endocrinol Metab Clin North Am* 21:859–875, 1992.

Miller M, Moses AM, Streeten DHP: Recognition of partial defects in antidiuretic hormone secretion. *Ann Intern Med* 73:721–729, 1970.

Quain R: Polyuria. In *A Dictionary of Medicine*. New York, NY: Appleton. 1883, pp 1239–1241.

Richardson DW, Robinson AG: Desmopressin. *Ann Intern Med* 103:228–239, 1985.

Robertson GL: Differential diagnosis of polyuria. *Am Rev Med* 39:425–442, 1988.

Vokes TJ, Robertson GL: Disorders of antidiuretic hormone. *Endocrinol Metab Clin North Am* 17:456–475, 1988.

Chapter 4

THE THYROID GLAND

Cary N. Mariash, M.D., and Jack H. Oppenheimer, M.D.

■ CHAPTER OUTLINE

Case Study:
Introduction

The patient is a 23-year-old woman who complained of feeling extremely tired and "jumpy" for the past 4 months. She also felt short of breath, and her heart "raced" whenever she exerted herself. Her symptoms have become progressively worse, and at the time of her first clinic visit, they occurred after she climbed one flight of stairs or carried her infant from the car to the house. She had taken medical leave from her construction job because she could not perform the strenuous tasks required. Her hands shook, and she was unable to handle a full cup of coffee without spilling it. She was irritable and argued constantly with her husband. The house always seemed hot to her. She lost 10 lbs despite a good appetite, and her menstrual flow had become much lighter.

Her medical history was unremarkable. Her review of systems was positive for frequent bowel movements.

Physical examination revealed a thin woman who fidgeted continuously throughout the interview. Her blood pressure was 130/58 mm Hg; her pulse was 126 beats/min and regular. Her skin was warm, velvety, and moist. She had a prominent stare and lid lag. Her thyroid gland was three times normal in size, diffusely enlarged, and soft. A prominent bruit was present over the gland. Her cardiac examination was normal except for the tachycardia. There were no rales on chest examination. Her abdominal examination was normal. Diplopia developed during upward and outward gaze. Muscle strength and tone were normal. Deep tendon reflexes revealed a rapid relaxation phase. Several tests were ordered.

■ STRUCTURE AND SYNTHESIS OF THYROID HORMONES

The thyroid hormone system consists of the hormones that regulate the secretion of thyroid hormone from the thyroid gland, the thyroid gland, which secretes thyroid hormones, and the peripheral tissues that respond to thyroid hormone. The two major thyroid hormones are thyroxine (T_4) and triiodothyronine (T_3), which are iodinated amino acids (Figure 4-1). T_4 contains four iodine molecules; T_3 contains three iodine molecules. The major secretory product of the thyroid is T_4. Approximately 15% of the T_3 produced is secreted by the thyroid; the remainder is produced in peripheral tissues by the deiodination of T_4, which results in T_3. T_3 is the physiologically active hormone.

FIGURE 4-1
MAJOR THYROID HORMONES AND METABOLITES. The thyroid hormone receptor has greater affinity for triiodothyronine (T_3) than thyroxine (T_4), so the relative activity of T_3 is greater than the relative activity of T_4.

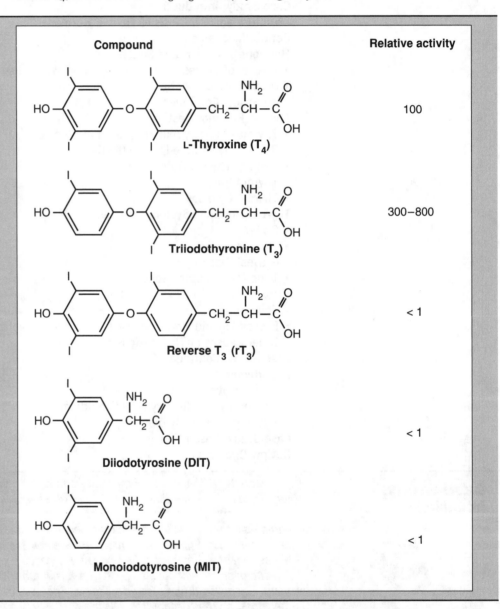

T_4 is made within the basic functional unit of the thyroid gland, the thyroid follicle (Figure 4-2). The follicle consists of a single layer of epithelial cells surrounding a sphere of colloid, which contains the protein thyroglobulin. T_4 is synthesized on and is covalently linked to thyroglobulin. The large capacity of thyroglobulin to store iodine-containing thyroid hormones is important given the decreased availability of iodine in certain geographic regions of the world.

The thyroid gland concentrates iodide to levels 30–40 times those in plasma to maintain adequate stores for thyroid hormone synthesis. The recommended intake of iodine to maintain thyroid hormone synthesis is 150 μg/d. Intake below 50 μg/d is

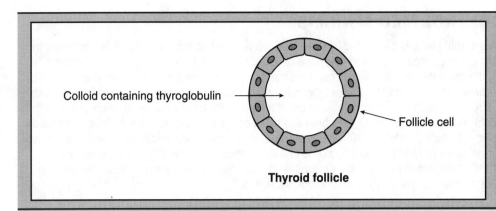

FIGURE 4-2
CROSS SECTION OF A THYROID FOLLICLE.

Colloid containing thyroglobulin →

← Follicle cell

Thyroid follicle

inadequate. Iodine is plentiful in foods obtained from the ocean and coastal areas, but in mountain and inland areas the supply may be very low. In the United States, iodide is added to foods, salt, and vitamin preparations; therefore, iodine deficiency is rare. Some medications and contrast media also contain very high concentrations of iodine.

The thyroid follicle traps inorganic iodide, transporting it against a concentration gradient. Iodide is transported by a recently discovered protein that transports sodium (Na) and iodide together, the Na/I symporter, which is located only in thyroid cells. During times of relative iodine insufficiency, this trapping mechanism is enhanced to assure optimal use of available iodine. Following the uptake of the iodide through specific pores in the epithelial cells, the trapped iodide is oxidized to iodine by the enzyme thyroid peroxidase. During this reaction, tyrosine residues on thyroglobulin are iodinated to produce monoiodotyrosine (MIT). Subsequent iodination of MIT produces diiodotyrosine (DIT). By mechanisms that are not fully understood, two DIT molecules are coupled on the thyroglobulin backbone to produce T_4. MIT and DIT can also be coupled to produce T_3. The hormones remain covalently bound to the thyroglobulin backbone; therefore, thyroglobulin in the thyroid follicle is replete with T_4, T_3, DIT, and MIT (see Figure 4-1).

Thyroid hormones must be released from thyroglobulin to be released into the circulation. Thyroglobulin undergoes endocytosis at the apical surface of the thyroid epithelial cell and is degraded within the lysosomes of the cell. The thyroid hormones are released from thyroglobulin and secreted into the circulation. At the same time, released MIT and DIT are deiodinated within the epithelial cell, and the iodide can be recovered. This highly efficient process assures that losses of free iodine are minimized.

Defects in any of these processes produce thyroid hormone deficiency (Table 4-1). Patients have been found with congenital defects due to abnormalities of the iodine pores, defective oxidation due to abnormal thyroid peroxidase, and inefficient iodine conservation due to deficiencies of thyroid deiodinase. Defects in the two subunits of the thyroglobulin molecule are associated with defective synthesis of thyroid hormones.

Steps in Thyroid Hormone Synthesis
Iodide trapping
Organification of iodide:
  I^- + peroxidase → I^0
Synthesis of thyroid hormones on thyroglobulin
I^0 + tyrosine → MIT
MIT + I^0 → DIT
DIT + DIT → T_4
DIT + MIT → T_3
Proteolysis of thyroglobulin to release thyroid hormones
Deiodinases remove iodide from remaining DIT and MIT

Iodide deficiency
Intrathyroid defects
  Iodide transporter defects
  Thyroid peroxidase defects
  Thyroglobulin defects
Intrathyroid and peripheral tissue defects
  Deiodinase deficiency

Table 4-1
Causes of Congenital Thyroid Hormone Deficiency

The secreted hormones eventually are deiodinated in peripheral tissues to release free iodide. Since the kidney can excrete the free iodide, the kidney and the thyroid compete for iodide in the circulation. When dietary iodine is sufficient, as in most American diets, the thyroid gland accumulates approximately 20% of the ingested iodine. The remainder is excreted by the kidney. However, when the iodine supply is low, the thyroid can increase the uptake and trapping of iodine. Under extreme circumstances, the thyroid can trap nearly 100% of ingested iodine. Because the thyroid gland can adapt to iodide needs, there is no need for a renal mechanism to alter clearance of iodide.

■ CONTROL MECHANISMS

The thyroid gland is controlled by the anterior pituitary and the hypothalamus, and they in turn are regulated by thyroid hormone feedback (Figure 4-3). Thyroid gland function is tightly regulated by thyroid-stimulating hormone (TSH) made by the thyrotrophs in the anterior pituitary gland. TSH is composed of two highly glycosylated subunits: the α-subunit, which is common to other pituitary glycoprotein hormones, and the β-subunit, which is specific for TSH. TSH binds to its specific receptor on the surface of thyroid epithelial cells. This is followed by activation of adenylate cyclase, which increases formation of intracellular cyclic adenosine monophosphate (cAMP). A rise in intracellular cAMP stimulates most of the processes in the thyroid cell described in the previous section and results in thyroid hormone secretion.

TSH stimulates nearly all reactions required for thyroid hormone synthesis.

FIGURE 4-3
HYPOTHALAMIC-PITUITARY-THYROID GLAND FEEDBACK CONTROL LOOPS. Thyrotropin-releasing hormone (TRH) from the hypothalamus stimulates release of thyroid-stimulating hormone (TSH) from the pituitary. TSH stimulates secretion of thyroxine (T_4) and triiodothyronine (T_3) from the thyroid gland. Circulating T_4 goes to the liver and other tissues where it is converted to T_3. T_3 inhibits hypothalamic secretion of TRH and pituitary secretion of TSH. + = stimulatory; − = inhibitory.

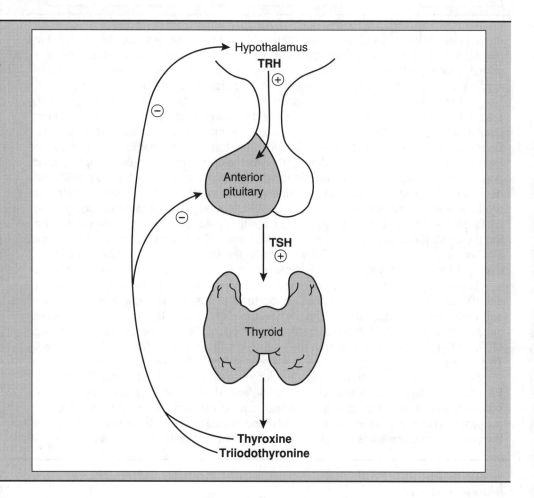

Secretion of TSH is regulated primarily by the pituitary T_3 level. As plasma thyroid hormone levels rise, the pituitary T_3 level also rises. An increase in pituitary T_3 inhibits synthesis and secretion of TSH by inhibiting the synthesis of the messenger RNA (mRNA) for both the α- and β-subunits of TSH.

TSH activity also is regulated by thyrotropin-releasing hormone (TRH), a cyclic tripeptide made from a larger precursor in the hypothalamus. TRH is released from the hypothalamus into the hypothalamic-pituitary portal system, which conveys it to the pituitary thyrotrophs. TRH plays an important role in modulating the pituitary response to feedback by T_3. When TRH secretion is increased, the pituitary set-point for feedback inhibition by T_3 is raised, making the pituitary less sensitive to T_3 inhibition. Conversely, when TRH is low, the pituitary is more sensitive to T_3 inhibition. TRH regulates both the acute release of TSH from the pituitary and glycosylation of the TSH molecule, which is required for TSH bioactivity.

Synthesis and release of TRH are regulated by negative feedback inhibition by T_3.

Control of Thyroid Hormone Synthesis
Level of iodide for hormone synthesis
Activity of deiodinases
Negative feedback regulation of hypothalamic-pituitary-thyroid axis

Functions of TRH
Regulates pituitary sensitivity to TSH
Stimulates acute TSH release
Regulates glycosylation of TSH

When plasma T_3 levels are elevated, hypothalamic TRH content is reduced, and when plasma T_3 levels are low, the content of hypothalamic TRH is high.

■ HORMONE TRANSPORT AND METABOLISM

Thyroid hormones are relatively water insoluble; therefore, they are transported in the plasma bound to carrier proteins. The three major carrier proteins are thyroxine-binding globulin (TBG), albumin, and transthyretin. The relative distribution of T_4 on these proteins is approximately 70%, 10%, and 20% respectively. T_3 also circulates bound to proteins, primarily to TBG and albumin. Approximately 99.9% of T_4 and 99.9% of T_3 are bound in plasma. Bound hormones are in equilibrium with free hormones in plasma. Only the small amount of unbound (free) hormone is available to move into the interstitial tissue fluid and ultimately into individual cells. Tissues respond to the concentration of free hormone, not the concentration of total thyroid hormone. The feedback inhibition discussed above refers to the free hormone concentration. A change in binding protein concentration alters the concentration of total plasma hormone, but the level of free hormone changes only transiently.

Inside cells, thyroid hormones are metabolized further. The *outer ring* of T_4 is 5'-deiodinated to produce the more potent T_3 (3,5,3'-triiodothyronine). This reaction occurs mostly in peripheral tissues, catalyzed by deiodinase enzymes. There are several deiodinases, which are unusual enzymes because they contain selenium. Type I 5'-deiodinase, which occurs mostly in liver and kidney but also in muscle, thyroid, and other tissues, provides T_3 to the plasma. Type I 5'-deiodinase activity is decreased by fasting and some drugs. Type II 5'-deiodinase is found primarily in the brain, adipose tissue, and the pituitary gland. Activity of type II 5'-deiodinase increases when the circulating T_4 level is low and decreases when the circulating T_4 level is high. This regulation maintains normal levels of T_3 within the nervous system and allows the pituitary and hypothalamus to respond to T_4 feedback from the thyroid gland. Type III 5'-deiodinase removes iodine from the inner ring of T_4. Its function is to inactivate T_3 and T_4. There may be other deiodinases as well.

Deiodinases also are involved in the ultimate degradation of thyroid hormones. T_4 can be 5'-deiodinated on the *inner* ring to produce inactive 3,3',5'-triiodothyronine (reverse T_3, or rT_3) [see Figure 4-1]. rT_3 can be deiodinated further by type I 5'-deiodinase to 3,3'-diiodothyronine (T_2). Continued deiodination of T_3 and T_2 leads to other inactive products. The iodine is recirculated for use by the thyroid gland or excreted in the urine. Other degradative processes include conjugation of T_4 with glucuronic acid or sulfate. The conjugated products are excreted in the bile.

EFFECTS OF ILLNESS ON THYROID HORMONE METABOLISM

Peripheral metabolism of thyroid hormones undergoes major changes in the presence of starvation, anorexia, carbohydrate deprivation, untreated diabetes mellitus, or non-thyroid systemic illness. In the presence of these illnesses, type I 5'-deiodinase is inhibited, and conversion of T_4 to T_3 is decreased, resulting in a low circulating T_3 level. Since degradation of rT_3 to T_2 also is decreased, the concentration of rT_3 is high. It is unclear whether the fall in the serum T_3 level is deleterious, protective, or simply represents an epiphenomenon. The lower concentration of T_3 should result in reduced energy expenditure in the setting of starvation or illness. TSH levels usually are normal, unless the patient is receiving glucocorticoids or dopamine, which suppress TSH. Thyroid hormone replacement is not indicated, as studies to date have failed to show any benefit from efforts to restore thyroid hormone levels to normal. Hormone levels return to normal when the illness subsides.

Major Plasma Carrier Proteins for Thyroid Hormones
Thyroxine-binding globulin (TBG)
Transthyretin (prealbumin)
Albumin

Sources of T_3
Thyroid gland, 15%
Peripheral tissue T_4 to T_3 conversion, 85%

■ THYROID HORMONE ACTION

Thyroid hormone action at the cellular level is initiated by the binding of thyroid hormone to a specific nuclear receptor. Thyroid hormone nuclear receptors belong to a family of transcription factors that regulate the transcription of specific genes.

There are three thyroid hormone receptor proteins (α_1, β_1, β_2), which are the products of two different genes. The distribution of these receptors differs among different tissues, and the response of the tissues to thyroid hormone depends on the relative occupancy of the receptors by thyroid hormone. The receptors preferentially bind T_3, which is why T_3 is more active than T_4. Once bound to the receptor, T_3 regulates the expression of different genes in different tissues.

Thyroid hormones exert major effects on growth and development. The role of thyroid hormone in prenatal development is still uncertain, but the absence of thyroid hormone in the early postnatal period is devastating. Thyroid hormone deficiency in the first few months of life leads to irreversible abnormalities in brain development. Prolonged and severe thyroid hormone deficiency in early infancy results in cretinism, which is characterized by marked mental retardation and short stature. If hypothyroidism develops later in childhood, growth is delayed, but normal growth can be restored by thyroid hormone replacement therapy.

Thyroid hormone increases oxygen consumption and heat production. This can be measured as changes in resting (basal) metabolic rate. At the cellular level, the increase in metabolic rate is associated with changes in many metabolic processes, including an increase in sodium–potassium adenosine triphosphatase ($Na^+–K^+$-ATPase) in liver and skeletal muscle, increases in lipid synthesis and lipid oxidation, and increases in protein synthesis and protein degradation. The effects on lipids and protein represent futile cycles in which there is no net change in end product (such as lipid content) at the expense of increased oxygen consumption and heat production.

Oxygen consumption and heat production are also regulated by conditioning, diet, genetics, and other hormones. The net result reflects the interaction of these factors and the thyroid hormone status. Thyroid hormone influences many other physiologic processes, including glucose absorption, insulin requirements, sensitivity to catecholamines, and the rate of drug metabolism (all increased in hyperthyroidism and decreased in hypothyroidism). Some effects of thyroid hormone on specific organ systems are listed in Table 4-2.

Effects of T_3 on Development
Normal postnatal brain development
Normal growth

Functions Increased by T_3
Oxygen consumption
Heat production
Metabolic rate
Lipid synthesis
Lipid oxidation
Cholesterol synthesis and degradation
Protein synthesis
Protein degradation
Drug metabolism
Catecholamine receptors (important only in hyperthyroidism)
Glucose absorption (important only in hyperthyroidism)
Gluconeogenesis (important only in hyperthyroidism)

Table 4-2
Effects of Thyroid Hormone on Organ Systems

ORGAN SYSTEM	HORMONE EXCESS	HORMONE DEFICIENCY
Heart	Increased heart rate Decreased contractility	Decreased heart rate Decreased cardiac output
Vascular	Vasodilatation	Hypertension
Skin	Warm, smooth, and moist	Rough and dry
Gastrointestinal	Increased motility and absorption	Decreased motility
Skeletal	Increased bone turnover	Decreased bone turnover
Neuromuscular	Hyperactivity Increased muscle contraction	Lethargy Slow muscle relaxation

Case Study:
Continued

The patient presented with heat intolerance, weight loss, palpitations, an increased heart rate, vasodilatation (warm, smooth, moist skin), increased gastrointestinal motility, and increased neuromuscular hyperactivity (lid lag, stare, irritability, hyperactivity, tremor, rapid relaxation of deep tendon reflexes), suggesting excessive thyroid hormone action on many organ systems. To confirm this diagnosis and to evaluate the cause and severity of her thyroid disease, laboratory tests were performed. These included measurements of circulating thyroid hormone levels; antibodies indicating autoimmune thyroid disease; the ability of the thyroid gland to take up iodide; and the distribution of iodine within the gland.

These studies revealed a high total T_4 of 15 μg/dL (normal: 5–11 μg/dL); an elevated *free T$_4$ index (FT$_4$I) of 19.5 μg/dL (normal: 5–11 μg/dL); an elevated free T$_3$ index (FT$_3$I) of 390 ng/mL (normal: 80–165 ng/mL); a TSH level of less than 0.04 μU/mL (normal: 0.4–5.0 μU/mL); and a high titer of thyroid-stimulating immunoglobulin. A thyroid uptake study revealed 60% uptake of radioactive iodine at 24 hours (normal: 10%–35%), and a thyroid scan showed an enlarged gland with diffuse uptake in a homogeneous pattern.*

■ THYROID FUNCTION TESTING

Early investigators at the turn of the twentieth century established a relationship between the rate of oxygen consumption under basal conditions and thyroid status. For several decades, measurement of the basal metabolic rate (BMR) was the only objective test for thyroid function. In the 1940s, measurement of protein-bound iodine (PBI) and radio-iodine uptake by the thyroid represented major advances in assessing thyroid function. However, the BMR and PBI are influenced by many factors other than thyroid status, and these tests are no longer used to assess thyroid function.

Symptoms and signs of thyroid hormone excess and deficiency often are not specific and can be confused with those of other disorders. Appropriate thyroid function testing provides an accurate assessment of the thyroid status of the patient, defines the pathogenesis of the dysfunction, and helps to assess the response to treatment.

THYROID-PITUITARY AXIS HORMONES IN BLOOD

Total and Free Serum T$_4$ and Free T$_4$ Index. Since the late 1960s, tests for the level of circulating T$_4$ have been based on the interaction of T$_4$ with antibodies directed to the T$_4$ molecule. Measurement of total serum T$_4$ is one of the classic tests of clinical thyroid status.

The level of total T$_4$ does not always reflect the actual thyroid status of the patient. The total T$_4$ level is a mixture of free T$_4$ (FT$_4$) [the active form] and T$_4$ attached to binding proteins. If binding protein concentrations are high or low, total T$_4$ will be high or low, reflecting the amount of T$_4$ bound, but the FT$_4$ may be within normal limits. For example, in pregnancy total T$_4$ is high because the increase in estrogen stimulates increased production of TBG, and TBG clearance is decreased. FT$_4$ concentrations are normal. Some clinically euthyroid individuals have high levels of total T$_4$ all their lives due to genetic overproduction of TBG. Families with a propensity toward increased transthyretin or an abnormal albumin that binds more than normal amounts of T$_4$ also have high total T$_4$ levels but normal FT$_4$ levels.

Conversely, patients treated with androgens and individuals with genetic underproduction of TBG have low levels of total T$_4$, normal levels of FT$_4$, and no symptoms of hypothyroidism. Table 4-3 lists conditions associated with altered plasma protein binding due to changes in TBG.

INCREASED BINDING	DECREASED BINDING
Pregnancy (↑ TBG synthesis, ↓ TBG clearance)	Nonthyroid illness[a]
Estrogen treatment (↑ TBG synthesis, ↓ TBG clearance)	Testosterone treatment (↓ TBG synthesis, ↑ TBG clearance
Acute hepatitis (damaged cells release TBG)	Hereditary decrease in TBG
Hereditary increase in TBG	Hyperthyroidism (↑ catabolism of TBG)
Hypothyroidism (↓ catabolism of TBG)	

[a] Decreased protein synthesis, increased protein loss (malnutrition, nephrotic syndrome, others).

Table 4-3
Major Conditions Associated with Changes in Thyroxine-Binding Globulin (TBG)

Since the total T$_4$ level does not always indicate the true thyroid status, it is necessary to assess the level of circulating FT$_4$. The FT$_4$ concentration can be measured by equilibrium or nonequilibrium dialysis (techniques to assess the fraction of free hormone) or by ultrafiltration. Reliable measurements of FT$_4$ have become more widely available and are being used instead of the indirect tests which measure the strength of T$_4$ binding to plasma proteins.

Indirect tests provide an estimate of the FT_4 level, the free T_4 index (FT_4I), by measuring the binding of radiolabeled thyroid hormone to resin, charcoal, or antibody that has been added to serum. This measurement makes it possible to determine the relative strength of plasma protein–binding. The FT_4I is calculated by multiplying the total T_4 concentration by the measurement of relative plasma protein–binding. This corrects the total T_4 concentration for abnormalities of binding proteins. The FTI is an excellent approximation of the true thyroid status except in patients with severe illness or very abnormal binding protein. In these situations it is better to obtain a direct measurement of the FT_4 level.

Total and Free Serum T_3. Total serum T_3 and free T_3 (FT_3) levels can be measured or estimated by methods similar to those used for total and free T_4 levels. Since T_3 is the active hormone, one would predict that the serum FT_3 level would be the best test of hormone action at the cellular level. However, the plasma FT_3 concentration may not reflect the tissue T_3 concentration accurately because local tissue T_3 concentrations are greatly influenced by local tissue conversion of T_4 to T_3. This may establish a tissue-to-plasma T_3 gradient that is specific for each organ. Also, the plasma half-life of T_3 is much shorter than that of T_4, and diurnal factors affect plasma measurements.

The major indication for determination of serum T_3 levels is suspected hyperthyroidism. In patients with early Graves' disease or a toxic adenoma, secretion of T_3 is increased even more than the secretion of T_4. In these patients, the serum concentration of T_3 can be high while the serum concentration of T_4 remains within the normal range.

In the hypothyroid state, the fall in serum T_4 levels stimulates deiodinase activity, leading to a compensatory increase in the conversion of T_4 to T_3. In the very early stages of hypothyroidism, T_3 values may still be within the normal range. Serum TSH levels together with serum T_4 levels or the FT_4 or FT_4I are better tests for the diagnosis of early thyroid failure.

Serum TSH. The radioimmunoassay for circulating TSH was introduced in the 1960s. The earliest TSH assays could measure accurately only the elevated levels of TSH in the hypothyroid state. However, progressive improvements in the immunoassays have made it possible to measure the level of TSH in the euthyroid range and to measure the low level of TSH due to negative feedback to the hypothalamus and pituitary in patients with hyperthyroidism.

The TSH level in euthyroid individuals ranges from approximately 0.5 to 5 μU/mL. However, clinical manifestations of hypothyroidism are difficult to demonstrate until TSH levels rise to 10 μU/mL or higher. Symptoms of hyperthyroidism do not generally become evident until the TSH level falls below 0.05 μU/mL. Finding abnormal TSH levels in patients who are asymptomatic may warrant careful follow-up rather than immediate treatment, but each situation should be evaluated on its clinical merits. The TSH assay is particularly helpful for following the results of treatment of hypothyroidism and hyperthyroidism.

The TSH level is low or low-normal if hypothalamic or pituitary disease is present. It is not clear why the TSH level is not uniformly low in pituitary insufficiency. The diagnosis of pituitary hypothyroidism can be made by finding a low FT_4I or FT_4 level in addition to deficits of other pituitary hormones. Radiographic studies can demonstrate structural damage in the pituitary-hypothalamic system.

Thyroid Function Testing in Patients with Nonthyroid Disease. Problems in the interpretation of thyroid function tests arise in patients with catabolic nonthyroid disease. The level of circulating thyroid hormones is depressed in patients with severe illness. Recent studies from intensive care units (ICUs) have shown that the lower the level of T_4, the higher the mortality rate. The level of T_3 also is low in these patients. Low T_3 concentrations also occur with a very high prevalence in patients who are dieting or who have only minor disease. These changes in T_4 and T_3 generally are not accompanied by alterations in steady-state levels of serum TSH. In this setting, a decreased level of FT_4 and FT_3 or a low FT_4I or FT_3I cannot be used to make the diagnosis of primary hypothyroidism. A substantial elevation of TSH above the normal range is essential for making the diagnosis.

Serum Thyroglobulin. Thyroglobulin mostly is contained in the colloid within thyroid follicles, but low concentrations of thyroglobulin can be detected in serum from euthyroid individuals. Serum thyroglobulin is increased in various forms of thyroiditis when the protein escapes from a damaged thyroid gland. The level also is elevated in patients with hyperthyroidism who have thyroid overactivity and in patients with large goiters and in patients with

The sensitive **TSH assay** has become the single most useful clinical test of thyroid function.

metastatic thyroid carcinomas. Patients with thyroid carcinomas who have undergone near total or total ablation of the thyroid gland have very low levels of thyroglobulin unless they have metastatic disease. A subsequent rise in serum thyroglobulin indicates a recurrence.

RADIOACTIVE IODINE UPTAKE (RAIU)

The RAIU by the thyroid remains a useful test of thyroid function. A tracer dose of radioactive iodine is administered orally, and the amount of tracer located in the thyroid gland is measured 6 or 24 hours later. The normal range for RAIU depends on dietary iodine intake. The RAIU is higher in areas where usual dietary iodine intake is low and is lower in areas where the usual iodine intake is high. RAIU is increased in hyperthyroid states such as Graves' disease or toxic multinodular goiter, where thyroid hormone synthesis is increased. However, RAIU is low in patients with thyroiditis who are hyperthyroid due to release of stored hormone from damaged cells. The injured or inflamed gland cannot take up iodine. RAIU is low in patients taking exogenous thyroid hormone whose TSH levels are suppressed. RAIU also is low following ingestion of drugs or administration of contrast material containing iodide because the thyroid gland is saturated with iodine.

Radioactive Iodine Uptake

High: Graves' disease
Multinodular goiter
Toxic nodule
TSH-producing tumors

Low: Thyroiditis
After ingestion of exogenous thyroid hormone
After ingestion of iodide-containing medications
After administration of iodide-containing contrast material
Ectopic thyroid tissue

TESTS OF THYROID AUTOIMMUNITY

Thyroid-Stimulating Immunoglobulin. This assay is useful in the diagnosis of Graves' disease, a form of hyperthyroidism caused by endogenously generated autoantibodies to the TSH receptor. When immortalized rat thyroid cells are exposed to serum containing these antibodies, cAMP is generated. The presence of such antibodies in a patient's serum is the hallmark of the disorder.

Antithyroid-Peroxidase and Antithyroglobulin Antibodies. These antibodies are elevated in patients with chronic lymphocytic thyroiditis (Hashimoto's disease) and reflect the autoimmune basis of this disorder. They do not cause the thyroid disease but are markers of thyroid damage. Continued elevation of these antibodies may foreshadow progressive reduction in thyroid function. Patients with increased titers of these antibodies need periodic evaluation for hypothyroidism.

THYROID IMAGING

A radioactive iodine ^{123}I or technetium scan provides information about the size and functioning areas of the thyroid gland (Figure 4-4). Functioning thyroid nodules that take up the isotope are called "hot" nodules; nonfunctioning or poorly functioning areas of the thyroid that take up little isotope are called "cold" areas. A tracer dose of ^{131}I, which has a longer half-life than ^{123}I, is used for total body scanning for thyroid cancer metastases.

Thyroid ultrasound is used primarily to follow changes in size of thyroid nodules and for differentiating cystic from solid nodules. Computed tomography (CT) scanning and magnetic resonance imaging (MRI) can be used to follow thyroid malignancies in the neck.

THYROID CYTOLOGY

The fine needle aspiration biopsy of thyroid nodules is simple, well tolerated, and provides a small amount of material for screening thyroid nodules for malignant cells. It is approximately 90% accurate in the hands of an experienced cytologist.

▌ THYROID HORMONE SYSTEM DISORDERS

GOITER

Goiters are enlargements of the thyroid gland which arise because of increased stimulation of the thyroid gland by TSH or by thyroid-stimulating immunoglobulins, resulting in multiplication of follicle epithelial cells and eventually new follicles. Other growth factors also may contribute.

Diffuse simple or nontoxic goiters may develop in response to inadequate synthesis of thyroid hormone. TSH secretion then increases and induces diffuse thyroid hyperplasia. Some areas outgrow their blood supply and become necrotic and then fibrotic, as other new

FIGURE 4-4
RADIOACTIVE IODINE SCANS. (A) Iodine uptake in a normal thyroid gland. (B) Little or no iodine uptake in a patient with thyroiditis. Only the marker indicating the sternal notch is seen. (C) An enlarged thyroid gland with increased iodine uptake in a homogeneous pattern in a patient with Graves' disease. (D) An area of decreased iodine uptake in a solitary "cold" nodule in the right lobe of the thyroid gland.

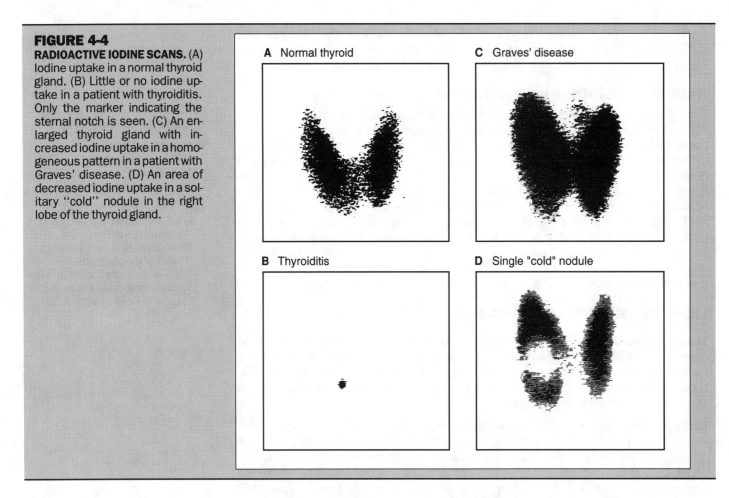

A   Normal thyroid

C   Graves' disease

B   Thyroiditis

D   Single "cold" nodule

Causes of Nontoxic Goiter
Iodine deficiency
Genetic defects in thyroid hormone synthesis
Drugs or chemicals impairing thyroid hormone synthesis
Goitrogens in the diet

areas are becoming hyperplastic. Some follicles become autonomous; their growth is no longer dependent on TSH. Eventually, the goiter becomes filled with nodules of different sizes and varying capacity for thyroid hormone synthesis. The diffuse goiter has been transformed into a multinodular goiter. If the goiter becomes large enough, patients may complain of neck pressure and difficulty swallowing. Treatment with T_4 to suppress TSH into the normal range may cause these goiters to regress, but autonomous areas and necrotic, hemorrhagic, or fibrotic areas do not respond. Sometimes surgery is necessary for cosmetic reasons or symptom relief.

Patients with these goiters are euthyroid if thyroid hyperplasia compensates for the defect in thyroid hormone synthesis, and their FT_4, FT_4I, and TSH levels are normal. If the increased follicle growth is not enough to compensate for the defect in hormone synthesis, patients are hypothyroid. These goiters also can be associated with hyperthyroidism, if autonomous follicle growth is accompanied by excessive thyroid hormone secretion. In these cases, the nontoxic goiters have been transformed into toxic multinodular goiters (see below).

THYROTOXICOSIS

Thyrotoxicosis results from the actions of excess thyroid hormone from any cause on peripheral tissues. The terms *thyrotoxicosis* and *hyperthyroidism* often are used interchangeably, but *hyperthyroidism* refers specifically to overproduction of thyroid hormone by the thyroid gland. Major causes of thyrotoxicosis are listed in Table 4-4.

Common symptoms of thyrotoxicosis include hyperactivity, nervousness, generalized fatigue, palpitations, excessive sweating, hyperdefecation, and heat intolerance. Menstruating women often have decreased menstrual flow or oligomenorrhea. Signs of thyrotoxicosis include weight loss despite a good appetite, if the increase in caloric intake does not match the increase in caloric expenditure, lid lag and stare due to spasm of the upper eyelid, sinus tachycardia, atrial fibrillation or high cardiac output, warm and moist skin, fine tremor of the outstretched hands, muscle weakness, and muscle wasting.

These symptoms and signs reflect the effects of excess thyroid hormone on several

	RAIU	IODINE SCAN
Graves' disease	High	Diffuse uptake
Toxic multinodular goiter	High	Patchy uptake
Toxic adenoma	High	Hot nodule

Thyroiditis
  Subacute granulomatous (de Quervain's thyroiditis)
  Chronic lymphocytic (Hashimoto's thyroiditis)
  Acute bacterial thyroiditis
  Radiation-induced thyroiditis
	Low	Little uptake

Exogenous thyroid hormone
  Thyroid hormone pills
  Meat contaminated with thyroid tissue
	Low	Little uptake

Rare causes of thyrotoxicosis
  TSH-secreting pituitary adenoma
  Metastatic thyroid cancer
  Ectopic thyroid tissue (struma ovarii)
  Trophoblastic tumor
	
	High
	High
	High
	High
		
		Diffuse uptake
		Uptake in metastases
		Uptake in pelvis only
		Diffuse uptake

Note. RAIU = radioactive iodine uptake; TSH = thyroid-stimulating hormone.

Table 4-4
Causes of Thyrotoxicosis

organ systems (Table 4-5). For example, excessive sweating is due to increased total body heat production (from liver and muscle) accompanied by increased cardiac output (heart contractility and heart rate), vasodilatation (peripheral vascular system), and increased sympathetic tone to the sweat glands (nervous system).

ORGAN SYSTEM	SIGNS AND SYMPTOMS
General	Fatigue, hyperactivity, and nervousness Heat intolerance and weight loss
Cardiovascular	Palpitations and rapid heart rate Increased cardiac output Atrial fibrillation
Gastrointestinal	Increased appetite and hyperdefecation
Musculoskeletal	Muscle weakness and muscle wasting Increased bone turnover and bone loss
Nervous	Hyperkinesia Lid lag and stare Fine tremor Rapid relaxation of deep tendon reflexes
Reproductive	Oligomenorrhea
Skin	Smooth, warm, and moist Excessive sweating
Growth (childhood)	Rapid growth Accelerated bone maturation

Table 4-5
Signs and Symptoms of Thyrotoxicosis

The combination of nervousness, tachycardia, sweating, lid lag, stare, and tremor suggests catecholamine excess. Plasma epinephrine levels are normal, but their effects are increased because the number of catecholamine receptors is increased. β-Blockers suppress the symptoms but do not treat the underlying disease.

In older patients, manifestations of thyrotoxicosis often are very subtle. These patients may present with weight loss, fatigue, lethargy, and depression, rather than with signs of catecholamine excess. This presentation is called apathetic hyperthyroidism. This diagnosis should be considered in elderly patients who develop a new mood disorder.

Thyrotoxicosis can be treated with the antithyroid drugs methimazole or propylthiouracil. These are sulfonamide derivatives that act primarily by inhibiting thyroid hormone synthesis. Drug treatment often must be continued for many years, and the incidence of permanent remission is low (35%). Major side effects of these drugs include rash, a hepatitis-like reaction, and agranulocytosis (in approximately 1/1000 patients).

Patients also can be treated with radioactive iodine since iodine is selectively taken up by the thyroid gland without causing significant damage to other tissues. It is difficult

Typical Presentation of Thyrotoxicosis
Young patients: symptoms and signs of catecholamine excess
Elderly patients: apathetic hyperthyroidism

to destroy the amount of thyroid tissue needed to restore the euthyroid state without causing hypothyroidism. At least 50% of patients successfully treated with radioactive iodine eventually will require thyroid hormone supplementation.

Surgical treatment (subtotal thyroidectomy) can be performed after patients have been made euthyroid with antithyroid drugs. Major complications include damage to the recurrent laryngeal nerve with vocal cord paralysis and hoarseness, and damage to the parathyroid glands resulting in hypoparathyroidism. If too little thyroid tissue is removed, patients remain hyperthyroid; if too much is removed, patients develop hypothyroidism.

GRAVES' DISEASE

Graves' disease, an autoimmune disorder, is the most common cause of hyperthyroidism. It occurs in approximately 0.5% of the population and is more common in women than men. T lymphocytes become sensitized to thyroid antigens and stimulate B cells to produce antibodies. Nearly all patients with Graves' disease have a high titer of an immunoglobulin of the IgG class which is directed against the TSH receptor. Interaction of the autoantibody with the TSH receptor stimulates the release of thyroid hormone from the thyroid gland. The autoantibody acts like TSH to stimulate the thyroid cell but does not cross-react with TSH in TSH immunoassays. This autoimmune disease often runs in families, with a very high concordance among monozygotic twins. The prevalence of Graves' disease is higher in Caucasians who carry the human leucocyte antigens (HLA) HLA-B8 and HLA-DRw3, indicating that part of the genetic predisposition to Graves' disease is linked to the HLA complex.

The autoantibody causes excess production of T_4 and T_3 independent of TSH. TSH is suppressed by the high levels of T_3 and T_4 since the normal feedback regulation of the pituitary remains intact. The stimulatory action of the Graves' immunoglobulin G (IgG) causes the thyroid gland to take up a large fraction of radioactive iodine in spite of the suppressed TSH. A radioactive iodine scan shows that the iodine is taken up diffusely throughout an enlarged gland.

Graves' disease is of particular concern during pregnancy because the IgG readily crosses the placenta. The antibody can stimulate the fetal or neonatal thyroid gland. If a woman with a history of Graves' disease still has a positive Graves' IgG titer prior to delivery, her physician should be concerned about possible neonatal hyperthyroidism.

A smooth, diffuse goiter is almost always present although it may be difficult to palpate in elderly patients. Vascularity of the thyroid gland is increased, and a bruit may be heard over the goiter. Other specific signs include Graves' eye signs (Graves' ophthalmopathy) and a rare dermopathy known as pretibial myxedema.

Graves' ophthalmopathy can be demonstrated in nearly all patients with Graves' disease if sensitive tests are used. Lymphocytes directed to an unknown antigen infiltrate into the orbital tissues, especially the eye muscles. Lymphocyte infiltration is associated with production of cytokines and inflammation. The infiltration and inflammation produce congestion and swollen eye muscles. This causes forward displacement of the eyeball (proptosis), protrusion of the globe because there is no room in the bony orbit for additional tissue and fluid, and periorbital edema. The protrusion is known as exophthalmos (Figures 4-5 and 4-6). Eventually the eye muscles can become fibrotic. This leads to diplopia, which is most common on upward, outward gaze due to involvement of the inferior rectus muscle. Excessive intraorbital pressure can cause optic nerve compression and blindness in severe cases that are not treated appropriately.

Dermopathy occurs in only 2%–3% of patients. The skin becomes markedly thickened over the pretibial areas due to the accumulation of glycosaminoglycans. Patients with Graves' disease also can have separation of their fingernails from their beds (onycholysis).

Treatment of Graves' disease is directed toward reducing secretion of thyroid hormone. There is no way to target immune suppression for Graves' IgG, and general immune suppression is unwarranted unless the ophthalmopathy is severe. If symptoms of thyrotoxicosis are severe, β-adrenergic blockade can be used until an antithyroid drug, radioactive iodine, or surgery has treated the underlying disease. The ophthalmopathy may not respond to the treatment for thyrotoxicosis, and patients with ophthalmopathy should be treated by ophthalmologists. Severe eye disease may require glucocorticoid therapy, external x-ray therapy, or surgery.

Treatment Options for Thyrotoxicosis
Antithyroid drugs
Radioactive iodine
Partial thyroidectomy

Hallmarks of Graves' Disease
Smooth diffuse goiter
Graves' ophthalmopathy
Dermopathy (rare)
High FT_3 and FT_4
Suppressed TSH
High RAIU

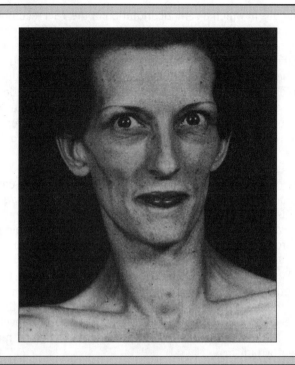

FIGURE 4-5
A PATIENT WITH GRAVES' DIS-EASE. Note the presence of ex-ophthalmos and evidence of weight loss and goiter. (*Source:* Reprinted with permission from Volpe R: Graves' disease. In *Thyroid Function and Disease.* Edited by Burrow GN, Oppen-heimer JH, Volpe R. Philadel-phia, PA: W. B. Saunders, 1990, p 220.)

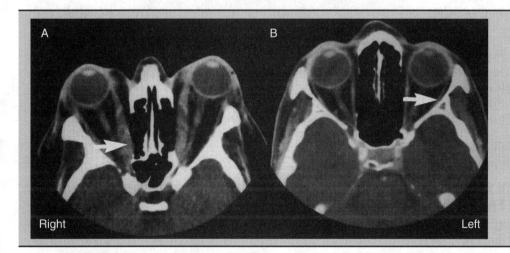

FIGURE 4-6
GRAVES' OPHTHALMOPATHY. Computed tomographic scans of the orbits in a patient with Graves' opthalmopathy (panel A) and a normal subject (panel B). Note the enlarged extraocu-lar muscles in panel A. The *arrow* points to an enlarged me-dial rectus muscle. In panel B the *arrow* points to a normal lateral rectus muscle. (*Source:* Reprinted with permission from Bahn RS, et al: Pathogenesis of Graves' ophthalmopathy. *N Engl J Med* 329: 1469, 1993.)

TOXIC MULTINODULAR GOITER

Toxic multinodular goiter (also called Plummer's disease) usually occurs in patients older than 50 years of age. These patients often have a long history of a benign goiter and normal thyroid tests. Hyperthyroidism develops gradually and usually is less severe than that seen in Graves' disease. The precise mechanism that leads to autonomous function of multiple nodules is unknown. In some cases, the hyperthyroidism is precipitated by the ingestion of large quantities of iodide, especially iodide-containing drugs like am-iodarone or contrast dye.

The goiter may extend substernally, making it difficult to appreciate the full size of the gland. The FT_4, the FT_3, and the radioactive iodine uptake are high, and the TSH level is suppressed. A radioactive iodine scan reveals diffuse patchy uptake, with the more active areas taking up iodine more intensely. Treatment options for multinodular goiters are the same as those for Graves' disease: antithyroid drugs, radioactive iodine, or surgery.

TOXIC ADENOMA (TOXIC NODULE)

This condition is similar to multinodular goiter except that a single nodule accounts for the hyperthyroidism. Recent reports indicate that some of these nodules represent a clonal expansion of cells in which a somatic mutation in the TSH receptor has occurred. The mutation is associated with activation of the receptor in the absence of TSH. The excess thyroid hormone secreted by the nodule results in suppression of TSH.

A radioactive iodine scan reveals a single "hot" toxic nodule. These patients may be ideal candidates for radioactive iodine treatment. Since most of the gland is suppressed and will not take up the radioactive iodine, only the nodule is destroyed. After destruction of the nodule, TSH is no longer suppressed, and the rest of the gland can resume normal function. The incidence of hypothyroidism following radioactive iodine treatment for a toxic nodule is much lower than the incidence of hypothyroidism after similar treatment for Graves' disease.

THYROIDITIS

Several forms of thyroiditis are associated with thyrotoxicosis, which is caused by release of stored thyroid hormone from a damaged gland. *Painful, subacute thyroiditis* (de Quervain's thyroiditis or granulomatous thyroiditis) is an inflammatory disorder often associated with a viral infection. In addition to a painful, tender thyroid gland, patients have systemic symptoms such as fever, muscle aches, and a high erythrocyte sedimentation rate (ESR).

The FT_4 and FT_3 are high, and TSH is suppressed. However, since the thyroid gland is damaged, radioactive iodine uptake is very low. A radioactive iodine scan would reveal very little uptake throughout the gland. As the gland becomes depleted of stored hormone, circulating levels of T_3 and T_4 drop, and the suppressed TSH level begins to rise. Patients may then pass through a hypothyroid phase until the gland recovers and the patients return to euthyroidism.

No treatment is needed for the hyperthyroidism, which is self-limited, but β-adrenergic blockers can alleviate some of the symptoms. Aspirin is used for relief of fever and muscle aches. Glucocorticoid therapy may be necessary if the inflammation is severe.

Chronic lymphocytic thyroiditis (Hashimoto's thyroiditis) is an autoimmune disease that usually is associated with hypothyroidism (see below) but also can be associated in its early phase with transient hyperthyroidism. Autoimmune destruction of the thyroid gland leads to release of preformed hormone and transient hyperthyroidism. During the hyperthyroid phase, TSH and radioactive iodine uptake are suppressed. Many of these patients have ongoing destruction of the thyroid gland, leading to eventual hypothyroidism.

Acute bacterial thyroiditis and *radiation thyroiditis* can cause hyperthyroidism. The mechanism of hyperthyroidism is the same as the other forms of thyroiditis: release of preformed hormone from a damaged gland. These forms of thyroiditis are rare.

EXCESS THYROID HORMONE INGESTION (THYROIDITIS FACTITIA)

This condition can be self-induced, usually by patients trying to lose weight, or can be due to overtreatment of hypothyroidism. There is no goiter, since TSH is suppressed by exogenous hormone. Both ingestion of exogenous thyroid hormone and thyroiditis are associated with a high FT_4, low TSH, and suppressed radioactive iodine uptake. However, thyroiditis usually causes an elevation of serum thyroglobulin, which is released from the damaged gland. The thyroglobulin level is normal or low after exogenous hormone ingestion because TSH and endogenous hormone release are suppressed.

An epidemic of exogenous hyperthyroidism due to hamburger made from neck muscle contaminated with thyroid tissue was reported several years ago. Ground meat containing neck muscle can no longer be sold for human consumption.

OTHER CAUSES OF THYROTOXICOSIS

Other forms of thyrotoxicosis listed in Table 4-4 are very rare and can be difficult to diagnose. Hyperthyroidism caused by a TSH-producing tumor is distinguished by a high TSH level. In all other forms of thyrotoxicosis, TSH is suppressed. Metastatic thyroid carcinoma occasionally is able to produce sufficient thyroid hormone to cause thyrotoxicosis. Women with struma ovarii have mild thyrotoxicosis due to oversecretion of thyroid hormones by thyroid tissue within an ovarian teratoma. The ovarian thyroid tissue takes up iodine, but, since TSH is suppressed, thyroid tissue does not. A trophoblastic tumor (hydatidiform mole) produces human chorionic gonadotropin (HCG), which has some TSH-like activity. If tumor production of HCG is very high, the thyroid gland is stimulated to overproduce its hormones.

While many of the individual signs or symptoms in this patient can be associated with a number of different diseases, the overall constellation of signs and symptoms clearly suggested thyrotoxicosis. The differential diagnosis of the causes of thyrotoxicosis is relatively limited in this case. She had a soft, diffusely enlarged, nontender goiter, suggesting Graves' disease. Graves' disease is the most common cause of hyperthyroidism, especially in young women. The presence of a goiter also means that exogenous use of excess thyroid hormone is unlikely.

Some of her eye findings were specific for Graves' ophthalmopathy. Lid lag and stare can be seen with thyrotoxicosis of almost any cause because they reflect the increased sympathetic tone associated with thyrotoxicosis. However, the diplopia with movement of the eye to the upper-outer quadrant indicates restriction of eye muscles. This suggests that she has lymphocytic infiltration of the inferior rectus muscle, as described with Graves' ophthalmopathy.

The diagnosis of thyrotoxicosis was confirmed by the laboratory tests. She had elevated FT_4 and FT_3I. Her low TSH level shows that normal feedback inhibition is intact and that the excess thyroid hormone production is independent of the pituitary and hypothalamus. The elevated RAIU shows that the source of excess thyroid hormone is from the thyroid gland. The constellation of physical findings—elevated thyroid hormone levels, suppressed TSH, elevated RAIU diffusely over an enlarged gland—indicates Graves' disease. The diagnosis was confirmed by the elevated level of thyroid-stimulating immunoglobulin, the IgG responsible for the development of Graves' disease.

She was treated with ^{131}I to destroy some of her thyroid tissue after a pregnancy test confirmed that she was not pregnant (radioactive iodine crosses the placenta). Two months later, she felt much better and returned to her construction job. She did not return for follow-up because she felt well and did not think that further visits were necessary.

Two years after her treatment she felt fatigued again. Her skin had become unusually dry, she was constipated, and her menses had been irregular and unusually heavy for several months. She returned for further evaluation.

■ HYPOTHYROIDISM

Hypothyroidism is the syndrome that results from a lack of thyroid hormone action on tissues and organ systems. Hypothyroidism can be classified as primary hypothyroidism, which results from failure of the thyroid gland, secondary hypothyroidism, which is due to pituitary failure, or tertiary hypothyroidism, which is caused by disorders of the hypothalamus. There are rare cases of hypothyroidism due to peripheral resistance to thyroid hormones. Affected individuals have abnormal thyroid hormone receptors or postreceptor defects.

The consequences are most severe when hypothyroidism presents in infancy. Untreated neonatal hypothyroidism results in irreversible cretinism. This syndrome includes mental retardation, growth failure, puffy hands and face, and often deaf-mutism. Hypothyroidism that develops later in childhood is associated with slowed mentation, retardation of bone development, decreased longitudinal growth, and delayed sexual maturation. These are reversible with treatment of the hypothyroidism.

More than 90% of patients with hypothyroidism complain of lethargy, weakness, slow speech, and dry, coarse skin. Fatigue, cold intolerance, and hoarseness occur frequently. Additional symptoms and signs are listed in Table 4-6. Hyperthyroidism causes weight loss, but hypothyroidism is not a common cause of obesity. Patients with hypothyroidism rarely gain more than 10% of their premorbid weight, and the weight gain primarily is due to accumulation of glycosaminoglycans and interstitial edema, not adipose tissue (Figure 4-7). The interstitial edema may account, in part, for the association of hypertension with hypothyroidism. Hypothyroidism results in delayed absorption of nutrients and drugs, slower metabolism of drugs and anesthetics, decreased clearance of circulating enzymes (aspartate aminotransferase [AST], alanine aminotransferase [ALT], and creatine kinase [CK] often are elevated), and decreased catabolism of low-density lipoprotein (LDL) cholesterol (see Chapter 9).

Type of Hypothyroidism and Site of Defect
Primary hypothyroidism: thyroid gland
Secondary hypothyroidism: pituitary gland
Tertiary hypothyroidism: hypothalamus
Thyroid hormone resistance: peripheral tissues

Major deposition of glycosaminoglycans and interstitial edema in patients with hypothyroidism is referred to as **myxedema.**

Table 4-6
Signs and Symptoms of
Hypothyroidism

ORGAN SYSTEM	SIGNS AND SYMPTOMS
General	Fatigue, lethargy, and cold intolerance
Cardiovascular	Slow heart rate and enlarged heart Decreased cardiac output and pericardial effusion Hypertension
Gastrointestinal	Constipation
Nervous	Slow speech Delayed relaxation of deep tendon reflexes Mental retardation (neonatal, untreated) Dementia in elderly and depression
Musculoskeletal	Muscle cramps
Circulatory	Anemia
Renal	Impaired water excretion and mild hyponatremia
Reproductive	Irregular menses and menorrhalgia Ovulatory failure Oligospermia Decreased libido
Skin	Cool, dry, and coarse skin and puffy face
Interstitial tissue	Accumulation of glycosaminoglycans Capillary leak and loss of albumin
Growth (childhood)	Delayed bone age and short stature

FIGURE 4-7
PATIENTS WITH HYPOTHYROID-ISM BEFORE (PANELS A AND C) AND AFTER (PANELS B AND D) TREATMENT. (*Source:* Reprinted with permission from Shapiro LE, et al: Hypothyroidism. In *Principles and Practices of Endocrinology and Metabolism.* Edited by Becker KL. Philadelphia, PA: J. B. Lippincott, 1990, p 369.)

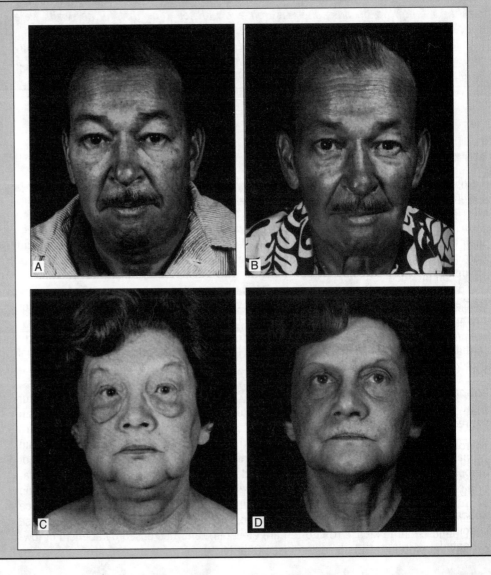

Very severe, untreated hypothyroidism results in weakness, hypothermia, hypoventilation, water retention, hyponatremia, hypoglycemia, bradycardia, pericardial effusion, shock, depression, and severe stupor (sometimes called myxedema coma).

PRIMARY HYPOTHYROIDISM

Primary hypothyroidism is characterized by a low FT_4 or FT_4I and a low or low-normal FT_3 or FT_3I. The TSH level is high, as the pituitary gland responds to the low level of circulating thyroid hormones. Major causes of primary hypothyroidism are listed in Table 4-7.

TYPE OF HYPOTHYROIDISM	CAUSES

Primary hypothyroidism	Autoimmune disease
	    Chronic lymphocytic thyroiditis (Hashimoto's thyroiditis)
	    Antibodies inhibiting the TSH receptor
	Gland destruction
	    Surgery
	    Radioactive iodine
	    External radiation
	Dietary goitrogens
	Drugs
	Iodine deficiency
	Congenital defects

Secondary hypothyroidism	Pituitary disease
Tertiary hypothyroidism	Hypothalamic disorders
Peripheral resistance to thyroid hormone	

Table 4-7
Causes of Hypothyroidism

Note. TSH = thyroid-stimulating hormone.

Chronic Lymphocytic Thyroiditis (Hashimoto's Thyroiditis). This is the most common cause of hypothyroidism in the United States. This disease is due to autoimmune destruction of the thyroid gland. The specific thyroid antigens that activate the T lymphocytes and lead to destruction of the thyroid are unknown. Hashimoto's disease is associated with the production of specific antibodies directed against thyroglobulin and thyroid peroxidase, but the evidence suggests that these antibodies are the result rather than the cause of thyroid damage. They are useful markers of Hashimoto's thyroiditis, and their presence in high titers helps to confirm the diagnosis.

Destruction of the thyroid gland occurs slowly over the course of many years. As the gland is destroyed and the serum T_4 level falls, a compensatory rise in the serum TSH level often allows the serum T_3 level to remain normal, and the patient to remain symptom free. The constellation of a low T_4 level, an elevated TSH level, and a normal T_3 level is known as the "failing gland" syndrome. Although the patients are clinically euthyroid during this phase, the rise in TSH and the lymphocytic infiltration of the thyroid gland can produce very firm goiters that can become quite large.

Patients who develop overt hypothyroidism have low FT_4 and FT_3 index and high TSH levels. Radioactive iodine uptake is low.

Hashimoto's thyroiditis and Graves' disease are autoimmune diseases. They may be familial, they are associated with specific HLA haplotypes, and they may be associated with autoimmune destruction of other endocrine glands. Some patients have features of both Graves' disease and Hashimoto's disease (a condition known as Hashitoxicosis).

Antibodies to the TSH Receptor. Antibodies to the TSH receptor have been found in some patients. These autoantibodies are inhibitory, not stimulatory like the antibodies to the receptor associated with Graves' disease. They lead to thyroid gland atrophy.

Thyroid Ablation. Another common cause of hypothyroidism is ablation of the thyroid gland secondary to surgery or radioactive iodine therapy. Radioactive iodine damages thyroid cell DNA. Hypothyroidism may develop over several weeks, or it may take as long as 30 years to develop. External radiation to the neck also can destroy the thyroid gland.

Subacute Thyroiditis (Resolving Phase). Patients in the resolving phase of subacute thyroiditis may develop hypothyroidism (see above). This usually is temporary, but some patients fail to recover fully and remain hypothyroid.

Dietary Goitrogens and Drugs. Foods such as cassava, cabbage, bamboo shoots, and sweet potatoes contain compounds that interfere with the synthesis of thyroid hormones in the thyroid. Foods grown in soils that contain natural goitrogens or goitrogens from industrial wastes may accumulate enough of these compounds to cause goiters and hypothyroidism. Medications also can do this. Lithium, for example, inhibits thyroid hormone synthesis. Drugs which contain excess iodine, like amiodarone, cause hypothyroidism in some patients. The antithyroid drugs propylthiouracil and methimazole, which interfere with thyroid hormone synthesis, also produce hypothyroidism.

Iodine Deficiency. This is a common cause of hypothyroidism worldwide, although it is rare in the United States, where many foods and salt are supplemented with iodine. Because there is no underlying destruction of the thyroid gland, the associated rise in TSH leads to the development of a goiter. If the iodine deficiency persists for many years, the goiter may remain even after successful iodine replacement.

Congenital Defects. A number of congenital defects of the thyroid gland are associated with decreased synthesis or secretion of thyroid hormones and hypothyroidism (see Table 4-1). In response to negative feedback, pituitary secretion of TSH increases and causes development of a goiter. Administration of iodine may exacerbate the defect in thyroid hormone synthesis or secretion. Congenital hypothyroidism also can be due to congenital absence of a thyroid gland.

SECONDARY AND TERTIARY HYPOTHYROIDISM

Primary pituitary or hypothalamic disease (secondary and tertiary hypothyroidism, respectively) can result in TSH insufficiency. Usually this is associated with other pituitary hormone deficiencies. The thyroid gland does produce some thyroid hormone in the absence of TSH, so secondary hypothyroidism usually is not severe. The serum TSH level is low or low-normal and is not a reliable marker for hypothyroidism. In these patients, the diagnosis is based on symptoms and signs of hypothyroidism, a low FT_4I, and evidence (clinical, laboratory, x-ray) of other defects in pituitary function.

THERAPY OF HYPOTHYROIDISM

Primary hypothyroidism is almost always treated by administration of T_4. The plasma half-life of T_4 is 7–10 days, so daily administration of replacement hormone does not cause large fluctuations in the plasma concentration of T_4. Peripheral tissue conversion of T_4 to T_3 supplies the active hormone. The dose of T_4 is increased gradually until the serum TSH level is within the normal range. Adjustments in the dose should be made at 4- to 6-week intervals, after steady-state concentrations of the hormone are attained.

Secondary hypothyroidism also is treated with replacement of T_4. In these patients, the serum TSH level cannot be used to titrate the replacement dose of hormone. Rather, the physician must rely on changes in signs and symptoms while monitoring the serum FT_4I. Most patients' TSH levels will be appropriately replaced at a time when the FT_4I is near the upper limits of normal.

When the patient returned to the clinic, her blood pressure was 140/90 mm Hg, her heart rate was 55 beats/min, and her temperature was 97.2°F. Her skin was dry, and her hair was thinning. She had no lid lag, but the diplopia was still present. She had no goiter. Her heart sounds were normal but distant. Deep tendon reflexes showed a marked delay in the relaxation phase.

Laboratory tests revealed the following: total T_4, 2.8 µg/dL; FT_4I, 1.4 (normal: 5–11); and TSH, 90 µU/mL. The electrocardiogram (ECG) showed a sinus bradycardia and low voltage. Her total cholesterol level was higher than before.

The patient's signs and symptoms suggest hypothyroidism. Insufficient thyroid hormone causes decreased bowel motility (constipation), slow heart rate, and dry skin. In addition, she now has mild hypertension, distant heart sounds, and low voltage ECG. Accumulation of fluid in interstitial spaces has resulted in pericardial fluid accumulation and decreased vascular compliance.

The low FT_4I confirmed the hypothyroidism. The high TSH shows that the hypothyroidism is due to failure of the thyroid gland and that the pituitary-hypothalamic feedback axis is intact. Metabolic processes, including cholesterol catabolism, are decreased in patients with hypothyroidism; this might explain her increased cholesterol level.

The patient's hypothyroidism is most likely due to destruction of her gland by previous radioiodine therapy. The high incidence of subsequent hypothyroidism emphasizes the need for continued follow-up in patients treated for Graves' disease. The patient can be treated with T_4 replacement.

▌REVIEW QUESTIONS

Directions: For each of the following questions, choose the **one best** answer.

Questions 1 and 2

Joyce L. is a 20-year-old university undergraduate student who comes to the clinic because she has been unable to concentrate for several months and her test scores have decreased significantly. Her appetite has increased, she has trouble sleeping because the apartment is too hot, and she is awakened by palpitations. Her physical examination reveals the following: heart rate, 120 beats/min; slight lid lag; a goiter three times the size of a normal thyroid gland; and warm skin. The physician suspects that she has Graves' disease and orders several tests.

1. Which of the following results are most consistent with Graves' disease?

   (A) Low free thyroxine index (FT_4I), low free triiodothyronine index (FT_3I), and low thyroid-stimulating hormone (TSH)
   (B) High FT_3I, low TSH, and high radioactive iodine uptake (RAIU)
   (C) High FT_4I, high TSH, and low RAIU
   (D) High FT_3I, high TSH, and high RAIU

2. Eighteen years later, Joyce L. returns to the physician's office for medical care. She is now 38 years old and feels older than her age. She complains of fatigue and dry skin, and her menses are longer and heavier than usual. Physical examination reveals that her pulse is 58 beats/min, her thyroid gland is not palpable, and her deep tendon reflexes show a slow relaxation phase. Screening laboratory tests reveal the following: TSH, 58 μU/mL (normal: 0.4–5.0 μU/mL); and FT_4I, 2.7 (normal: 5–11.5). Her chart confirms that she was treated with radioactive iodine for Graves' disease 18 years ago, and she had normal thyroid tests for several years after that treatment. You now suspect that she has

   (A) recurrent hyperthyroidism
   (B) chronic lymphocytic thyroiditis
   (C) abnormal TSH receptors
   (D) pituitary failure (secondary hypothyroidism)
   (E) hypothyroidism due to previous radioactive iodine

3. A fourth-year medical student is on an international medicine rotation in the hills of Peru. The student has noticed that many of the local residents have large goiters. According to the elders in the community, the goiters developed after a new commercial mining operation opened. The student wonders if the mining operation is discharging a chemical into the town's water supply which is preventing thyroxine (T_4) and triiodothyronine (T_3) attached to thyroglobulin from being hydrolyzed. If the student's hypothesis is correct, one would expect

   (A) a high thyroid-stimulating hormone (TSH) level because the circulating level of T_4 is too low to inhibit the pituitary
   (B) a high serum T_4 level because the thyroid is large and full of thyroglobulin
   (C) a low TSH level because the excess intrathyroidal T_4 inhibits hypothalamic thyrotropin-releasing hormone (TRH) release
   (D) a high serum T_3 level and a low TSH level because the chemical enhances the action of T_3

4. Barbara S. presents to the clinic for a routine 4-month pregnancy examination. This is her first pregnancy. She no longer has morning sickness, but she is feeling more tired than usual. She does not have a goiter, and the remainder of her examination suggests that her thyroid status is normal. However, the physician orders thyroid tests to be sure that she does not have hyperthyroidism. If she is euthyroid, the physician anticipates

    (A) a normal thyroid-stimulating hormone (TSH) level and a low total triiodothyronine (T_3) level
    (B) a low total thyroxine (T_4) level and a high TSH level
    (C) a low free thyroxine index (FT_4I) and a normal TSH level
    (D) a high total T_4 level and a normal FT_4I

5. John Y. has lost weight despite a good appetite. His eyes have become more prominent (proptosis), and he has developed lid lag, stare, and double vision. Further examination reveals tachycardia, a goiter, muscle weakness, and rapid relaxation of his deep tendon reflexes. The physician suspects

    (A) a diet high in thyrotoxic goitrogens
    (B) decreased tissue response to β-agonists such as epinephrine
    (C) antibodies stimulating the thyroid-stimulating hormone (TSH) receptor
    (D) infiltration of extraocular muscles by malignant cells

6. James A. is a 66-year-old man who complains of fatigue. He has mild weight loss and his heart rate has increased over the past 3 years. Physical examination reveals an enlarged, bilaterally irregular, nontender thyroid gland, which is slowly increasing in size. His free T_4 index (FT_4I) also has been increasing slowly, and his TSH level now has dropped below the normal range. Further evaluation would most likely reveal

    (A) a strong family history of thyroid disease
    (B) increased patchy uptake of radioactive iodine
    (C) increased iodine uptake by a toxic nodule
    (D) low radioactive iodine uptake due to thyroiditis
    (E) hyperthyroidism due to thyroid cancer

■ ANSWERS AND EXPLANATIONS

1. The answer is B. The FT_4I and the FT_3I should be elevated in hyperthyroidism. Graves' disease is characterized by hyperfunction of the thyroid gland due to autoantibodies directed to the TSH receptor which stimulate thyroid cells. This leads to a high radioactive iodine uptake. The TSH level should be suppressed (low) rather than high, since the pituitary and hypothalamus respond to normal feedback inhibition from the hyperfunctioning thyroid gland.

2. The answer is E. This question emphasizes the development of hypothyroidism in the natural history of radioactive iodine–treated Graves' disease. The patient's symptoms and signs and her low FT_4I indicate hypothyroidism, not recurrent hyperthyroidism. The high TSH level indicates the normal pituitary response to primary hypothyroidism. If she had secondary hypothyroidism, the TSH level would be low or low-normal. If she had recurrent hyperthyroidism, the pituitary and hypothalamus would respond to normal feedback inhibition by the elevated T_3 level, and the TSH level would be suppressed. Patients with Graves' disease have antibodies directed to TSH receptors, but the TSH receptors are normal. It is possible that she has developed chronic lymphocytic thyroiditis, which is an autoimmune disease, but the absence of a goiter makes this unlikely.

3. The answer is A. If thyroglobulin in the thyroid gland cannot be hydrolyzed, the thyroid gland is unable to release thyroid hormones from sites of synthesis on the thyroglobulin molecule. Circulating thyroid hormone levels in the serum will be low, and the pituitary should increase the synthesis and secretion of TSH leading to a high serum TSH concentration. Feedback inhibition is based on the amount of thyroid hormone reaching the hypothalamus, not the amount of thyroid hormone in the thyroid gland. If T_4 cannot be released from the thyroid gland, the serum T_3 level will also be low because most of the serum T_3 level comes from peripheral deiodination of T_4.

4. The answer is D. There is no reason for the total T_3 level to be low. She is eating normally and has no systemic illness. The total T_4 level should be high, and the total T_3 level may be elevated because pregnancy is associated with an increase in plasma thyroid hormone–binding proteins due to the increase in circulating estrogen. The FT_4I should be normal. The TSH level should be within normal limits.

5. The answer is C. John Y. has symptoms and signs of hyperthyroidism. Thyrotoxicosis from any cause increases receptors for β-agonists, which increases the effect of circulating epinephrine. This results in increased contraction of palpebral muscles of the eyelid, lid lag, and stare. The proptosis and double vision are the result of Graves' ophthalmopathy, in which the extraocular muscles are infiltrated with lymphocytes and mucopolysaccharides. The Graves' ophthalmopathy indicates autoimmune hyperthyroidism due to antibodies that stimulate the TSH receptor. A diet high in goitrogens toxic to thyroid tissue would result in hypothyroidism.

6. The answer is B. James A. has the findings often associated with a multinodular goiter—older age, an enlarged, irregular thyroid gland, and gradual development of hyperthyroidism due to autonomous nodules. This is not an autoimmune disorder; therefore, a strong family history would not be expected. Thyroid cancer tissue does not produce thyroid hormones efficiently, so hyperthyroidism is rare unless the tumor burden is very large. His slow, mild clinical course does not suggest this. The clinical course and physical findings are more compatible with multinodular goiter than thyroiditis. Because the entire gland is irregular, more than one nodule is probably present.

▮ REFERENCES

Bahn RS, Heufelder AE: Pathogenesis of Graves' ophthalmopathy. *N Engl J Med* 329:1468–1475, 1993.

Boyages SC: Iodine deficiency disorders. *J Clin Endocrinol Metab* 77:587–591, 1993.

Ekholm R: Biosynthesis of thyroid hormones. *Int Rev Cytol* 120:243–288, 1990.

Freake HC, Oppenheimer JH: Thermogenesis and thyroid function. *Ann Rev Nutrition* 15:263–291, 1995.

Hay ID: Thyroiditis: a clinical update. *Mayo Clin Proc* 60:836–843, 1985.

LiVolsi VA: The pathology of autoimmune thyroid disease: a review. *Thyroid* 4:333–339, 1994.

Paschke R and Ludgate M: The thyrotropin receptor in thyroid diseases. *N Engl J Med* 337(23):1675–1681, 1997.

Singer PA, Cooper DS, Levy ES, et al: Treatment guidelines for patients with hyperthyroidism and hypothyroidism. *JAMA* 273:808–812, 1995.

Staub J-J, Althaus BU, Engler H, et al: Spectrum of subclinical and overt hypothyroidism: effect on thyrotropin, prolactin and thyroid reserve, and metabolic impact on peripheral target tissues. *Am J Med* 92:631–642, 1992.

Surks MI, Chopra IJ, Mariash CN, et al: American Thyroid Association guidelines for use of laboratory tests in thyroid disorders. *JAMA* 263:1529–1532, 1990.

Chapter 5

THE ADRENAL CORTEX

John P. Bantle, M.D.

■ CHAPTER OUTLINE

Case Study:
Introduction

A 16-year-old boy first noted easy fatiguability during summer vacation from high school. By the following November, he had to stop and rest after climbing two flights of stairs. He found himself exhausted after his school day and usually went to bed upon arriving home from school. He was frequently nauseated and occasionally vomited. His weight had decreased 8 lbs since the summer.

In December, he was hospitalized due to weakness. He was unable to get out of bed without assistance. He experienced continuous nausea and intermittent vomiting and was noted to have episodes of confusion and disorientation. Physical examination was remarkable for blood pressure of 90/70 mm Hg supine and 60/40 mm Hg upright. He had a "dark" complexion, but his examination was otherwise normal. Laboratory tests revealed a low serum sodium (Na^+) level and a high serum potassium (K^+) level. His physician told his parents that he might not live beyond Christmas. A diagnostic test was performed.

■ ADRENAL PHYSIOLOGY

INTRODUCTION

The adrenal glands are located just above and medial to the upper poles of the kidneys. They are triangular in shape and are composed of an outer cortex and an inner medulla. Although the cortex and the medulla are contained within the same capsule, they are derived from different tissues and function as separate entities. The adrenal medulla is an extension of the sympathetic nervous system and is discussed in Chapter 6. The adrenal cortex produces three types of steroid hormones: glucocorticoid hormones, so-called because of their influence on glucose metabolism; mineralocorticoids, which regulate Na+ and K+ balance; and androgens. The major hormones are: cortisol (hydrocortisone), a glucocorticoid; aldosterone, a mineralocorticoid; and dehydroepiandrosterone (DHEA), an androgen.

The adult adrenal cortex is composed of three zones. The outer zona glomerulosa produces aldosterone and is regulated primarily by the renin-angiotensin system. The thicker middle zona reticularis, with its columns of cells, and the compact innermost zona fasciculata produce cortisol and androgens and are regulated by adrenocorticotropic hormone (ACTH) from the pituitary gland as described below.

STEROID HORMONE BIOSYNTHESIS AND REGULATION

Secretion of cortisol and adrenal androgens is regulated by the hypothalamic-pituitary-adrenal axis (Figure 5-1). The hypothalamic and pituitary components of this axis are corticotropin-releasing hormone (CRH) and ACTH.

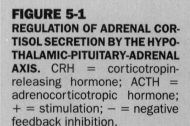

Major Adrenal Cortex Hormones
Glucocorticoid: cortisol (hydrocortisone)
Mineralocorticoid: aldosterone
Androgen: dehydroepiandrosterone (DHEA)

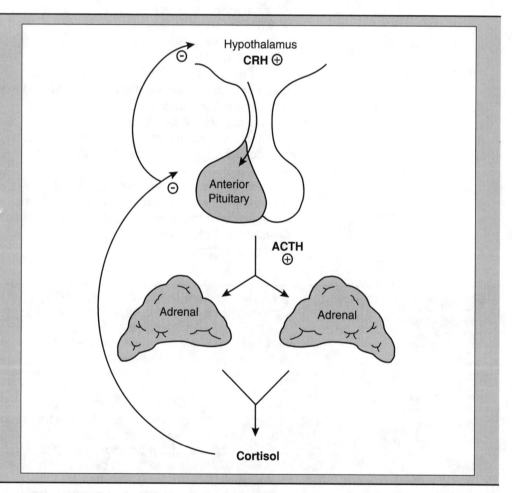

FIGURE 5-1
REGULATION OF ADRENAL CORTISOL SECRETION BY THE HYPOTHALAMIC-PITUITARY-ADRENAL AXIS. CRH = corticotropin-releasing hormone; ACTH = adrenocorticotropic hormone; + = stimulation; − = negative feedback inhibition.

Corticotropin-Releasing Hormone. CRH is a 41–amino acid peptide produced in the hypothalamus. It is also present in other areas of the brain, the pancreas, and the intestinal tract, but its purpose in these areas is not understood. CRH produced in the hypothalamus is secreted into the portal vessels of the pituitary. CRH stimulates ACTH synthesis and secretion by the pituitary gland.

Stress of all kinds (e.g., major illness, surgery, injury, exercise, hypoglycemia, starva-

Regulators of ACTH Secretion
CRH pulses
Superimposed stress (via CRH)
Negative feedback from cortisol

tion) *increases* CRH secretion. CRH is under negative feedback control from cortisol, which *decreases* CRH synthesis and secretion.

Adrenocorticotropic Hormone. ACTH is produced by pituitary corticotrophs, which comprise approximately 15% of pituitary cells and are clustered in the central pituitary. ACTH is a 39–amino acid peptide derived from a larger precursor molecule called pro-opiomelanocortin. Pro-opiomelanocortin is cleaved to yield ACTH and β-lipotropin, which are secreted together.

ACTH is secreted in pulses with a diurnal rhythm superimposed upon the pulses. The highest plasma ACTH concentrations occur in the early morning (4:00–6:00 A.M.); the lowest ACTH concentrations occur at night. This diurnal rhythm is abolished by stress, which causes increased ACTH secretion at all times of the day or night. ACTH has a half-life in the circulation of less than 10 minutes.

ACTH *stimulates* the adrenal gland to secrete cortisol. In turn, cortisol *inhibits* ACTH synthesis and secretion by negative feedback. ACTH also stimulates adrenal aldosterone secretion, but the renin-angiotensin system is the primary regulator of aldosterone. ACTH, β-lipotropin, or one of their subfragments stimulate melanocytes to produce melanin and thereby increase skin pigmentation.

Biosynthesis of Cortisol and Adrenal Androgens. Pituitary ACTH is the primary regulator of adrenal cortisol production. ACTH binds to specific receptors on the surface of adrenal cortical cells. This receptor binding activates adenyl cyclase via a stimulatory Gs protein, leading to an increase in cyclic adenosine monophosphate (cAMP). cAMP then activates protein kinases, which initiate ACTH action.

Acutely, ACTH stimulates removal of the six-carbon side chain from cholesterol to form pregnenolone, which is the first and rate-limiting step in cortisol synthesis (Figure 5-2). This effect occurs minutes after ACTH secretion by the pituitary. Chronically, ACTH stimulates the formation of all of the enzymes involved in steroid synthesis.

ACTH is also the primary regulator of adrenal androgen production. Although adrenal androgens such as DHEA and androstenedione are produced in substantial amounts, they are considerably less potent than the gonadal androgen testosterone.

Biosynthesis of Aldosterone. Aldosterone secretion is under the primary control of the renin-angiotensin system. Renin is a proteolytic enzyme produced by the juxtaglomerular (JG) cells of the kidney. The JG cells surround glomerular afferent arterioles. The substrate for renin is angiotensinogen, which is converted by renin to angiotensin I. Angiotensin I is converted to angiotensin II by angiotensin-converting enzyme, which is present primarily in the pulmonary vascular endothelium. Angiotensin II stimulates adrenal aldosterone secretion and, in addition, is a potent pressor that acts directly on arteriolar smooth muscle. Adrenal aldosterone secretion is stimulated by:

1. Reduced renal afferent arteriolar pressure, which stimulates renin secretion by the JG cells. The increased secretion of aldosterone results in renal Na$^+$ retention and expansion of extracellular fluid volume, which tends to raise blood pressure.
2. Increased delivery of filtered Na$^+$ to the macula densa cells of the renal distal convoluted tubules, which stimulate renin secretion by the JG cells. The secretion of renin decreases the glomerular filtration rate (GFR) and reduces the filtered load of Na$^+$.
3. Increased sympathetic nervous system activity.
4. Increased serum K$^+$, which stimulates aldosterone secretion directly.
5. ACTH, which also stimulates aldosterone secretion directly.

Figure 5-2 summarizes the synthetic pathways for adrenal steroid production. Note that there are three major pathways leading to cortisol, aldosterone, and adrenal androgens such as DHEA and androstenedione.

STEROID HORMONE TRANSPORT IN BLOOD

After cortisol is secreted into the bloodstream, approximately 90% of cortisol molecules become protein bound. Cortisol's primary transport protein is cortisol-binding globulin (CBG). However, cortisol is in dynamic equilibrium between protein bound and free

Stimulators of Aldosterone Secretion
Renin-angiotensin system
Sympathetic nervous system
Increased serum K$^+$
ACTH

FIGURE 5-2
SYNTHETIC PATHWAYS OF AD-RENAL STEROID PRODUCTION. These pathways lead to three products: cortisol (glucocorticoid), aldosterone (mineralocorticoid), and dehydroepiandrosterone (androgen).

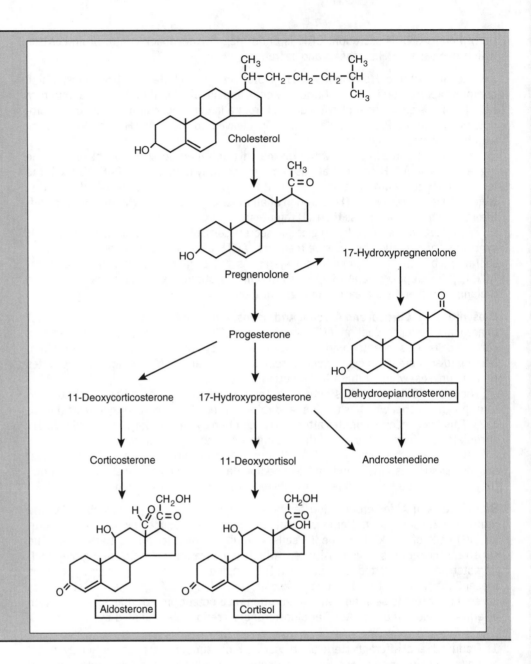

forms. It is the free cortisol that is able to leave the vascular compartment, enter cells, and initiate hormone actions. Aldosterone and androgens also are bound to transport proteins.

MECHANISM OF ACTION OF ADRENAL STEROID HORMONES

Adrenal cortex hormones are typical steroid hormones. Free cortisol molecules in the circulation enter cells of target tissues and bind to specific glucocorticoid receptors present in the cytosol. The binding of cortisol to its receptor causes a modification in the receptor molecule, changing it to a protein with high affinity for DNA. This process is called activation. The cortisol receptor complex then moves to the nucleus (translocation) and binds specific sites on specific genes. This binding causes increased transcription of specific RNA sequences, which then leads to increased messenger RNA (mRNA) formation and increased translation of specific proteins. These proteins become the mediators of the biologic effects of cortisol.

Binding of the cortisol-receptor complex to other specific genes results in decreased transcription of RNA sequences and decreased translation of the related proteins. Thus, cortisol causes an increase in the synthesis of certain proteins and a decrease in the synthesis of other proteins. The mechanism of action of cortisol is summarized in Figure 5-3.

BIOLOGIC EFFECTS OF ADRENAL HORMONES

Metabolic Effects of Cortisol. Cortisol is the principal glucocorticoid hormone of the adrenal cortex. It promotes the conversion of amino acids to glucose (gluconeogenesis) in the liver by stimulating enzymes of the gluconeogenic pathway. Cortisol also increases protein catabolism, which increases the supply of amino acids for gluconeogenesis. Cortisol inhibits glucose uptake by muscle and fat, resulting in insulin resistance. Cortisol promotes glycogen deposition by stimulating the enzymes required for glycogen synthesis, but the net effect of cortisol is to increase the blood glucose concentration.

In adipose tissue cortisol stimulates lipolysis, which releases free fatty acids into the circulation. Free fatty acids supply energy for muscle and other non–glucose-dependent tissues.

When cortisol is present in excess as a result of stress, adrenal hyperfunction, or pharmacologic administration, it has many additional effects. It stimulates appetite, causing increased energy intake and weight gain. Cortisol suppresses inflammation and immune function, the primary reasons why cortisol and its analogs are used pharmacologically. Cortisol suppresses bone formation and has catabolic effects on bone, connective tissue, and muscle, which result in loss of bone mass, poor wound healing, easy bruising, loss of muscle mass, and weakness. Cortisol inhibits linear growth in children. Excess cortisol also can alter mood, sometimes resulting in euphoria, insomnia, and even psychosis.

Cortisol has mineralocorticoid activity, although it is a much less potent mineralocorticoid than aldosterone. Excess cortisol increases blood pressure due to increased salt and water retention.

Aldosterone. Aldosterone is the principal adrenal mineralocorticoid. It promotes Na+ retention by reducing urinary Na+ excretion by the distal renal tubule and collecting ducts. Aldosterone also increases urinary K+ and hydrogen ion (H+) excretion.

DHEA and Other Adrenal Androgens. These are weak androgens. They do not have any known important effects in adult males because of the presence of more potent testicular androgens, such as testosterone. However, adrenal androgens are important in the maintenance of female axillary and pubic hair. If present in excess, adrenal androgens can cause hirsutism (abnormal facial and body hair) and masculinization of females and prepubertal males.

Major Metabolic Effects of Cortisol

Carbohydrate metabolism
    Increases gluconeogenesis
    Increases insulin resistance
    Increases blood glucose
    Increases glycogen synthesis
Fat metabolism
    Increases lipolysis and free fatty acids
Protein metabolism
    Increases protein breakdown
    Increases urinary nitrogen excretion

Major Biologic Effects of Increased Cortisol

Weight gain and truncal obesity
Na+ and water retention
Suppressed inflammation
Suppressed immune system
Inhibited fibroblasts, loss of connective tissue, thin skin, easy bruising, abdominal stria, and impaired wound healing
Growth failure in children
Decreased calcium absorption
Bone loss
Altered mood, behavior, and cognition

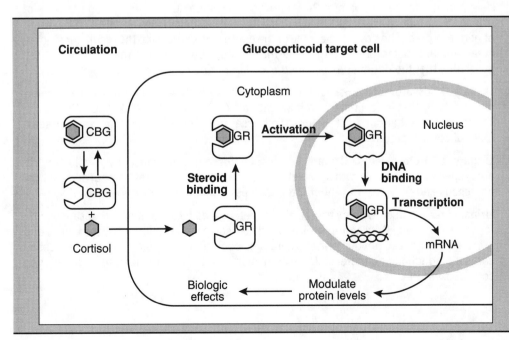

FIGURE 5-3
MECHANISM OF CELLULAR CORTISOL ACTION. CBG = cortisol-binding globulin; GR = glucocorticoid receptor. (*Source:* Reprinted with permission from Feldman D: Mechanism of action of cortisol. In *Endocrinology*, 2nd ed. Edited by DeGroot LJ. Philadelphia, PA: W. B. Saunders, 1989, p 1558.)

■ TESTS OF ADRENAL FUNCTION

PLASMA HORMONE LEVELS

Although it is possible to measure plasma levels of ACTH and a variety of adrenal cortical hormones, such measurements often are not very helpful. Many of these hormones are secreted in pulses with a diurnal rhythm and demonstrate substantial variation with time of day. In addition, hormones such as ACTH and cortisol are secreted in response to stress, so their concentrations can fluctuate substantially. Cortisol, in particular, is best measured under defined conditions, such as after ACTH stimulation or dexamethasone suppression. This is discussed further below. Aldosterone secretion is dependent in large part on Na^+ intake; thus, it is also best measured under defined conditions. Tests of adrenal function are listed in Table 5-1.

Table 5-1 **Tests of Adrenal Function**	**Plasma hormone levels** ACTH Cortisol Aldosterone 17-Hydroxyprogesterone 11-Deoxycortisol Dehydroepiandrosterone Dehydroepiandrosterone sulfate Androstenedione **Urinary 24-hour steroid excretion** 17-Hydroxysteroids 17-Ketosteroids Urinary free-cortisol	**ACTH stimulation test** **Dexamethasone suppression tests** One-mg overnight test (screening) Formal 6-day test (differential diagnosis) **Tests of ACTH production** CRH stimulation test Metyrapone test Insulin hypoglycemia test **Tests of aldosterone overproduction** Aldosterone suppression test

Plasma levels of androgens may be helpful in cases of apparent androgen excess in boys and girls or women. DHEA and its metabolite dehydroepiandrosterone-sulfate (DHEAS) are the adrenal androgens usually measured.

When a congenital adrenal enzyme defect is suspected, measuring the serum level of the precursor just prior to the block can help to make the diagnosis. For instance, measurement of 17-hydroxyprogesterone can be used to make the diagnosis of 21-hydroxylase deficiency.

URINARY STEROID EXCRETION

Three urinary steroids are commonly measured to assess adrenal cortex hormone production. These are urinary 17-hydroxysteroids, 17-ketosteroids, and free cortisol. All are best determined after collection of a 24-hour urine specimen and are expressed per gram of urinary creatinine. Measuring urinary steroids over 24 hours gives an integrated picture of hormone production over the course of the entire day. Expressing the result per gram of creatinine allows the physician to take into account body muscle mass as well as the possibility that the patient has provided a 24-hour urine collection that is not complete.

Urinary 17-Hydroxysteroids. Urinary 17-hydroxysteroids are determined by a colorometric assay that is specific for steroids with a 17,21-dihydroxy, 20-keto configuration. These are cortisol and its metabolites. This assay provides a 24-hour integrated assessment of cortisol production.

Urinary 17-Ketosteroids. Urinary 17-ketosteroids are determined by a colorometric assay specific for steroids with a 17-keto group. This assay measures adrenal and gonadal androgens and provides a 24-hour integrated assessment of androgen production.

Urinary Free Cortisol. Urinary free cortisol is determined by a radioimmunoassay specific for cortisol in urine. Only non–protein-bound cortisol in blood is filtered by the kidney and excreted unchanged in the urine. Therefore, conditions in which there is increased cortisol production and increased free cortisol in blood cause an increase in urinary free cortisol excretion.

ACTH STIMULATION TESTS

The ACTH stimulation tests assess the ability of the adrenal cortex to increase cortisol secretion in response to ACTH. Two ACTH stimulation tests are commonly used: the 4-hour ACTH stimulation test and the rapid ACTH stimulation test.

The 4-hour test is performed as follows: at approximately 8:00 A.M., a plasma sample for cortisol is obtained. For the next 4 hours, synthetic ACTH (cosyntropin) is infused intravenously. At approximately noon, a second plasma sample for cortisol is obtained. In a normal individual, plasma cortisol levels will increase to a value greater than 25 µg/dL after ACTH infusion. In someone with adrenal insufficiency, the adrenal glands do not respond normally, and the rise in plasma cortisol is subnormal.

Sometimes a shortened version of the ACTH stimulation test is performed for screening purposes. In this "rapid" ACTH stimulation test, a bolus of ACTH is administered intravenously, and plasma cortisol is checked 60 minutes later. If the rapid test is abnormal, the 4-hour ACTH test should be performed to establish the diagnosis of adrenal insufficiency.

DEXAMETHASONE SUPPRESSION TESTS

Dexamethasone suppression tests are used to determine whether there is cortisol overproduction. Dexamethasone is a long-acting cortisol analog which suppresses ACTH secretion but is not measured in the radioimmunoassay for cortisol. Suppression of ACTH secretion by dexamethasone causes a decrease in adrenal cortisol synthesis, and plasma cortisol decreases. Two dexamethasone suppression tests are in common use: the 1-mg overnight dexamethasone suppression test and the formal 6-day dexamethasone suppression test.

One-mg Overnight Dexamethasone Suppression Test. The 1-mg overnight dexamethasone suppression test is used to detect the overproduction of cortisol (Cushing's syndrome). To perform this test, 1 mg of dexamethasone is administered at 11:00 P.M. At 8:00 A.M. the next morning, a blood sample is obtained to determine the plasma cortisol level. In a healthy individual, 1 mg of dexamethasone is enough to suppress pituitary ACTH secretion overnight, and by the next morning, plasma cortisol should be suppressed to less than 5 µg/dL. There are virtually no false-negative results (patients who suppress normally do not have Cushing's syndrome). However, stress of any kind can cause a false-positive result. For instance, patients with malnutrition, obesity, depression, renal failure, and many other medical conditions may not suppress plasma cortisol normally after dexamethasone administration; the stress associated with these conditions probably increases ACTH secretion.

Formal 6-Day Dexamethasone Suppression Test. The formal 6-day dexamethasone suppression test is used to determine the *cause* of Cushing's syndrome (cortisol hypersecretion). For 6 consecutive days, 24-hour urine collections are obtained for measurement of 17-hydroxysteroids. Sometimes urinary 17-ketosteroids and urinary free cortisol are measured also. On days 1 and 2, the patient receives no dexamethasone—these are collections to determine the patient's baseline steroid production; on days 3 and 4, the patient receives "low-dose dexamethasone" (0.5 mg every 6 hours). On days 5 and 6, the patient receives "high-dose dexamethasone" (2 mg every 6 hours). Expected results from this test are summarized in Table 5-2.

In a healthy individual, urinary 17-hydroxysteroid excretion is normal on days 1 and 2 and is suppressed to subnormal levels with low-dose dexamethasone and remains suppressed with high-dose dexamethasone. Patients who are obese may have slightly

SITUATION	URINARY 17-HYDROXYSTEROIDS					
	Day 1	Day 2	Day 3	Day 4	Day 5	Day 6
Normal health	N	N	S	S	S	S
Simple obesity	I	I	S	S	S	S
Pituitary Cushing's	I	I	I	I	S	S
Adrenal tumor	I	I	I	I	I	I
Ectopic ACTH	I	I	I	I	I	I

Note. N = normal; I = increased; S = suppressed.

Table 5-2
Formal 6-Day Dexamethasone Suppression Test Results

increased urinary 17-hydroxysteroids on days 1 and 2 because obesity may cause increased clearance of cortisol. However, with low-dose dexamethasone administration on days 3 and 4, urinary 17-hydroxysteroid excretion is suppressed normally in obese patients.

Patients with a pituitary tumor producing ACTH have increased urinary 17-hydroxysteroid excretion on days 1 and 2. With administration of low-dose dexamethasone on days 3 and 4, urinary 17-hydroxysteroid excretion remains increased because the pituitary tumor does not have normal sensitivity to dexamethasone. However, with high-dose dexamethasone on days 5 and 6, ACTH secretion and urinary 17-hydroxysteroid excretion are finally suppressed.

In patients who have cortisol-secreting adrenal tumors, cortisol production is not ACTH-dependent. Urinary 17-hydroxysteroid excretion is increased on days 1 and 2 and remains high after low-dose and high-dose dexamethasone. Increased urinary 17-hydroxysteroid excretion without suppression also occurs with ectopic ACTH production by neoplasms like lung carcinomas. Such ACTH production is autonomous and is not influenced by dexamethasone administration.

TESTS OF ACTH PRODUCTION

Overproduction of ACTH can be determined by the 6-day dexamethasone suppression test described above. If it is unclear whether excess ACTH is from the pituitary gland or is ectopic ACTH produced by a nonpituitary tumor, a CRH stimulation test can be helpful. In this test, the plasma ACTH response to an infusion of CRH is measured. Pituitary tumors respond to CRH, but most ectopic ACTH-producing tumors do not.

The metyrapone test and the insulin-induced hypoglycemia test are used to determine pituitary ACTH reserve. Metyrapone blocks the last step in cortisol synthesis. If the pituitary is able to respond to a low cortisol level by increasing production of ACTH, there will be an abrupt increase in 11-deoxycortisol, which is the immediate precursor of cortisol. Hypoglycemia due to a controlled insulin infusion is a stress that should elicit a burst of ACTH followed by cortisol secretion. Patients with ACTH deficiency will not have an adequate cortisol response. These tests usually are ordered only by specialists in endocrinology and metabolism.

TESTS OF ALDOSTERONE OVERPRODUCTION

A patient who has hyperaldosteronism should have a high plasma aldosterone level, and the Na^+ and water retention caused by the high aldosterone should suppress plasma renin activity. Therefore, a high plasma aldosterone:plasma renin activity ratio indicates hyperaldosteronism.

Hyperaldosteronism also can be assessed by the aldosterone suppression test. Normal saline is infused into the patient for 4 hours. This expands the extracellular volume, which suppresses plasma renin, thereby suppressing aldosterone. Patients with hyperaldosteronism do not have normal suppression of aldosterone in response to volume expansion.

▌ COMMONLY USED PHARMACOLOGIC ADRENAL ▌ STEROID PREPARATIONS

Since cortisol (hydrocortisone) is the principal naturally occurring glucocorticoid, it is the preferred drug for treatment of adrenal insufficiency. Hydrocortisone replacement is given in divided doses, usually two-thirds in the morning and one-third at noon, in an attempt to mimic the natural diurnal rhythm of cortisol secretion. Cortisone is also used to treat adrenal insufficiency, but cortisone must be converted in vivo to cortisol by 11-hydroxylation before it becomes biologically active. This conversion is not complete, so cortisone is slightly less potent per unit weight than is cortisol.

Cortisol replacement provides considerable mineralocorticoid activity, but patients with adrenal insufficiency may require additional mineralocorticoid replacement to maintain Na^+ and water balance. This can be provided by synthetic fluorinated mineralocorticoids such as fludrocortisone.

Glucocorticoids frequently are prescribed for their anti-inflammatory and anti-immune properties rather than for treatment of adrenal insufficiency. In these situations, pharmacologic rather than physiologic doses are required. Prednisone and dexamethasone are synthetic glucocorticoid analogs used to treat a variety of medical conditions. Cortisol in large doses would have the same anti-inflammatory and anti-immune effects but would also have unwanted mineralocorticoid activity. When large doses of prednisone or dexamethasone are used chronically to treat a disease process, serious side effects are likely. These include opportunistic infections, hypertension, unmasking of latent diabetes mellitus, loss of bone mass (osteoporosis), psychiatric disorders, and growth retardation in children. Thus, the lowest effective dose of glucocorticoid should be used. Table 5-3 provides a summary of commonly used steroid preparations.

Table 5-3
Commonly Used Pharmacologic Steroid Preparations

NAME	RELATIVE GLUCOCORTICOID POTENCY	RELATIVE MINERALOCORTICOID POTENCY	DURATION OF BIOLOGIC ACTIVITY
Cortisol (hydrocortisone)	1	1	< 12 hr
Cortisone	0.8	0.8	< 12 hr
Prednisone[a]	4–5	0.25	24 hr
Dexamethasone[a]	30–40	Negligible	48 hr
Fludrocortisone[a]	10	140	24 hr

[a] Not naturally occurring.

Case Study: Continued

In the case of the critically ill high school student, the best diagnostic test would have been an ACTH stimulation test, as his fatigue, weakness, weight loss, nausea, vomiting, hypotension, hyperpigmentation, hyponatremia, and hyperkalemia all indicated adrenal insufficiency. However, a urinary 17-hydroxysteroid determination, rather than an ACTH stimulation test, was performed. The patient excreted 0.1 mg 17-hydroxysteroids in 24 hours (normal: 4–14 mg/24 hr).

When the patient's low urinary 17-hydroxysteroid value was reported, he was treated with cortisol immediately. He demonstrated remarkable improvement. Within 24 hours, he was thinking clearly, walking without assistance, and eating all food served to him. He was referred to a university hospital for further evaluation.

∎ DISORDERS OF THE ADRENAL GLANDS

PRIMARY ADRENAL INSUFFICIENCY (ADDISON'S DISEASE)

Adrenal insufficiency is rare, with a prevalence of 4–6 per 100,000 people. Until recently, tuberculosis was the most common cause of adrenal insufficiency. Now the most common cause is bilateral destruction of the adrenal glands by autoimmune adrenalitis. This often is associated with other autoimmune endocrine disorders such as type 1 diabetes mellitus, chronic lymphocytic thyroiditis, and vitiligo (patches of white, depigmented skin). Vitiligo is due to a concomitant autoimmune process that attacks melanocytes and may be a clue to the presence of autoimmune adrenalitis. Autoimmune adrenalitis is more common in women, as are other autoimmune disorders.

Tuberculosis is still the major infectious cause of primary adrenal insufficiency. Adrenal gland destruction due to cytomegalovirus and other infections occurs as part of the acquired immunodeficiency syndrome (AIDS). Other causes of primary adrenal insufficiency include treatment with antifungal drugs such as ketoconazole, adrenal hemorrhage, metastatic carcinoma, and surgical removal of the adrenal glands.

Fatigue and weakness are common in patients with primary adrenal insufficiency, and adrenal insufficiency should always be considered in patients with unexplained weight loss. Nausea, anorexia, and abdominal pain are common symptoms. Women often have amenorrhea.

Hyperpigmentation occurs frequently because the high levels of ACTH, β-lipotropin, or one of their subfragments that occur in response to the low level of cortisol stimulate melanocytes and increase the production of melanin. Hyperpigmentation is present everywhere, but it is particularly prominent over pressure points, such as elbows and

Major Diseases of the Adrenal Cortex
Adrenal insufficiency
Adrenal hyperfunction
Hyperaldosteronism
Congenital adrenal hyperplasia

Major Causes of Adrenal Insufficiency
Autoimmune adrenalitis
Infection
Hemorrhage
Metastases
Surgery

Primary Adrenal Insufficiency

Symptoms and Signs	Percent of Patients
Weakness and fatigue	99
Hyperpigmentation	98
Unexplained weight loss	97
Anorexia, nausea, and vomiting	90
Hypotension (blood pressure < 110/70 mm Hg)	88
Hyponatremia (low serum Na+)	88
Hyperkalemia (high serum K+)	64

Primary versus Secondary Adrenal Insufficiency

Manifestations	Primary	Secondary
Hyperpigmentation	Yes	No
Pallor	No	Yes
Low Na+	Yes	No
High K+	Yes	No
Hypotension	Yes	No
Cortisol level	Low	Low
ACTH level	High	Low

Symptoms and Signs of Adrenal (Addisonian) Crisis
Volume depletion
Hypotension and shock
Fever
Nausea and vomiting
Weakness
Hypoglycemia

Major Causes of Cushing's Syndrome
Exogenous glucocorticoids (cortisol, prednisone, dexamethasone)
ACTH-producing pituitary tumors
Cortisol-secreting adrenal adenoma or adrenal carcinoma
Ectopic ACTH production by nonpituitary tumors
Ectopic CRH production by nonhypothalamic tumors

knees. The buccal mucosa and palmar creases are other places to look for hyperpigmentation. The degree to which a change in pigmentation is detectable depends upon the underlying skin pigmentation of the patient.

Hypoglycemia also can be present. Hyponatremia and hyperkalemia are caused by aldosterone deficiency and are accompanied by orthostatic hypotension.

Patients are treated with cortisol (hydrocortisone). They also may require a mineralocorticoid such as fludrocortisone.

SECONDARY (PITUITARY) ADRENAL INSUFFICIENCY

Adrenal insufficiency can be due to inadequate secretion of ACTH by the pituitary gland. Pituitary insufficiency can be caused by pituitary tumors, postpartum pituitary infarction (see Chapter 12), pituitary irradiation or surgery, head trauma, or withdrawal of long-term exogenous glucocorticoid therapy that has suppressed pituitary ACTH production. It may take months after withdrawal of exogenous glucocorticoid for ACTH production to recover after chronic suppression.

Symptoms and signs are similar to those of primary adrenal insufficiency *except* that patients exhibit pallor instead of hyperpigmentation. ACTH and β-lipotropin secretion are low, and melanocyte stimulation is decreased. Usually, there are no electrolyte abnormalities because the renin-angiotensin-aldosterone system remains intact. Patients lose axillary and pubic hair if both ACTH and gonadotropin secretion are defective and total androgen production is low.

Diagnosis of secondary adrenal insufficiency is indicated by low plasma cortisol and ACTH levels and low urine 17-hydroxysteroids. Other pituitary hormone deficiencies almost always are present. Patients are treated with cortisol, but fludrocortisone usually is not necessary because the renin-angiotensin-aldosterone axis should be intact. The underlying pituitary disorder must also be treated and other hormone deficiencies should be corrected if present.

ACUTE ADRENAL CRISIS

Individuals with a normal hypothalamic-pituitary-adrenal axis respond to stress (e.g., infection, surgery) with acute increases in CRH, ACTH, and cortisol. Patients receiving treatment for adrenal insufficiency must compensate by increasing their dose of cortisol above the usual maintenance level during stress. If they do not, they may present with acute adrenal crisis: a combination of extreme weakness, dehydration, hypotension, fever, nausea, vomiting, and hypoglycemia, which can be fatal if untreated. They must be given high doses of cortisol plus fluids, saline, and glucose. The cause of the underlying stress must also be treated.

Patients with undiagnosed adrenal insufficiency can present for the first time in adrenal crisis. Patients who have been on chronic glucocorticoid therapy for immunosuppression or suppression of inflammation can also present with adrenal crisis if their glucocorticoid dose is discontinued abruptly. Their hypothalamic-pituitary-adrenal axis will be suppressed and unable to resume cortisol production acutely.

ADRENAL HYPERFUNCTION (CUSHING'S SYNDROME)

Cortisol excess due to any cause results in a characteristic constellation of symptoms and signs that is referred to as Cushing's syndrome. Cushing's syndrome most often is the result of long-term use of pharmacologic doses of exogenous glucocorticoids (cortisol, prednisone, dexamethasone) prescribed for treatment of chronic inflammation or immune suppression. CRH and ACTH production are suppressed by the high plasma glucocorticoid concentration.

Tumors also cause Cushing's syndrome. ACTH-producing pituitary tumors cause bilateral adrenal hyperplasia and excess cortisol secretion. Cushing's syndrome due to an ACTH-producing pituitary tumor is referred to specifically as Cushing's disease. ACTH production by pituitary tumors remains partially responsive to feedback inhibition by high doses of glucocorticoids (see dexamethasone suppression test above).

ACTH production by nonpituitary neoplasms such as carcinomas of the lung (ectopic ACTH) is unregulated by CRH and does not respond to feedback inhibition by high-dose dexamethasone. CRH production by neoplasms (ectopic CRH) stimulates excess pituitary ACTH production, resulting in bilateral adrenal hyperplasia. This is rare.

Adrenal adenomas or carcinomas can produce cortisol without ACTH stimulation. CRH and ACTH production are suppressed by the high cortisol levels.

Patients with Cushing's syndrome lose the classic diurnal rhythm of cortisol secretion. Their cortisol levels are high day and night. Symptoms and signs of cortisol excess include weight gain with a typical body habitus due to fat deposition in the face (round face or "moon" facies), neck, and trunk, especially the abdomen. Excess connective tissue catabolism results in purple abdominal striae (stretch marks with visible subcutaneous blood vessels), pink cheeks, and easy bruising. Weakness and muscle wasting due to protein catabolism are common. Osteoporosis (loss of bone mass) due to suppressed bone formation, decreased calcium absorption, and increased urinary calcium excretion results in vertebral compression fractures and other fractures. Women develop hirsutism and amenorrhea due to excess adrenal androgen production. Growth retardation occurs in children. Hypertension and hypokalemia result from the mineralocorticoid activity of cortisol. Hyperglycemia and sometimes overt diabetes are due to increased gluconeogenesis and insulin resistance.

Patients with tumors producing ACTH ectopically often are very ill from the underlying neoplasm, and weight loss and weakness are common. ACTH levels are very high, resulting in hyperpigmentation. Hypertension and hypokalemia often are the prominent problems in these patients. These tumors progress rapidly, and often there is not enough time for the other manifestations of glucocorticoid excess to develop.

If the physical examination suggests Cushing's syndrome, the best screening test is the 1-mg (overnight) dexamethasone suppression test. If this or other screening tests are positive, the patient should be referred to an endocrinologist for a formal 6-day dexamethasone suppression test and other tests as necessary (magnetic resonance imaging [MRI] of the pituitary gland, computed tomography [CT] scan of the adrenal glands, CRH stimulation test).

Treatment of Cushing's syndrome depends upon the cause. The dose of exogenous glucocorticoid should be reduced, if possible. An ACTH-producing pituitary adenoma can be removed by transsphenoidal pituitary adenomectomy, and an adrenal adenoma or carcinoma can be treated with adrenal surgery. Tumors producing ectopic ACTH are treated surgically, if possible, or with chemotherapy. If tumors causing Cushing's syndrome cannot be controlled with surgery or chemotherapy, cortisol synthesis can be blocked pharmacologically with aminoglutethimide or ketoconazole.

PRIMARY HYPERALDOSTERONISM (CONN'S SYNDROME)

Hyperaldosteronism accounts for hypertension in about 1% of hypertensive patients. Excess production of aldosterone most often is due to an adrenal adenoma or bilateral adrenal hyperplasia. The cause or causes are unknown. Cortisol production remains normal. Hypertension usually is the only clinical sign. Unexplained hypokalemia often is an important diagnostic clue.

Serum K^+ levels and plasma renin activity are measured to make the diagnosis. Plasma renin activity should be suppressed because the high aldosterone level causes Na^+ retention and expansion of plasma volume. The aldosterone suppression test is abnormal. An abdominal CT scan can be obtained to determine if an adenoma is present.

An adrenal adenoma can be removed surgically. If this is not possible, the hypertension and hyperkalemia can be treated with spironolactone, an aldosterone antagonist. Spironolactone is the treatment of choice for bilateral adrenal hyperplasia.

CONGENITAL ADRENAL HYPERPLASIA DUE TO 21-HYDROXYLASE DEFICIENCY

Congenital adrenal hyperplasia (CAH) is due to an inborn error of metabolism with a specific deficiency in one of the enzymes involved in cortisol synthesis. The most common is a deficiency in 21-hydroxylase. Because of the deficiency in the 21-hydroxylase enzyme, there is a block in cortisol production. This causes a compensatory increase in ACTH secretion and intense stimulation of the adrenal cortex. With this stimulation it often is possible to produce adequate amounts of cortisol. However, cortisol precursors proximal to the block are produced in large quantities. As depicted in Figure 5-4, excess 17-hydroxyprogesterone and other precursor steroids are shunted into the androgen pathway and result in increased adrenal androgen secretion.

Cushing's Syndrome

Symptoms and Signs	Percent of Patients
Weight gain, round facies, and truncal obesity	97
Weakness	87
Hypertension (blood pressure > 150/90 mm Hg)	82
Hirsutism (in women)	80
Amenorrhea	77
Cutaneous striae (stretch marks)	67
Ecchymoses (bruises)	65
Osteoporosis (loss of bone mass)	Common
Hyperglycemia	Common
Growth retardation (in children)	Common

Differential Diagnosis of Cushing's Syndrome

Diagnosis	ACTH	Cortisol
Pituitary tumor	High	High
Ectopic ACTH	High	High
Adrenal tumor	Low	High
Exogenous cortisol	Low	High
Exogenous prednisone or dexamethasone	Low	Low

Symptoms and Signs of Hyperaldosteronism

Hypertension
Hypokalemia
Suppressed plasma renin activity
Abnormal aldosterone suppression

FIGURE 5-4
ADRENAL STEROID PRODUC-TION IN CONGENITAL ADRENAL HYPERPLASIA DUE TO 21-HY-DROXYLASE DEFICIENCY. Because of the block in cortisol production and the increased adrenocorticotropic hormone (ACTH) stimulation that results, 17-hydroxyprogesterone and other precursors accumulate and are shunted into the androgen pathway.

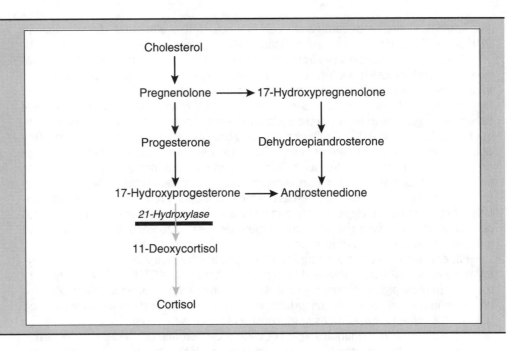

Symptoms and signs of CAH include masculinization of external genitalia in female infants, precocious sexual development of male infants, and rapid early growth but final short stature due to premature closure of the epiphyses (see Chapters 13 and 14). In cases where there also is a block in aldosterone production, there is excessive urinary Na^+ loss. This usually presents in early infancy as an adrenal crisis. Women with the adult-onset type of CAH may develop hirsutism, oligomenorrhea, and infertility.

The diagnosis of CAH is made by measuring serum 17-hydroxyprogesterone, which is very high. Urinary 17-ketosteroids also are increased. Patients with CAH are treated with cortisol, prednisone, or dexamethasone in physiologic amounts sufficient to suppress ACTH secretion, thereby preventing excess androgen production.

Case Study:
Resolution

When the patient was hospitalized 1 month later for additional testing, he reported feeling 100% normal. He was noted to be hyperpigmented. Blood pressure was 125/75 mm Hg. Plasma cortisol levels were 2 μg/dL at 8:00 A.M. (normal: > 5 μg/dL). After infusion of synthetic ACTH, plasma cortisol remained 2 μg/dL, demonstrating a grossly deficient cortisol response. The diagnosis of adrenal insufficiency was confirmed.

His physical examination and laboratory tests suggested that this was primary, not secondary, adrenal insufficiency. He was hyperpigmented, indicating that ACTH was high. His initial hypotension, low Na^+, and high K^+ suggested concomitant aldosterone deficiency. This would be expected with adrenal destruction but not with ACTH deficiency because aldosterone is regulated primarily by the renin-angiotensin system, not ACTH. There was no evidence of tuberculosis or other infectious problems, and the cause of his adrenal insufficiency was thought to be immune adrenalitis.

The patient was placed on maintenance therapy with cortisol (hydrocortisone) and fludrocortisone and has had a normal, productive life. He was instructed to increase his maintenance dose of cortisol when he became ill. Several years later, he developed chronic lymphocytic thyroiditis, providing additional support for the diagnosis of an autoimmune cause for his adrenal insufficiency.

Twenty-five years after his medical close call, this patient is married with two children, is the full-time manager of an automobile dealership, and enjoys running approximately 20 miles a week.

■ REVIEW QUESTIONS

Directions: For each of the following questions, choose the **one best** answer.

1. A 27-year-old man with adrenal insufficiency is being treated with cortisol. He can expect cortisol to do which one of the following?

    (A) Increase corticotropin-releasing hormone (CRH) secretion
    (B) Increase adrenocorticotropic hormone (ACTH) secretion
    (C) Increase conversion of amino acids to glucose
    (D) Increase inflammation and wound healing
    (E) Increase sensitivity to insulin in muscle

2. A 43-year-old woman complains of fatigue, intermittent vomiting, and a weight loss of 15 lbs. Physical examination is remarkable for a blood pressure of 100/60 mm Hg supine and 80/40 mm Hg standing. She has a large patch of white, depigmented skin on the right side of her neck. Her diagnostic evaluation should include which of the following tests?

    (A) Corticotropin-releasing hormone (CRH) stimulation test
    (B) Adrenocorticotropic hormone (ACTH) stimulation test
    (C) Aldosterone suppression test
    (D) One-mg (overnight) dexamethasone suppression test
    (E) Formal 6-day dexamethasone suppression test

Questions 3 and 4

A 40-year-old woman complains of fatigue, weight gain of 30 lbs, cessation of menstruation, and recent growth of dark facial, chest, and abdominal hair. Physical examination is remarkable for a blood pressure of 160/95 mm Hg, a round face, obesity, hirsutism involving the face and trunk, multiple ecchymoses, and purplish abdominal striae.

3. Which of the following tests should be the next step in her evaluation?

    (A) Corticotropin-releasing hormone (CRH) stimulation test
    (B) Adrenocorticotropic hormone (ACTH) stimulation test
    (C) Aldosterone suppression test
    (D) One-mg (overnight) dexamethasone suppression test
    (E) Formal 6-day dexamethasone suppression test

4. After demonstrating abnormal screening tests, the patient undergoes a formal 6-day dexamethasone suppression test. Twenty-four hour urine collections for 17-hydroxy-steroids are obtained on 6 consecutive days. On days 3 and 4, she receives low-dose dexamethasone; on days 5 and 6, she receives high-dose dexamethasone. Her urinary 17-hydroxysteroid excretion is elevated on days 1 and 2, remains elevated on days 3 and 4, decreases on day 5, and suppresses to a subnormal level on day 6. What is the most likely cause of this patient's Cushing's syndrome?

    (A) A pituitary tumor producing adrenocorticotropic hormone (ACTH)
    (B) A lung carcinoma producing ACTH ectopically
    (C) An adrenal adenoma
    (D) An adrenal carcinoma
    (E) Surreptitious use of the medication prednisone

5. A 47-year-old man with diabetic nephropathy and end-stage renal disease received a kidney transplant 4 months ago. His post-transplant immunosuppressant medications include prednisone, 15 mg twice daily. Renal function is now normal. Evaluation of his hypothalamic-pituitary-adrenal axis would most likely yield which of the following results?

   (A) Decreased plasma adrenocorticotropic hormone (ACTH), decreased plasma cortisol, increased urinary free cortisol
   (B) Decreased plasma ACTH, increased plasma cortisol, decreased urinary free cortisol
   (C) Increased plasma ACTH, increased plasma cortisol, decreased urinary free cortisol
   (D) Increased plasma ACTH, decreased plasma cortisol, decreased urinary free cortisol
   (E) Decreased plasma ACTH, decreased plasma cortisol, decreased urinary free cortisol

6. A 42-year-old man is discovered to be hypertensive during a routine examination. He is taking no medications. Physical examination is normal except for blood pressure of 156/95 mm Hg. Several additional blood pressure readings are elevated. Laboratory evaluation demonstrates normal renal function but a low serum potassium (K+) level. Further evaluation of his hypertension should include which test?

   (A) Plasma cortisol
   (B) Plasma adrenocorticotropic hormone (ACTH)
   (C) Plasma renin activity
   (D) Plasma 17-hydroxyprogesterone
   (E) Plasma 11-deoxycortisol

ANSWERS AND EXPLANATIONS

1. The answer is C. Cortisol is called a *gluco*corticoid because it increases gluconeogenesis. Cortisol also decreases glucose uptake by muscle and adipose tissue by increasing resistance to insulin. The net result is to make more glucose available to non–insulin-requiring tissues. Cortisol decreases CRH and ACTH secretion by feedback inhibition. Cortisol decreases inflammation and retards wound healing. This is the major reason for pharmacologic administration of cortisol or one of its analogs.

2. The answer is B. The combination of fatigue, vomiting, weight loss, and postural hypotension should suggest the possibility of adrenal insufficiency. The patch of depigmented skin is probably vitiligo, a condition that occasionally accompanies adrenal insufficiency. The diagnosis is best established by demonstrating an inadequate cortisol response following ACTH administration. CRH stimulation tests and dexamethasone suppression tests are used to diagnose Cushing's syndrome. Aldosterone suppression tests are used in the evaluation of hyperaldosteronism.

3. The answer is D. The combination of hypertension, obesity, hirsutism, ecchymoses, and abdominal striae strongly suggests the possibility of Cushing's syndrome. A good screening test for Cushing's syndrome is the 1-mg (overnight) dexamethasone suppression test. Normally, dexamethasone would suppress pituitary ACTH secretion, thereby causing suppression of plasma cortisol. However, in Cushing's syndrome, ACTH and cortisol do not suppress normally following dexamethasone administration.

4. The answer is A. Pituitary tumors that produce ACTH are not completely autonomous. Although ACTH production and, therefore, cortisol production and urinary 17-hydroxysteroid excretion do not suppress normally after low-dose dexamethasone administration, they are suppressed by the administration of high-dose dexamethasone. Ectopic ACTH production by a lung carcinoma would not be decreased by dexamethasone administration. Production of glucocorticoids by adrenal adenomas and adrenal carcinomas is not ACTH-dependent and, therefore, is unaffected by dexamethasone administration. Surreptitious administration of prednisone would cause suppression of ACTH and cortisol production, and urinary 17-hydroxysteroid excretion would be suppressed in the baseline state and after both high- and low-dose dexamethasone.

5. The answer is E. Prednisone administration would suppress CRH and ACTH secretion and, thereby, plasma cortisol and urinary free cortisol excretion.

6. The answer is C. The finding of hypertension in association with low serum K+ suggests the possibility of hyperaldosteronism. A good screening test for hyperaldosteronism is plasma renin activity, which should be suppressed. Hyperaldosteronism decreases urinary sodium (Na+) excretion, causes Na+ retention and volume expansion, and because of volume expansion, suppresses plasma renin activity. Measurement of plasma ACTH, cortisol, 17-hydroxyprogesterone, or 11-deoxycortisol would not help determine the cause of his hypertension.

REFERENCES

Chrousos GP: The hypothalamic-pituitary-adrenal axis and immune-mediated inflammation. *N Engl J Med* 332:1351–1362, 1995.

Cutler GB, Laue L: Congenital adrenal hyperplasia due to 21-hydroxylase deficiency. *N Engl J Med* 323:1806–1813, 1990.

Grinspoon SK, Biller BMK: Laboratory assessment of adrenal insufficiency. *J Clin Endocrinol Metab* 79:923–931, 1994.

Orth DN: Cushing's syndrome. *N Engl J Med* 332:791–803, 1995.

White PC: Disorders of aldosterone biosynthesis and action. *N Engl J Med* 331:250–258, 1994.

Williams GH, Dluhy RG: Diseases of the adrenal cortex. In *Harrison's Principles of Internal Medicine*, 13th ed. Edited by Isselbacker KJ, Braunwald E, Wilson JD, et al: New York, NY: McGraw-Hill, 1994, pp 1953–1976.

Chapter 6
THE ADRENAL MEDULLA

J. Michael Gonzalez-Campoy, M.D., Ph.D., and

Christopher H. Sorli, M.D., Ph.D.

Case Study: *Introduction*	*At age 27, K. Roberts began complaining of heat intolerance, excessive sweating, palpitations, and occasional headaches. These symptoms came in paroxysms and often lasted for days. Despite careful consideration, she could not identify any precipitating events. At times her symptoms were accompanied by chest pain, abdominal pain, nausea, vomiting, and pallor. Her physician documented an elevated blood pressure, but it was attributed to anxiety.* *Ms. Roberts continued to have episodic symptoms. Four years later, at the age of 31, she again sought medical care and was found to have an elevated blood glucose. She was given a diagnosis of diabetes and was encouraged to follow a weight reduction diet.*

■ EMBRYOLOGIC ORIGIN OF THE ADRENAL MEDULLA

There are two adrenal glands, one superior to each kidney. Each adrenal gland consists of two morphologically and functionally distinct endocrine tissues: the outer cortex and the inner medulla. The adrenal cortex secretes steroid hormones and is the subject of Chapter 5.

The adrenal medulla is derived embryologically from pheochromoblasts, which migrate from the neural crest. During differentiation, pheochromoblasts give rise to modified neuronal (gland) cells, not neurons. After birth, extra-adrenal pheochromoblast derivatives degenerate, and adrenomedullary cells mature. These mature cells turn brown when treated with oxidizing agents and thus are referred to as *chromaffin cells*.

Chromaffin cells are confined to the adrenal medulla and the paraganglia of the sympathetic nervous system.

HORMONES OF THE ADRENAL MEDULLA

CATECHOLAMINE SYNTHESIS

Adrenal Medulla Catecholamine Hormones
Epinephrine
Norepinephrine
Dopamine

The adrenal medulla secretes amine hormones and may be considered a modified sympathetic ganglion whose cell bodies do not send out nerve fibers but, rather, directly release hormones into the circulation. The two major amines released from the adrenal medulla are *epinephrine* and *norepinephrine*. *Dopamine* is also released but in smaller quantities. Together, this group of compounds constitutes the catecholamines. They all contain a catechol ring (i.e., a six-sided carbon ring with two adjacent hydroxyl groups). They also contain an amine group. Figure 6-1 shows the biochemical structures of the major catecholamines; tyrosine, their common precursor; and their major metabolites. The rate-limiting enzyme in the catecholamine synthesis cascade is tyrosine hydroxylase, which converts tyrosine to dihydroxyphenylalanine (dopa).

The adrenal *medulla contains large amounts of the enzyme phenylethanolamine-N-methyltransferase (PNMT)*, which catalyzes the conversion of norepinephrine to epinephrine. High glucocorticoid concentrations that result from the adrenal cortico-medullary portal system induce PNMT activity. Thus, the normal adrenal secretion of

FIGURE 6-1
CATECHOLAMINE SYNTHETIC AND METABOLIC PATHWAYS.
The conversion of tyrosine to dopa is the rate-limiting step in catecholamine synthesis. MAO = monoamine oxidase; COMT = catechol-*O*-methyltransferase.

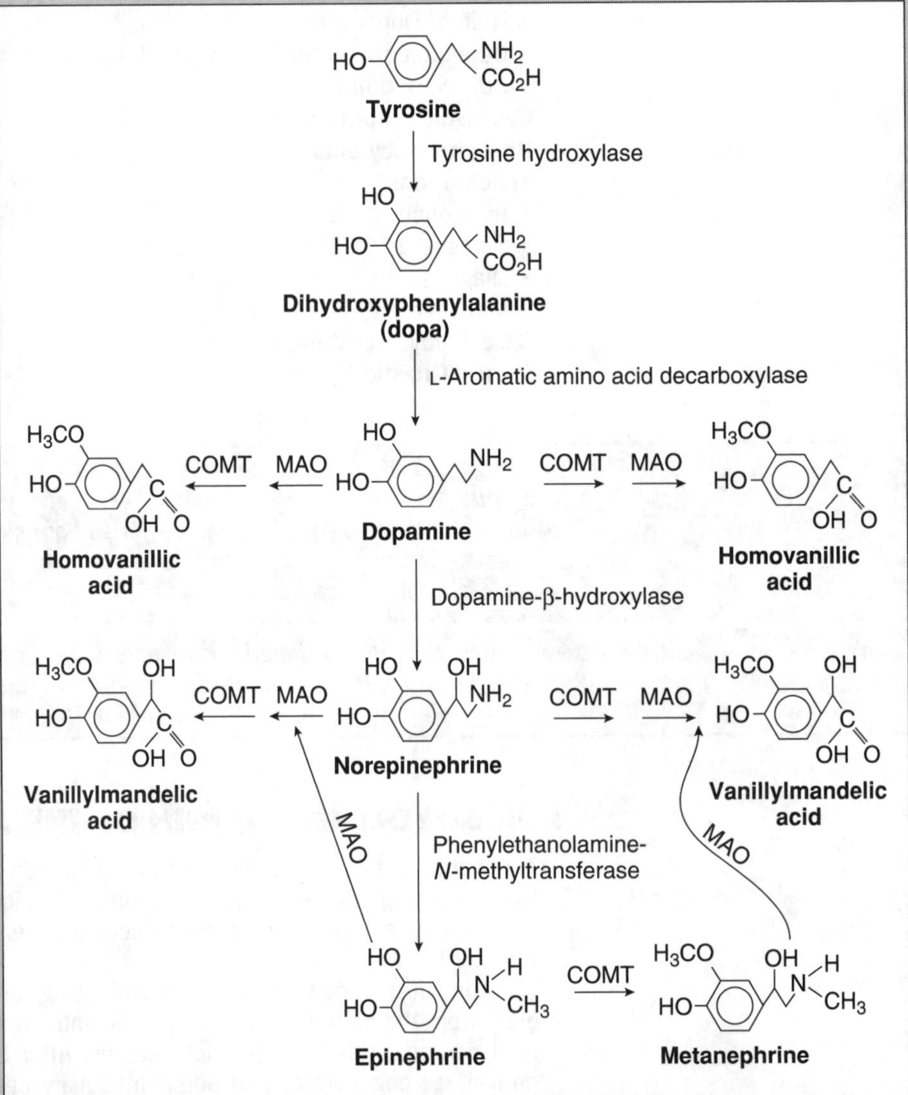

epinephrine is four times more than that of norepinephrine. (Basal circulating levels of norepinephrine are higher due to neurotransmitter release by postganglionic sympathetic neurons and are not due to secretion by the adrenal medulla.) The secretion of dopamine is negligible by comparison.

The adrenal medulla is functionally an amplifier of the sympathetic nervous system. The adrenal medulla is innervated by preganglionic sympathetic axons, which use acetylcholine (ACh) as a neurotransmitter. ACh depolarizes the chromaffin cells by increasing plasma membrane permeability to sodium (Na^+). This results in an influx of calcium (Ca^{2+}), a rise in the cytoplasmic Ca^{2+} level, and the exocytotic release of catecholamines. Adenosine triphosphate (ATP), enkephalins, chromogranins, neuropeptide Y, and dopamine β-hydroxylase are released from the exocytotic vessels at the same time.

> The **adrenal medulla** is an amplifier for the sympathetic nervous system.

SIGNALS FOR CATECHOLAMINE RELEASE

Anything that stimulates or decreases sympathetic outflow from the central nervous system (CNS) leads to altered catecholamine release seconds to minutes later from storage granules in the adrenal medulla. Major conditions associated with changes in catecholamine release from the adrenal medulla are listed in Table 6-1. Significant changes in circulating adrenal medulla hormone concentrations occur primarily in response to stress, such as a change in intravascular volume or marked hypoglycemia (blood glucose < 50 mg/dL). In most of these situations, secretion of epinephrine increases more than secretion of norepinephrine. The hormones circulate as free hormones or are loosely bound to plasma protein.

> **Major Signals for Catecholamine Release**
> Decreased blood pressure
> Decreased blood volume
> Decreased blood glucose
> Severe illness
> Severe emotional stress

CATECHOLAMINES INCREASED	CATECHOLAMINES DECREASED
Change in posture (supine to standing)	Change in posture (standing to supine)
Low intravascular volume	Bilateral adrenal hemorrhage
Hypoglycemia	Bilateral adrenal damage
Severe illness	Bilateral adrenalectomy
Emotional stress	
Fear (initiating fight or flight response)	
Rage	
Tumors	
Pheochromocytoma	
Paraganglioma	

> **Table 6-1**
> **Major Conditions Affecting Plasma Catecholamine Levels**

CATECHOLAMINE-RECEPTOR INTERACTION

Catecholamines released from the adrenal medulla and catecholamines released from sympathetic nerve endings bind to the same family of receptors, which are located on cell membranes throughout the body. Five different types of receptors have been identified for epinephrine and norepinephrine: the α-adrenergic receptors, α_1 and α_2, and the β-adrenergic receptors, β_1, β_2, and β_3. Three α_1- and three α_2-receptor subtypes also have been identified. Epinephrine is slightly more active than norepinephrine at α_2-receptors, but they have similar potency at β_1-receptors; however, epinephrine is much more potent than norepinephrine at β_2-receptors. The adrenergic receptors are part of the dual innervation of most tissues, with parasympathetic or cholinergic receptors representing the other half. Adrenergic and cholinergic effects on tissues often oppose each other.

Receptor binding by catecholamines triggers a complex series of intracellular events. The catecholamine-receptor complex associates with membrane-bound G proteins, which, in turn, activate intracellular effector molecules, commonly termed second messengers. Beta-adrenoreceptor activation results in the generation of the second messenger cyclic adenosine monophosphate (cAMP). Stimulation of α-adrenoreceptors results in the activation of either phospholipase C or cAMP and may also directly affect Ca^{2+} and potassium (K^+) channels.

A significant change in the number of catecholamine receptors obviously affects the response elicited by the hormones. For example, patients with hyperthyroidism have increased cardiac epinephrine receptors. The effects of circulating epinephrine are magnified in these patients, even if plasma epinephrine is within the normal range.

> **Receptor:Hormone Affinity**
> α_1, α_2: epinephrine > norepinephrine
> β_1: epinephrine = norepinephrine
> β_2: epinephrine >>> norepinephrine

Four dopamine receptor types have been characterized. By convention the CNS dopaminergic receptors are denoted as D_1, D_2, D_3, and D_4; the peripheral dopaminergic receptors are DA_1, DA_2, DA_3, and DA_4. All known dopamine receptors are coupled to adenylate cyclase via G proteins. DA_1 and D_1 activate stimulatory Gs proteins and adenylate cyclase. DA_2 and D_2 activate inhibitory Gi proteins and inhibit adenylate cyclase.

ACTIONS OF EPINEPHRINE AND NOREPINEPHRINE

Norepinephrine and epinephrine secreted by peripheral sympathetic nerves act as local regulators of glucose and fat metabolism, visceral function, cardiovascular responses, and response to stress. Since the adrenal medulla secretes these hormones into the circulation rather than locally, the responses are more general. Tables 6-2 and 6-3 list the major effects of adrenergic stimulation on various tissues and metabolism. A fully activated sympathetic response is called the "fight-or-flight" response, since the hormones increase skeletal muscle blood flow and contraction at the expense of blood flow to visceral organs and skin. The accompanying increase in glycogenolysis, gluconeogenesis, and lipolysis provides the fuel for the increased oxygen consumption required.

Major Actions of Catecholamines
- ↑ Blood glucose
- ↑ Lipolysis
- ↑ Skeletal muscle blood flow, and contractility
- ↑ Heart rate, contractility, and cardiac output
- ↑ Blood pressure
- ↓ Visceral blood flow
- ↓ Gastrointestinal tract motility
- ↓ Urine output

Table 6-2
Major Physiologic Effects of Increased Epinephrine and Norepinephrine

ORGAN	RECEPTOR TYPE	EFFECT
Skeletal muscle	β_2	Increased contractility
Heart	β_1	Increased heart rate, conduction velocity, and contractility
Arterioles	α (norepinephrine effect) β_2 (epinephrine effect)	Constriction (abdominal viscera) Vasodilatation (skeletal muscle)
Lungs	β_2	Bronchodilatation
Stomach and intestine	α_1 and β_2	Decreased motility and increased sphincter contraction
Gallbladder	β_2	Relaxation
Kidney	β_1	Increased renin causing increased blood pressure
Ureter	α	Increased motility
Urinary bladder	β α	Detrusor relaxation Sphincter contraction
Uterus	β_2	Relaxation
Penis	α	Ejaculation
Skin	α	Increased pallor and sweating (palms)
Posterior pituitary	β_1	Increased antidiuretic hormone secretion causing decreased urine output

Table 6-3
Major Metabolic Effects of Increased Epinephrine

ORGAN	EFFECT
Liver	Increased gluconeogenesis and glycogenolysis
Skeletal muscle	Increased glycogenolysis
Adipose tissue	Increased lipolysis
Overall	Increased oxygen consumption and thermogenesis

ROLE OF DOPAMINE

Although dopamine is a critical neurotransmitter in the CNS and plays a crucial role in the modulation of prolactin release from the pituitary gland, the action of dopamine on peripheral tissues is much less important than the actions of epinephrine and norepinephrine. Dopamine is the most abundant free catecholamine in the urine. The kidneys synthesize it from L-dopa (levodopa), and renal excretion of dopamine exceeds its renal clearance. This is not true of the other catecholamines.

CATECHOLAMINE METABOLISM AND DISPOSAL

Secreted catecholamines have a short half-life of a few minutes. Catecholamines secreted by sympathetic nerves usually are taken up again and metabolized in the sympathetic nerve terminals. Adrenal medulla hormones mostly are metabolized to inactive compounds by the enzymes catechol-O-methyltransferase (COMT) or monoamine oxidase (MAO) [see Figure 6-1] in peripheral tissues such as liver and kidney. Some catecholamine is conjugated with sulfate ion. Free and conjugated catecholamines and their metabolites are excreted in the urine. Since catecholamines are secreted in bursts in response to changing situations, plasma concentrations are highly variable, and a single blood level may not provide an accurate picture of catecholamine secretion. In clinical practice, measurement of catecholamine levels in a timed urine collection is more useful. A 24-hour urine collection indicates the total daily production of catecholamines. Table 6-4 indicates the normal concentrations of catecholamines and their major metabolites in plasma and urine and shows the effects of upright posture on plasma epinephrine and norepinephrine concentrations.

Table 6-4
Normal Plasma and Urine Values of Catecholamines in Adults

PLASMA		
Norepinephrine	Supine	70–750 pg/mL
	Standing	200–1700 pg/mL
Epinephrine	Supine	< 110 pg/mL
	Standing	< 140 pg/mL
Dopamine	Supine	< 30 pg/mL
	Standing	< 30 pg/mL
URINE (24 HOUR)		
Epinephrine		0–20 µg
Norepinephrine		15–80 µg
Dopamine		65–400 µg
Metanephrines		< 1.3 mg
Vanillylmandelic acid		< 9 µg/mg creatinine

ADRENOMEDULLIN

Adrenomedullin (AM) is a regulatory peptide identified in a human chromaffin cell tumor that has been located in various human tissues, including the adrenal gland, heart, lung, kidney, and aorta. AM is generated from a larger 185–amino acid prehormone through consecutive enzymatic cleavage and amidation, ultimately resulting in a 52–amino acid, biologically active peptide. AM is a vasodilatory agent and a natriuretic factor. It acts through specific receptors identified in heart, lung, spleen, liver, muscle, and spinal cord. On interaction with its receptor, AM activates adenylate cyclase and modulates Ca^{2+} flux in target cells.

The precise physiologic role of AM is yet to be defined. Individuals with congestive heart failure (CHF) exhibit progressively elevated levels of AM, which correlate with the clinical severity of their disease, and AM may play a role in the cardiovascular abnormalities associated with sepsis. In addition to its vasodilatory effects in the periphery and

Case Study:
Continued

The patient's symptoms and signs of increased sweating and palpitations (increased cardiac contractility), hypertension, headaches (perhaps due to episodic hypertension), and hyperglycemia are not specific when considered alone but should suggest epinephrine excess when taken together. Two years later, her symptoms increased in frequency and severity. Her blood pressure was elevated at 180/100 mm Hg. She was referred to an endocrinologist for further evaluation.

Her medical history was otherwise unremarkable. She had no history of illicit drug use. She denied regular use of any over-the-counter medications. Her maternal grandfather had surgery for a "gland" tumor.

On physical examination, her blood pressure while sitting was 192/104 mm Hg measured on the right arm. Her heart rate was 92 beats/min and regular. Examination of her head, ears, eyes, nose, throat, lungs, heart, abdomen, and pelvis were normal. Neurologic and peripheral vascular examinations were also normal. Her thyroid gland was normal in size, and there were no nodules. She had no cutaneous lesions, ecchymoses, café-au-lait spots, or mucosal neuromas. A 24-hour urine collection revealed a metanephrine level five times the upper limit of normal, a vanillylmandelic acid (VMA) level three times the upper limit of normal, a norepinephrine level fifteen times the upper limit of normal, and a dopamine level in the normal range.

natriuretic actions in the kidney, AM is an inhibitor of adrenocorticotropic hormone (ACTH) secretion by pituitary cells and is a regulatory factor in insulin secretion.

PHEOCHROMOCYTOMA

DEFINITIONS

Catecholamine-Secreting Tumors of Chromaffin Cells
Pheochromocytoma: tumor arising from adrenal medulla
Paraganglioma: tumor arising from sympathetic paraganglia

Pheochromocytoma is a catecholamine-secreting tumor of chromaffin cells arising from the adrenal medulla. *Paraganglioma* is a catecholamine-secreting tumor of chromaffin cells arising from the sympathetic paraganglia. In the literature, these terms are used interchangeably, and pheochromocytoma denotes any catecholamine-secreting tumor of neural crest origin. These tumors are described as either adrenal or extra-adrenal pheochromocytomas.

INCIDENCE

Disorders Associated with Pheochromocytoma
MEN IIA and IIB
Neuroectodermal syndromes

Pheochromocytoma is a rare tumor. The incidence rate is approximately 1 in 100,000 person years. It is found in less than 0.1% of patients with hypertension, the hallmark of the disease. The peak prevalence is in the third to fourth decades, but it may occur in all age groups. There is no race or sex predisposition.

Over 90% of pheochromocytomas are located in the abdomen; 90% of these arise within the adrenal glands, and approximately 10% are extra-adrenal. Figure 6-2 shows

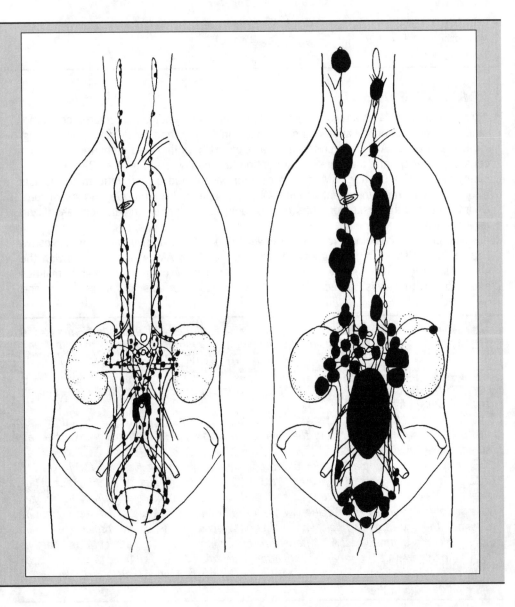

FIGURE 6-2
The anatomic distribution of chromaffin tissue (the paraganglia) in the newborn (*left*) and the similar location of paragangliomas (extra-adrenal pheochromocytomas) reported in the literature. (*Source:* Reprinted with permission from Page LB, Copeland RB: Pheochromocytoma. In *Disease-a-Month* (January). Edited by Dowling HF, et al. St. Louis, MO: Year Book, 1968, p 7.)

the reported locations of paragangliomas (extra-adrenal pheochromocytomas). The most common locations for paragangliomas are the aortic bifurcation, the bladder wall, and the organ of Zuckerkandl, but these tumors also are found in the chest. About 10% of pheochromocytomas are bilateral and multicentric, especially when they occur as part of the familial multiple endocrine neoplasia (MEN) syndromes (i.e., MEN types IIA and IIB). Pheochromocytomas are also associated with neurofibromatosis, cerebelloretinal hemangiomatosis, tuberous sclerosis, and the Sturge-Weber syndrome. Table 6-5 summarizes the pathologic conditions associated with pheochromocytoma, and highlights the need for a thorough family history in the evaluation of these patients.

Multiple endocrine neoplasia type IIA
Pheochromocytoma, medullary carcinoma of the thyroid, and hyperparathyroidism
Multiple endocrine neoplasia type IIB
Pheochromocytoma, mucosal neuromas, and hyperparathyroidism (rare)
Neurofibromatosis
Cerebelloretinal hemangiomatosis
Tuberous sclerosis
Sturge-Weber syndrome

Table 6-5
Disorders Associated with Pheochromocytoma

Approximately 3%–14% of pheochromocytomas are malignant, with metastases most often to regional lymph nodes, liver, bone, lung, and the CNS. Malignant pheochromocytomas are more likely to have disproportionately increased urinary excretion of dopamine, homovanillic acid, or both and a tumor size greater than 6 cm.

SIGNS AND SYMPTOMS

The hallmark of pheochromocytoma is either paroxysmal or sustained hypertension, which is often labile and resistant to treatment. Hypertension is found in 95% of cases. Other signs and symptoms classically associated with pheochromocytoma are headache, sweating, palpitations, chest or abdominal pain, nausea, vomiting, pallor, anxiety, glucose intolerance, increased metabolic rate, and funduscopic changes (Table 6-6). The classic triad of sudden severe headache, diaphoresis, and palpitations carries a high degree of specificity (94%) and sensitivity (91%) for pheochromocytoma in a hypertensive population. The absence of all three symptoms makes the diagnosis of pheochromocytoma extremely unlikely. Paroxysmal attacks may be triggered by a variety of stimuli, which are summarized in Table 6-7. A careful review of the medical history and family history is essential, as indicated above.

Hypertension: sustained or paroxysmal	Tremor
Headache	Pallor
Sweating	Hyperglycemia
Palpitations	Nausea, vomiting, and abdominal pain
Anxiety and nervousness	

Table 6-6
Signs and Symptoms of Pheochromocytoma

Activity: postural change, exertion, and sexual intercourse
Meals, alcohol, and smoking
Urination and straining at stool
Emotional stress
Trauma and pain
General anesthesia and barbiturates
Hormones/drugs: glucagon, adrenocorticotropic hormone, and histamine

Table 6-7
Stimuli Causing Paroxysmal Catecholamine Release

DIAGNOSIS

The diagnosis of pheochromocytoma depends on the demonstration of excessive amounts of catecholamines in plasma or urine or of degradation products of catecholamines, such as metanephrines or VMA, in urine. A 24-hour urine collection for metanephrine and catecholamines is a good screening test for pheochromocytoma.

Diagnostic Tests for Pheochromocytoma
Measurement of 24-hour urine catecholamines (first choice)
Clonidine suppression test
Glucagon stimulation test (higher risk)

Levels of plasma catecholamines greater than 2000 pg/mL at rest suggest the presence of a pheochromocytoma.

Cases in which screening tests are equivocal warrant a clonidine suppression test. Clonidine is a centrally active α_2-agonist. In individuals with essential hypertension in whom increased catecholamine secretion is due to neurogenic stimulation rather than a tumor, 0.3 mg of orally administered clonidine suppresses catecholamine release, and plasma catecholamines decrease to less than 500 pg/mL. Patients with pheochromocytoma, on the other hand, fail to suppress catecholamine release.

Glucagon stimulation, a provocative test for pheochromocytoma in patients who have infrequent symptoms and signs, is also available. Following an intravenous bolus of 1–2 mg glucagon, patients with pheochromocytoma manifest a threefold increase in plasma catecholamines and a rise in blood pressure of 20/15 mm Hg. This rise in blood pressure is hazardous to patients, and this test should not be used in patients with severe symptoms during attacks. Other diagnostic tests that should be considered in patients in whom MEN II (A and B) is suspected include a plasma calcitonin level to exclude medullary thyroid cancer and plasma parathyroid hormone (PTH) and Ca^{2+} levels to exclude hyperparathyroidism.

Imaging studies are necessary to determine whether the catecholamine-secreting tumor is adrenal or extra-adrenal. Magnetic resonance imaging (MRI) is preferable to computerized axial tomography (CAT) scanning for locating very small or extra-adrenal tumors because pheochromocytomas have a characteristic hyperintense image on T_2-weighted scans. Use of MRI is limited by availability and cost. Scintigraphic localization with ^{131}I-metaiodobenzylguanidine (MIBG) can be used when CAT scanning and MRI imaging are inconclusive, but this type of imaging is available only at selected tertiary care centers.

MANAGEMENT

Definitive treatment of pheochromocytoma is surgical resection. Preoperative α-receptor blockade is indicated to reduce the risk of intraoperative hypertensive crisis or postoperative hypotension. Phenoxybenzamine (10–20 mg 2–3 times/d, advanced to 80–100 mg/d) or prazosin (1 mg 3 times/d, advanced to 5 mg 3 times/d) are the preferred agents for α-receptor blockade. The goals of therapy are a blood pressure of 160/90 mm Hg or less, normalization of the electrocardiogram if previously abnormal, and a decrease in the frequency of premature ventricular contractions to no more than one every 15 minutes. α-Receptor blockade is typically achieved over the 2 weeks immediately preceding surgical resection. β-Receptor blockade to control tachycardia should be instituted only after α-receptor blockade because unopposed α-stimulation as a consequence of β-receptor blockade could lead to increased vasoconstriction and even worse hypertension. Postoperative hypotension following removal of vasoconstricting tumor hormones requires intravascular volume expansion.

Case Study:
Resolution

K. Roberts's symptoms and signs and elevated urinary catecholamines and their metabolites indicated that she had a pheochromocytoma. She had no signs of a neuroectodermal disorder, but her family history of a "gland" tumor made it imperative to rule out MEN II. Her plasma calcitonin, PTH, and Ca^{2+} values were all within the normal range. Her grandfather's hospital records eventually were located and indicated that he had had a pheochromocytoma removed.

A CAT scan of the patient's abdomen revealed a 5 × 5.3-cm right adrenal mass. She was treated preoperatively with the α-blocker phenoxybenzamine for 2 weeks. The tumor was removed successfully, and a brief period of postoperative hypotension was easily managed with intravenous fluids. The tumor was indeed a pheochromocytoma. Her hyperglycemia also resolved after the tumor was removed. The presence of hypertension accompanied by paroxysmal headaches and palpitations over a period of years should have prompted an evaluation for pheochromocytoma much earlier.

▌REVIEW QUESTIONS

Directions: For each of the following questions, choose the **one best** answer.

1. Catecholamine levels are high in a 60-year-old man who has just had a severe myocardial infarction. Which of the following physiologic responses is most likely to result from his increased catecholamine secretion?

   (A) Decreased lipolysis to reduce circulating free fatty acids
   (B) Increased glycogen synthesis to increase fuel stores in the myocardium
   (C) Hyperglycemia due to increased gluconeogenesis and glycogenolysis
   (D) Decreased oxygen consumption to protect the remaining myocardium

2. A 44-year-old man suddenly finds himself in a terrifying situation inducing both fear and rage. His appropriate catecholamine response elicits

   (A) an increased urine output
   (B) an increased blood flow to muscles and less to viscera
   (C) an increased blood flow to skin so that he can remain cool
   (D) a decreased cardiac output and heart rate to help him remain calm

Questions 3–6

A 20-year-old woman comes to the physician's office with a history of paroxysmal hypertension, palpitations, headache, and profuse sweating. Her father died from a thyroid cancer, and a paternal aunt has hypercalcemia and hypertension.

3. What would be the most appropriate first step in evaluating this woman?

   (A) Draw blood samples for norepinephrine and epinephrine following an overnight fast
   (B) Perform a clonidine suppression test by drawing blood for catecholamines before and 3 hours after the oral administration of clonidine
   (C) Collect urine for 24 hours and measure levels of epinephrine and norepinephrine, metanephrines, or vanillylmandelic acid
   (D) Perform a glucagon stimulation test by administering an intravenous bolus of glucagon and monitoring any rise in catecholamines and blood pressure

4. In view of this woman's family medical history, the physician would be most likely to measure serum levels of

   (A) calcitonin, calcium, and glucose
   (B) glucagon, insulin, and cholesterol
   (C) thyroid hormone, adrenomedullin, and phosphorus
   (D) nerve growth factor, gastrin, and renin

5. The woman's test results are consistent with a pheochromocytoma. After a careful history and physical examination her physician would be most likely to order

   (A) surgical exploration of the adrenal glands
   (B) magnetic resonance imaging (MRI) or computerized tomography (CT) scanning
   (C) surgical exploration of the thyroid and parathyroid glands
   (D) a radioactive iodine scan of the thyroid gland

6. Surgery to remove this woman's pheochromocytoma is scheduled. Appropriate management is most likely to include which of the following?

   (A) Medical preparation with the β-adrenergic blocker metoprolol before surgery followed by α-adrenergic blockade with phenoxybenzamine at the time of surgery
   (B) Treatment of postoperative hypertension with a diuretic to promote salt and water loss
   (C) Aggressive volume replacement for treatment of hypotension after removal of the tumor
   (D) A glucagon stimulation test to check for residual tumor immediately after surgery

■ ANSWERS AND EXPLANATIONS

1. The answer is C. In response to stress, catecholamine-induced oxygen consumption increases, and catecholamines stimulate both fat and glycogen catabolism to provide fuel.

2. The answer is B. Increased blood flow to muscles and less to viscera would theoretically aid the man's escape in this "fight or flight" situation.

3. The answer is C. The patient in the question presents with the classic symptoms of catecholamine excess characteristic of a pheochromocytoma: paroxysmal hypertension, palpitations, headache, and sweating. The diagnosis of pheochromocytoma is based on the measurement of elevated catecholamines or their metabolites in the urine. Familial forms of pheochromocytoma are more likely to overproduce epinephrine than norepinephrine. Since catecholamine secretion by these tumors can be episodic, a 24-hour urine specimen that integrates catecholamine production over a 24-hour period is a better diagnostic test than a single plasma catecholamine measurement. The clonidine suppression and glucagon stimulation tests are reserved for patients whose other test results are equivocal. The glucagon stimulation test can be dangerous because it induces additional hypertension.

4. The answer is A. The family history of the woman described in the question suggests familial multiple endocrine neoplasia type IIA (MEN IIA). If this is correct, her father's thyroid cancer was a medullary carcinoma of the thyroid, which produced calcitonin. Her aunt's history of hypercalcemia suggests hyperparathyroidism, and her hypertension might be due to a pheochromocytoma. Excess epinephrine secretion by a pheochromocytoma stimulates gluconeogenesis and glycogenolysis and can result in hyperglycemia.

5. The answer is B. The next step in the management of this woman is to localize the pheochromocytoma, not to search for a calcitonin-producing tumor or parathyroid hyperplasia, which are components of MEN IIA. A careful history and physical examination may yield important clues as to the location of a pheochromocytoma, as in the case of postmicturition hypertension secondary to pheochromocytoma of the urinary bladder. MRI and CT scans are useful for locating the tumor. Because pheochromocytomas have a characteristic hyperintense image on T_2-weighted scans, MRI is preferable but more expensive. Scanning with ^{131}I-metaiodobenzylguanidine is less widely available, but it reveals 80%–95% of pheochromocytomas and can be particularly useful with familial pheochromocytoma where bilateral and extra-adrenal involvement are more common.

6. The answer is C. In the management of the pheochromocytoma patient, β-adrenergic blockade should never precede α-blockade. The result would be an exacerbation of epinephrine-induced vasoconstriction (mediated through α-adrenergic receptors) because of a pharmacologic block of the vasodilatory effects mediated through β-adrenergic receptors. Life-threatening hypertension might result. β-Receptor blockades are used in the treatment of pheochromocytoma only if the patient develops significant tachycardia or catecholamine-induced arrhythmia. After removal of the tumor, the sudden loss of excessive α-adrenergic–induced vasoconstriction results in vasodilatation and hypotension, which can be treated with fluids. Further volume depletion with a diuretic would only exacerbate the hypotension. If hypertension persists after surgery, urine collection for catecholamines should be done after the patient has recovered from the stress of surgery. (Surgical stress would be expected to increase catecholamine secretion.)

■ REFERENCES

Gifford RW, Manger WM, Bravo EL: Pheochromocytoma. *Endocrinol Metab Clin North Am* 23:387, 1994.

Goldstein DS: Physiology of the adrenal medulla and the sympathetic nervous system. In *Principles and Practice of Endocrinology and Metabolism*. Edited by Becker KL: Philadelphia, PA: J. B. Lippincott, 1995, pp 753–762.

Hull CJ: Phaeochromocytoma: diagnosis, preoperative preparation and anaesthetic management. *Br J Anaesthiol* 68:1305, 1986.

Manger WM, Gifford RW Jr: Pheochromocytoma: current diagnosis and management. *Cleveland Clin J Med* 60:365, 1993.

Martinez A, Weaver C, Lopez J, et al: Regulation of insulin secretion and blood glucose metabolism by adrenomedullin. *Endocrinology* 137(6):2626–2632, 1996.

Neumann HPH, Berger DP, Sigmund G, et al: Pheochromocytomas, multiple endocrine neoplasia type 2, and von Hippel-Lindau disease. *N Engl J Med* 329:1531, 1993.

Chapter 7

CALCIUM-REGULATING HORMONES AND METABOLIC BONE DISEASE

Catherine B. Niewoehner, M.D.

▮ CHAPTER OUTLINE

Case Study:
Introduction

Ms. A. R. was found to have hypercalcemia at age 53 when she volunteered for an exercise study. She had been healthy, experiencing two normal pregnancies and undergoing menopause at age 50. She was very active, working as a trail guide. She drank two glasses of milk daily, and her only medication was a daily multivitamin containing 400 units of vitamin D. She had stopped smoking 20 years before and drank only an occasional glass of wine. Her mother had osteoporosis and died at age 65 in an automobile accident. Her father had a kidney stone and hypertension and died after a myocardial infarction at age 65. Two sisters and two daughters were healthy. Her physical examination revealed mild hypertension. She weighed 128 lbs and was 66 in tall. Her chest x-ray was unremarkable; an abdominal x-ray showed no kidney stones. Her serum albumin, creatinine, and magnesium levels were normal, but she had several abnormal values: calcium, 10.9 (normal: 8.5–10.5 mg/dL); phosphorus, 2.2 (normal: 2.3–4.5 mg/dL); parathyroid hormone (PTH), high; urine calcium and phosphorus, high; 1,25-dihydroxyvitamin D (1,25(OH)$_2$D), upper limit of normal. Ms. A. R. agreed to keep herself well hydrated. She stopped her multivitamin tablet and started taking antihypertensive medication and estrogen and a progestin for osteoporosis prophylaxis.

Seven years later, Ms. A. R. was hit by a snowmobile while cross-country skiing. The accident resulted in a head injury and seizures, fractured cervical vertebrae, and a badly fractured pelvis, femurs, and right tibia. She developed pneumonia with a temperature of

103°F. Increasing anorexia and constipation originally were attributed to opiates given for pain, but laboratory studies revealed a serum calcium level of 14.9 mg/dL, a phosphorus level of 2.0 mg/dL, a normal albumin level, and a high PTH level. After rehydration, her calcium level was still high (12.5 mg/dL). A parathyroid adenoma was removed, and her calcium and phosphorus levels returned to normal. She was discharged to a long-term rehabilitation facility. Medications given at that time were phenytoin for seizures and acetaminophen with codeine for pain. She stopped taking the estrogen and progestin.

CALCIUM AND PHOSPHORUS HOMEOSTASIS

Problems for Calcium Homeostasis
Narrow normal range for extracellular calcium
Extracellular:intracellular calcium concentration ~1000:1
Extra calcium for growth, pregnancy, and lactation
Preserving circulating calcium without excessive bone loss

Calcium is critically important for a wide range of body functions. Extracellular calcium is essential for blood clotting, nerve and muscle function, and maintaining the skeletal system. Intracellular calcium regulates cell secretion, cell motility, and cell differentiation. Calcium ions are cofactors for enzymes and act as intracellular second messengers. Calcium homeostasis is jealously guarded, and the extracellular calcium concentration normally changes very little over an entire lifetime, despite major fluctuations in dietary calcium, calcium entering and leaving the skeleton, renal calcium excretion, and the extra demands of pregnancy and lactation (Table 7-1). The intracellular calcium concentration can change dramatically as a result of release of calcium from intracellular stores or an influx of extracellular calcium, but generally it is maintained at a level 1000 times lower than the extracellular calcium.

Table 7-1
Calcium and Phosphorus Levels in Plasma and Bone

MEASUREMENT	CALCIUM	PHOSPHORUS
Total plasma concentration (mg/dL)	8.6–10.2	2.5–4.5
Total plasma concentration (mmol/L)	2.1–2.5	0.8–1.4
Plasma ionized concentration (mg/dL)	4.1–4.7	2.1–3.8
Plasma ionized concentration (mmol/L)	1.0–1.2	0.68–1.2
Bound to plasma proteins	45%	15%
Percent of total body stores in bone	99%	85%

Phosphorus, the major intracellular anion, is required for the generation of adenosine triphosphate (ATP), is an essential component of the phospholipids in all membranes, and directly regulates enzyme action and protein function. Both calcium and phosphorus are required to form hydroxyapatite ($Ca_{10}[PO_4]_6[OH]_2$), the major mineral of bone. The extracellular concentration of phosphorus is less tightly regulated than the extracellular concentration of calcium, and the normal plasma concentration can vary by almost 100% (see Table 7-1). The levels of calcium and phosphorus are regulated together, sometimes in opposite directions. A low calcium × phosphorus product (< 20 mg/dL or 0.7 mmol/L) indicates a major deficiency; a high calcium × phosphorus product (> 70 mg/dL or 2.2 mmol/L) increases the propensity for deposition of insoluble $CaPO_4$ in soft tissues.

Phosphorus is widely available in foods, and most of the ingested phosphorus (70%–80%) normally is absorbed from the small bowel. The kidneys play a major role in protecting the plasma phosphorus concentration in the face of dietary deficiency.

Calcium traffic is more complex. It is more difficult to obtain adequate calcium from the diet because calcium is less ubiquitous than phosphorus, and absorption of calcium from the small bowel is less efficient. Healthy young adults absorb only 35%–50% of dietary calcium, and absorption efficiency decreases with age.

The optimum dietary calcium intake varies markedly with age (Table 7-2). Infants and adolescents require extra calcium for rapid growth. Pregnant women also require extra calcium, especially in the last trimester when the fetal skeleton develops. Lactating women require extra calcium to replace the calcium secreted in breast milk. These groups absorb dietary calcium from the intestine very efficiently, particularly when

Infants (birth–6 mo)	400	
Infants (6–12 mo)	600	
Children (1–5 yr)	800	
Children (6–10 yr)	800–1200	
Adolescent/young adult (11–24 yr)	1200–1500	
Adult men	1000	
Premenopausal adult women	1000	
Postmenopausal women taking estrogen	1000	
Pregnant/lactating women	1200–1500	
Pregnant/lactating women below age 19	1600	
Postmenopausal women not taking estrogen	1500	
Elderly (over age 65)	1500	

Table 7-2
Optimal Daily Calcium Intakes

Note. Intakes recommended by National Institutes of Health Consensus Conference, 1994. Units of measure are mg/d.

calcium intake is low. Postmenopausal women and the elderly require more calcium because they do not absorb dietary calcium as well, and their renal calcium losses are greater.

Dairy products are the best source of dietary calcium unless lactose intolerance is a problem. Fish with bones, nuts, and green vegetables also are good sources, but the amounts required can be rather daunting (Table 7-3). Dietary calcium can be augmented with oral calcium supplements (Table 7-4), if necessary. The calcium content and cost of these supplements differ markedly. Calcium carbonate is absorbed better if it is taken with meals.

Milk (8 oz)	300	Canned salmon (+ bones, 2 oz)	120
Yogurt (8 oz)	350	Sardines canned (2 oz)	220
Yogurt (low fat, 8 oz)	425		
Cottage cheese (1 cup)	150	Almonds, peanuts (1 cup)	200
Ice cream (1 cup)	175	Supplemented orange juice (8 oz)	300
Cheese (1 oz)	150–250	Supplemented cereal (¾ cup)	150
Kale (1 cup)	200		
Collards (cooked, ½ cup)	180		
Broccoli (cooked, ½ cup)	90	Some tofu (raw, firm, ½ cup)	250

Table 7-3
Dietary Sources of Calcium

Note. Calcium content measured in mg.

Calcium carbonate	40%
Tricalcium phosphate	39%
Calcium phosphate dibasic	31%
Calcium citrate	21%
Calcium lactate	13%
Calcium gluconate	9%

Table 7-4
Calcium Content of Oral Calcium Supplements

Calcium homeostasis for a healthy, young adult in calcium balance is shown in Figure 7-1. Only 55% of plasma calcium is available for metabolism, because 45% is bound to protein, mostly albumin (see Table 7-1). Most of the ionized calcium that is filtered by the kidneys is reabsorbed in the proximal tubules. Additional resorption in the distal tubules is highly regulated by hormones. Most of the calcium in the body is contained in the skeleton. Only 1% of skeletal calcium is readily exchangeable with plasma, but this constitutes a major calcium reserve that can be used to maintain the plasma calcium concentration when needed. Calcium entry and exit from the skeleton are highly regulated by the hormones described below.

Major Sites of Calcium Regulation
Absorption from the gastrointestinal tract
Reabsorption from the kidney
Resorption from bone

FIGURE 7-1
MAINTENANCE OF THE BODY'S CALCIUM BALANCE ON A DIETARY INTAKE OF 800 MG CALCIUM PER DAY.

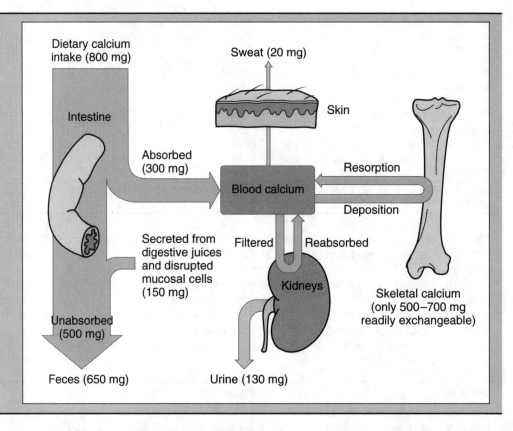

■ HORMONAL REGULATORS OF CALCIUM BALANCE

The two most influential hormones affecting calcium balance are PTH and $1,25(OH)_2D$. The roles of calcitonin and parathyroid hormone–related peptide (PTHrP) in normal human physiology are uncertain, but calcitonin is used therapeutically, and a high level of PTHrP is a major cause of hypercalcemia.

PARATHYROID HORMONE

PTH is an 84–amino acid polypeptide produced by the parathyroid glands in response to low extracellular calcium. PTH secretion and production are exquisitely responsive to any drop in the concentration of plasma ionic calcium, which is recognized by the calcium receptor protein on parathyroid cells. PTH interacts with receptors on bone and renal tubules. PTH-occupied receptors interact with membrane G proteins, resulting in increased cyclic adenosine monophosphate (cAMP). cAMP initiates a cascade of cellular phosphorylations that result in cellular action:

$$PTH \longrightarrow receptor \longrightarrow G\ protein \longrightarrow$$

$$cAMP\ and\ other\ messengers \longrightarrow \uparrow calcium$$

The major function of PTH is to correct hypocalcemia. In bone, PTH interacts with its receptors on osteoblasts, which elicits mononuclear cell cytokine release. Cytokines activate osteoclasts, the bone-resorbing cells. Osteoclast action releases calcium and phosphorus from bone. Stimulation by PTH also increases the number of osteoclasts. The dual action of PTH on the kidney to increase phosphorus excretion and calcium resorption at the distal tubule salvages calcium and prevents hyperphosphatemia. PTH-induced excretion of bicarbonate tends to produce acidosis, which inhibits binding of calcium to albumin and results in an increase in ionic calcium availability. Finally, PTH action increases the activity of the renal enzyme 1α-hydroxylase, which converts inactive 25(OH)D to the active $1,25(OH)_2D$. $1,25(OH)_2D$ acts on the intestinal mucosa cells to increase calcium absorption from the intestine.

PTH regulation by extracellular calcium involves feedback loops (Figure 7-2). Hypocalcemia stimulates PTH release and synthesis. Hypercalcemia suppresses PTH. Both

---

Major Hormonal Regulators of Calcium Balance
PTH
$1,25(OH)_2D$
Calcitonin
PTHrP

Major Actions of PTH
Increases release of calcium and phosphorus from bone
Increases renal tubular resorption of calcium
Increases renal phosphate excretion
Increases renal conversion of 25(OH)D to active $1,25(OH)_2D$
Net result: increased plasma calcium and decreased plasma phosphorus

PTH secretion and action are impaired if the magnesium concentration is very low, but magnesium is a much less important regulator of PTH than calcium.

PARATHYROID HORMONE–RELATED PEPTIDE

PTHrP is a 141–amino acid peptide, which is similar to PTH at the N-terminal (i.e., 8 of the first 13 amino acids are the same). PTHrP can bind to the PTH receptor and cause similar effects. In bone, PTHrP causes an increase in osteoclast activity with release of calcium and phosphorus. In the kidney, PTHrP stimulates an increase in urinary cAMP levels and causes increased calcium retention and increased phosphorus excretion. Patients with high PTHrP have much lower levels of $1,25(OH)_2D$ than patients with high PTH. The reason for this is unknown. Overall, PTHrP action results in increased plasma calcium and decreased plasma phosphorus.

Major Regulators of PTH

Stimulators
Low plasma ionized calcium

Inhibitors
High plasma ionized calcium and Very low plasma magnesium

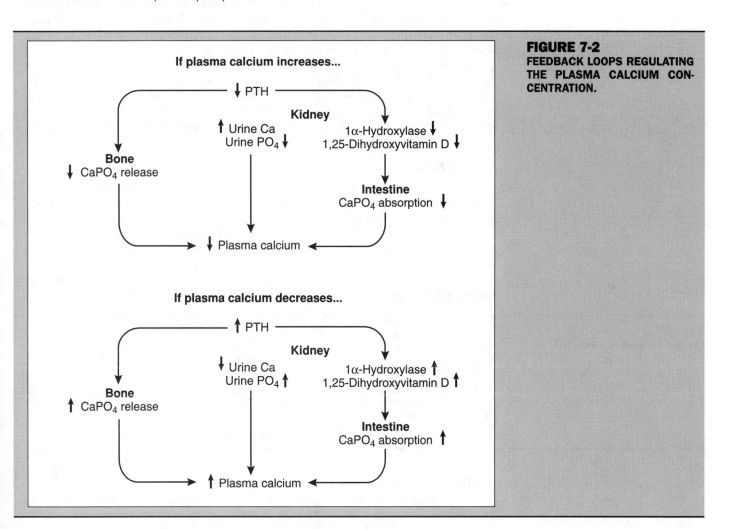

FIGURE 7-2
FEEDBACK LOOPS REGULATING THE PLASMA CALCIUM CONCENTRATION.

The PTHrP concentration is high in many fetal tissues, amnionic fluid, and breast milk, where it is presumed to affect calcium transport, cartilage development, and mineralization. PTHrP is the major cause of humoral hypercalcemia of malignancy (see below).

CALCITONIN

Calcitonin is a 32–amino acid peptide, which is secreted primarily by parafollicular C cells of the thyroid gland in response to an increase in extracellular calcium. The main action of calcitonin is to suppress osteoclasts, the bone-resorbing cells. After a meal, plasma calcium increases, calcitonin is secreted, bone resorption is suppressed, and calcium and phosphorus are retained in the bone. Calcitonin action opposes action of PTH (Table 7-5).

Table 7-5
Parathyroid Hormone (PTH) versus Calcitonin

HORMONE	SOURCE	RECEPTORS	EFFECTS
PTH	Parathyroid glands	Osteoblasts	Increased osteoclast action Increased bone resorption Increased plasma calcium
Calcitonin	Thyroid parafollicular cells	Osteoclasts	Decreased osteoclast action Decreased bone resorption Decreased plasma calcium (transiently)

Calcitonin and PTH should check and balance each other to maintain calcium homeostasis. However, it is unclear whether calcitonin has a significant effect on plasma calcium in adult humans. Thyroid C cells secrete calcitonin in response to acute changes in plasma calcium, but changes in calcitonin secretion in response to chronic hypercalcemia and hypocalcemia are uncertain. People who undergo total thyroidectomy and lose all of their thyroid C cells do not develop hypercalcemia, and patients with medullary carcinoma of the thyroid have extremely high plasma calcitonin levels but do not have hypocalcemia. Calcitonin levels are higher in men than in women and decrease with age, but whether this contributes to bone loss with aging is not known. Calcitonin is found in many other tissues, including the central nervous system, where it may have paracrine actions. Calcitonin can be used for the treatment of hypercalcemia, osteoporosis, and Paget's disease (see below).

VITAMIN D

Vitamin D is not a true vitamin since it can be made by action of sunlight on the skin. It is a fat-soluble hormone that increases the absorption of calcium from the intestine. When exposed to light in the ultraviolet B range (UVB), 7-dehydrocholesterol (7-DHC) in the epidermis is transformed to previtamin D_3, which isomerizes to vitamin D_3 over the course of several hours (Figure 7-3). Vitamin D_3 also is available in the diet, mostly from animal sources such as fatty fish, liver, egg yolk, and vitamin D–fortified milk (Table 7-6). Severe nutritional vitamin D deficiency has decreased markedly since fortified milk was introduced. Vitamin D_2 is a similar product found in plants and yeast.

Table 7-6
Dietary Sources of Vitamin D

Cod liver oil	125–625	Egg yolk	1.75
Herring	22.5	Butter	0.76
Mackerel	17.7	Liver	0.75
Salmon, canned	12.5	Cheese	0.25
Sardines, canned	7.5	Cows' milk[a]	0.01–0.10
Tuna	5.8	Human milk	0.01–0.25

Note. Units of measure are µg/100 g. 1 µg = 25 IU vitamin D. Vitamin D recommended daily allowances (RDAs): 400 IU/day for children, adolescents, pregnant or lactating women; 200 IU/day for adults; RDAs are higher if exposure to sunlight is low.
[a] Cows' milk in the USA is supplemented with vitamin D (400 IU/qt).

The recommended daily allowance (RDA) of dietary vitamin D (see Table 7-6) is higher for children, adolescents, and pregnant and lactating women because their calcium requirements are higher. The RDA is based on the assumption that much of the daily requirement will come from exposure to sunlight. This can be a major problem for those who are housebound and those who live in northern latitudes. The amount of UVB available from sunlight diminishes markedly as summer progresses into fall, and at the latitudes of Boston, Minneapolis, and Seattle, for example, very little skin production of vitamin D occurs between November and February. Clothing and sunblock prevent vitamin D formation even when more sunlight is available.

Obtaining adequate vitamin D from sunlight becomes more difficult with age as skin becomes thinner and skin content of 7-DHC decreases. Individuals over the age of 70 produce only 30% as much vitamin D as young adults do from the same amount of sunlight. Individuals with high melanin levels in the skin require longer sun exposure for the synthesis of vitamin D because melanin competes with 7-DHC for UVB.

Vitamin D supplements (Table 7-7) are available for those who are unable to obtain adequate vitamin D from their diet and sunlight. Some multivitamin tablets and oral

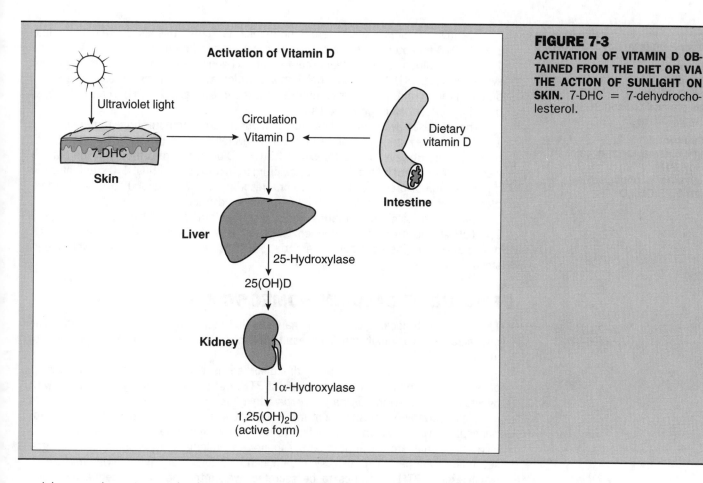

FIGURE 7-3
ACTIVATION OF VITAMIN D OBTAINED FROM THE DIET OR VIA THE ACTION OF SUNLIGHT ON SKIN. 7-DHC = 7-dehydrocholesterol.

calcium supplements contain vitamin D. It is important for most patients to avoid pharmacologic doses of vitamin D because excess vitamin D and its metabolites can be stored in body fat for a long time and cause prolonged hypercalciuria and hypercalcemia.

SUPPLEMENT	GENERIC NAME	DAILY DOSE
Vitamin D_3	Cholecalciferol	400–1000 units
Vitamin D_2	Ergocalciferol	400–1000 units
Reduced D_2 (DHT)	Dihydrotachysterol	200 µg
25(OH) vitamin D_3	Calcifediol	$\leq$ 20–50 µg
1,25(OH)$_2$ vitamin D_3	Calcitriol	0.25–1.0 µg

Table 7-7
Vitamin D Supplements

Vitamin D_3 and D_2 enter the circulation from the skin or intestine and are carried to the liver bound to vitamin D–binding protein. In the liver, they are hydroxylated to 25(OH)D (Figure 7-3). This step is poorly regulated, so any amount of vitamin D can be converted to 25(OH)D, the major storage form of the hormone. The best measurement of vitamin D status is the 25(OH)D level, which reflects vitamin D stores.

Eventually, 25(OH)D is transported to the kidney where it is hydroxylated to the active form, 1,25(OH)$_2$D, by the enzyme 1α-hydroxylase. The conversion of 25(OH)D to 1,25(OH)$_2$D is highly regulated by feedback loops. A decrease in plasma ionized calcium elicits an increase in PTH, which stimulates renal 1α-hydroxylase activity. PTH also stimulates renal excretion of phosphorus, and lower plasma phosphorus stimulates 1,25(OH)$_2$D production. 1,25(OH)$_2$D also regulates its own production. A low level of 1,25(OH)$_2$D stimulates its synthesis.

When plasma ionized calcium is increased, these pathways operate in reverse. High calcium suppresses PTH, 1α-hydroxylase activity decreases, and activation of 25(OH)D decreases. High plasma phosphorus and a high 1,25(OH)$_2$D level also suppress 1α-hydroxylase activity. These feedback loops normally insure an adequate supply of 1,25(OH)$_2$D while preventing hypercalcemia due to overproduction of the active hormone (see Figure 7-2).

Major Actions of 1,25(OH)$_2$D
Increases calcium absorption from the small intestine
Increases phosphorus absorption from the small intestine

Major Regulators of 1,25(OH)$_2$D

Stimulators

Low plasma ionized calcium → high PTH

Low plasma phosphorus

Low 1,25(OH)$_2$D

Inhibitors

High plasma ionized calcium → low PTH

High plasma phosphorus

High 1,25(OH)$_2$D

1,25(OH)$_2$D acts like a steroid hormone. Its target tissues contain a nuclear 1,25(OH)$_2$D receptor, which is similar to other steroid hormone receptors. When the 1,25(OH)$_2$D binds to its nuclear receptor, altered gene transcription results in protein synthesis. 1,25(OH)$_2$D increases calcium absorption by increasing synthesis of calcium-binding protein that transports calcium across the intestine. 1,25(OH)$_2$D also increases intestinal absorption of phosphorus.

The increased availability of calcium and phosphorus promotes bone mineralization. 1,25(OH)$_2$D also stimulates the synthesis of several proteins in osteoblasts, the bone-forming cells. However, the actions of 1,25(OH)$_2$D on bone are complex. If the plasma calcium level cannot be maintained by calcium from the diet, 1,25(OH)$_2$D stimulates the differentiation of precursor cells into bone-resorbing osteoclasts and stimulates osteoblasts to produce cytokines, which increase osteoclast activity.

Many non–calcium-regulating cells also contain 1α-hydroxylase activity and 1,25(OH)$_2$D receptors. They produce 1,25(OH)$_2$D, which acts locally to suppress cell proliferation and increase cell differentiation. These mechanisms are not well understood.

FAILURE OF CALCIUM HOMEOSTASIS

The elegant, interlocking control mechanisms that maintain plasma calcium within the normal range occasionally fail. This results in hypercalcemia, hypocalcemia, or failure to maintain normal bone.

The nomenclature of some of the disorders is confusing. For example, hyperparathyroidism indicates overproduction of PTH, but this is not always associated with hypercalcemia. The term *primary hyperparathyroidism* is used when the primary problem is excess parathyroid tissue secreting PTH that is not suppressed by high calcium. *Secondary hyperparathyroidism* refers to parathyroid hyperplasia and high-circulating PTH levels that are an appropriate response to prolonged hypocalcemia. Prolonged secondary hyperparathyroidism eventually can lead to *tertiary hyperparathyroidism*, in which excess PTH continues to be secreted even after the hypocalcemia has been corrected. Tertiary hyperparathyroidism results from a combination of excess parathyroid tissue and acquired defects in the parathyroid tissue response to calcium.

HYPERCALCEMIA

Hypercalcemia results from excessive resorption of bone or increased calcium absorption from the intestine with inadequate renal excretion of the excess calcium. In the past, when measuring the serum calcium level was impossible or uncommon, hypercalcemia went undiagnosed until the symptoms or signs were severe. Now hypercalcemia presents most often as an abnormal laboratory measurement in patients who are asymptomatic or who have symptoms (e.g., weakness and fatigue), which might be due to other causes. It is important to be sure that the calcium level is not falsely elevated due to dehydration or hemoconcentration during the blood drawing. These may result in high albumin and total calcium levels, but the ionized calcium level is normal. If this is suspected, subtracting 0.8 mg/dL per each gram of albumin over a level of 4.0 g/dL will provide a rough estimate of the true total calcium level.

Symptoms and Signs of Hypercalcemia. Hypercalcemia has been described as the disease of the "-ones" (rhymes with "stones").

- Stones: kidney stones, nephrocalcinosis, thirst, polyuria, and metabolic acidosis
- Bones: bone pain and fractures
- Groans: anorexia, dyspepsia, and constipation
- Moans: fatigue, myalgia, proximal muscle weakness, and joint pain
- Overtones: depression, memory loss, confusion, lethargy, and coma

Obviously, hypercalcemia affects many organ systems. Impaired renal concentrating ability causes the polyuria and thirst. The resulting dehydration makes the hypercalcemia worse. Bone pain and fractures occur only with severe or prolonged bone resorption.

Gastrointestinal symptoms occur more frequently. Hypercalcemia makes nerves and muscles hypoexcitable and results in the neuromuscular abnormalities listed above. The rate of cardiac repolarization is increased, and the electrocardiogram may show a short Q-T interval. Joint pain is due to calcium deposition in joints and tendons and to chondrocalcinosis. Patients with hypercalcemia have excess hypertension, but the mechanism is not known.

Causes of Hypercalcemia.

Primary hyperparathyroidism and hypercalcemia associated with malignancy account for 90% of hypercalcemia. Other causes include an abnormal calcium sensor protein, vitamin D excess, drugs, states associated with high bone turnover, and prolonged immobilization.

Hypercalcemia Due to Primary Hyperparathyroidism (excess PTH).

Eighty percent of primary hyperparathyroidism is due to hypersecretion of PTH from a single parathyroid adenoma. The remainder is due to parathyroid hyperplasia (all parathyroid glands are enlarged and overactive). Parathyroid carcinoma is very rare.

Hypercalcemia due to a parathyroid adenoma is common (incidence is 1 in 500–1000), especially in middle-aged women. Classic renal manifestations include hypercalciuria (24-hr calcium excretion greater than 240 mg in women, greater than 300 mg in men), increased urine phosphorus, and reduced creatinine clearance. Twenty percent of patients have kidney stones. Cortical bone mineral density may be low due to excess bone resorption. Surprisingly, trabecular bone often is spared. Complications of severe disease include subperiosteal bone resorption and erosion of the distal tufts of the fingers, which can be seen on industrial grade x-ray film (Figure 7-4). Bone cysts (osteitis fibrosa cystica) occur in less than 2% of cases. Most patients have mild hypercalcemia and are asymptomatic or have only vague, nonspecific complaints. The diagnosis is confirmed by the classic laboratory findings shown in Table 7-8. No treatment except maintaining good hydration is necessary for mild disease. Surgical removal of the adenoma is recommended for more severe disease, which is indicated by plasma calcium of 12 mg/dL or more, 24-hour urine calcium greater than 400 mg, history or presence of kidney stones, or cortical bone density more than 2 standard deviations (SD) below the mean for age and sex.

Major Causes of Hypercalcemia
Too much PTH
  Primary hyperparathyroidism
Too much PTHrP
  Hypercalcemia of malignancy
Abnormal calcium sensor protein
  Familial hypocalciuric hypercalcemia
  Infantile hypercalcemia
Too much vitamin D
  Exogenous: excess ingestion
  Endogenous: granulomatous diseases, malignancy
Tumor cytokines, which stimulate osteoclasts
Drugs
Miscellaneous causes
  High bone turnover
  Prolonged immobilization

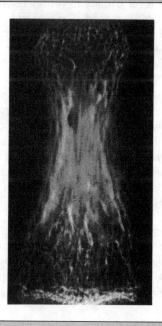

FIGURE 7-4
HIGH RESOLUTION VIEW OF THE MIDDLE PHALANX. This view shows marked subperiosteal and intracortical bone resorption as a result of primary hyperparathyroidism. (*Source:* Reprinted with permission from Genant HK: Radiology of osteoporosis and other metabolic bone diseases. In *Primer on the Metabolic Bone Diseases and Disorders of Mineral Metabolism*, 3rd ed. Edited by Favus MJ. Philadelphia, PA: Lippincott-Raven, 1996, p 161.)

Table 7-8
Abnormal Calcium States: Circulating Concentrations

DISORDER	CALCIUM	PHOSPHORUS	1,25(OH)$_2$D	PTH[a]
Hypercalcemia				
Hyperparathyroidism	High	Low	High	High
PTH-related peptide (PTHrP)	High	Low	Normal	Low
Vitamin D excess	High	High	High	Low
Hypocalcemia				
Hypoparathyroidism	Low	High	Low	Low
Pseudohypoparathyroidism	Low	High	Low	High
Vitamin D deficiency	Low	Low	Low	High
Resistance to 1,25(OH)$_2$D	Low	Low	High	High
Renal failure	Low	High	Low	High

[a] PTH = parathyroid hormone.

Hypercalcemia due to parathyroid hyperplasia occurs as part of two familial, autosomal dominant *multiple endocrine neoplasia* (MEN) syndromes. MEN I is the association of parathyroid hyperplasia with pituitary and pancreatic islet cell tumors. The abnormality has been mapped to chromosome 11. MEN IIA is the association of parathyroid hyperplasia with pheochromocytoma and medullary carcinoma of the thyroid. The MEN IIA gene is located on chromosome 10. The clinical and laboratory manifestations of hypercalcemia are the same as for a parathyroid adenoma. Treatment of the hypercalcemia associated with both MEN syndromes is surgical removal of most parathyroid tissue.

Causes of Malignancy-Induced Hypercalcemia
Tumor PTHrP
Tumor 1,25(OH)$_2$D
Tumor cytokines

Hypercalcemia Due to Malignancy. Tumors usually cause hypercalcemia by producing factors that affect bone resorption. Tumor production of circulating PTHrP is the most common cause of hypercalcemia associated with malignancy. This occurs most often with squamous cell cancers, usually late in the course, when the disease is severe. Patients have hypercalcemia, hypophosphatemia, high urine calcium and phosphorus, and high PTHrP. The PTH level is low because it is suppressed by the hypercalcemia (see Table 7-8). The 1,25(OH)$_2$D level usually is within normal limits, and absorption of calcium from the intestine is not increased. The reason for this is not known.

Some lymphomas produce enough 1,25(OH)$_2$D to cause hypercalcemia. This is thought to be due to excessive conversion of 25(OH)D to 1,25(OH)$_2$D by tumor cells. Laboratory values are similar to those expected for vitamin D excess (see Table 7-8). PTH is suppressed by the hypercalcemia.

Some tumors like multiple myeloma produce cytokines, which strongly stimulate osteoclasts. Release of both calcium and phosphorus from bone causes hypercalcemia and hyperphosphatemia, especially if tumor-associated kidney disease impairs calcium and phosphorus excretion. PTH is suppressed in response to the hypercalcemia, and 1,25(OH)$_2$D is low due to low PTH, high phosphorus, and renal disease.

Hypercalcemia due to bone destruction by invasive tumor metastases is likely to be due to local tumor production of cytokines or PTHrP. This is thought to be the mechanism causing hypercalcemia in patients with breast cancer.

Hypercalcemia Due to Excess Vitamin D. The amount of vitamin D in most over-the-counter multivitamin tablets is too small to cause hypercalcemia if taken as recommended. High doses of exogenous vitamin D can cause hypercalciuria and hypercalcemia, especially in patients taking calcium supplements or patients with another problem with calcium regulation. Since vitamin D is fat-soluble, depletion of accumulated body stores can take some time.

Hypercalcemia can be due to excessive endogenous 1,25(OH)$_2$D production. Conversion of 25(OH)D to 1,25(OH)$_2$D by some lymphomas has been described above. This also occurs with granulomatous diseases, including sarcoid, tuberculosis, leprosy, and silicone-induced granulomatosis. Levels of calcium, phosphorus, and 1,25(OH)$_2$D are high (see Table 7-8), despite PTH suppression by hypercalcemia. Macrophage 1α-hydroxylase does not respond to PTH and also is not down-regulated by high 1,25(OH)$_2$D levels. Patients with granulomas sometimes have worse hypercalcemia and hypercalciuria in the summer when sun exposure increases their 25(OH)D stores.

Hypercalcemia Due to Calcium-Sensing Receptor Mutations. Familial hypocalciuric hypercalcemia (FHH) is an autosomal dominant disorder caused by mutations in the calcium receptor gene located on chromosome 3. Under normal conditions, if plasma ionized calcium increases, more calcium occupies the calcium receptor on parathyroid cells, less PTH is released, and calcium decreases to normal. Families with FHH have defective calcium receptors so a higher level of calcium is required to lower PTH.

Patients with FHH have lifelong hypercalcemia that usually is asymptomatic. They have relatively low urine calcium considering the hypercalcemia (renal calcium clearance/creatinine clearance < 0.01) and borderline high serum magnesium. Serum phosphorus is mildly depressed. Their PTH levels are slightly high or normal (not suppressed as would be expected). They usually require no treatment. Hypercalcemia persists even after subtotal parathyroidectomy. Hypocalciuria also persists, due to the abnormal calcium receptor on the renal tubule cells. Total parathyroidectomy causes hypocalcemia.

Family screening should be done to prevent unnecessary surgery in other affected members. Occasionally newborns who are homozygous for the abnormal receptor gene develop severe neonatal hypercalcemia.

Other Causes of Hypercalcemia. Hydrochlorothiazide (HCTZ) increases calcium resorption by the kidney. This can cause hypercalcemia, particularly in the setting of very mild (often previously undiagnosed) hyperparathyroidism. Lithium can cause hypercalcemia by raising the setpoint for suppression of PTH by calcium. Vitamin A toxicity causes excessive osteoclast activation. High acute or chronic calcium ingestion can cause hypercalcemia, usually in the setting of renal impairment. The milk-alkali syndrome is the association of hypercalcemia, metabolic alkalosis, and renal impairment after ingestion of calcium plus an absorbable alkali such as calcium carbonate.

Immobilization, prolonged bed rest, and weightlessness in space flight are associated with marked bone resorption. Growing children and adults with an underlying disorder causing high bone turnover, such as hyperparathyroidism or hyperthyroidism, are particularly vulnerable to developing hypercalcemia in these settings.

Evaluation of Hypercalcemia

- Review symptoms, signs, and duration (a long course is more likely to be benign)
- Review family history to rule out MEN or FHH
- Physical examination
- Laboratory values: serum calcium, albumin, phosphorus, PTH, 25(OH)D, creatinine, magnesium; urine calcium and creatinine
- X-rays: abdomen for kidney stones and any site of bone pain
- Bone densitometry

All of this is not necessary in every case. It usually is not necessary to measure PTHrP. Most of the time, an underlying malignancy is obvious because humoral hypercalcemia is a late manifestation. A low PTH level rules out hyperparathyroidism.

Treatment of Hypercalcemia. Patients should keep themselves hydrated, discontinue any medications contributing to hypercalcemia, and avoid immobilization as much as possible. No other treatment may be necessary for patients with mild hypercalcemia who are asymptomatic.

Hydration and diuresis lower plasma calcium by increasing renal excretion. Oral phosphate binds ingested calcium but may cause diarrhea and hyperphosphatemia. The combination of hypercalcemia and hyperphosphatemia increases the risk of soft tissue calcification. Glucocorticoids inhibit tumor cytokine release. They also inhibit intestinal calcium absorption, which is useful in cases of vitamin D excess. Calcitonin suppresses osteoclast activity, but the effect is transient, perhaps due to down-regulation of receptors. Three other classes of drugs that strongly inhibit osteoclast activity can be used to treat hypercalcemia of malignancy: biphosphonates such as pamidronate, gallium nitrate, and mithramycin (plicamycin). Dialysis may be required if severe hypercalcemia is accompanied by renal failure.

Parathyroidectomy is the treatment of choice when a parathyroid adenoma or parathyroid hyperplasia causes symptomatic or severe hypercalcemia.

Case Study:
Continued

Ms. A. R. presented with asymptomatic primary hyperparathyroidism. The differential diagnosis included the MEN syndromes because her father had kidney stones and hypertension. However, these are common disorders in the general population. Neither Ms. A. R.'s daughters nor her sisters had hypercalcemia, and Ms. A. R. presented no evidence of another endocrine disorder. The high urine calcium ruled out FHH. There was no evidence of malignancy, and the high PTH level ruled out either PTHrP or vitamin D toxicity as the primary cause of the hypercalcemia. The small amount of vitamin D in her multivitamin tablets was not enough to cause hypercalcemia, but it could exacerbate hypercalcemia as a result of another condition. When her hypercalcemia worsened, Ms. A. R. underwent surgery, which confirmed the presence of a parathyroid adenoma.

Ms. A. R. spent 3 years in a rehabilitation center before she was able to resume modest activity at home. Two years later, she noted increasing weakness and pain in her arms and legs and occasional tingling in her fingers and toes and around her mouth. Her only medication was phenytoin to prevent seizures. Her physical examination revealed a tender sternum and tibia, proximal muscle weakness, positive Chvostek's sign, and slight hyperreflexia. Her electrocardiogram (ECG) showed a normal Q-T interval. Laboratory tests revealed: calcium, 7.0 mg/dL; PTH, high; albumin, normal; phosphorus, 2.1 mg/dL; 25(OH)D and 1,25(OH)$_2$D, low; and urine calcium and phosphorus, low.

HYPOCALCEMIA

Symptoms and Signs of Hypocalcemia.
Most symptoms of hypocalcemia are due to increased neuromuscular irritability. Numbness and tingling occur around the mouth and in the fingertips and toes. More severe or rapidly developing hypocalcemia elicits muscle cramps and pain, irritability, impaired mentation, and seizures. Severe hypocalcemia causes congestive heart failure, a prolonged Q-T interval on the ECG, laryngospasm, bronchospasm, and tetany (spontaneous spasms of the muscles of the face and extremities). Panicky patients may hyperventilate and become hypocapnic and alkalotic, which makes the problem worse. Alkalosis causes increased binding of calcium to albumin, decreasing ionized calcium even further. Prolonged hypocalcemia causes intestinal malabsorption, posterior cataracts, basal ganglia calcifications, and extrapyramidal neurologic symptoms. Defective dentition occurs if hypocalcemia begins in childhood.

Latent tetany can be elicited by tapping over the facial nerve in front of the ear lobe (facial spasm = Chvostek's sign) or by inflating a blood pressure cuff above the systolic pressure for 2 minutes (carpal spasm = Trousseau's sign).

If hypocalcemia presents as an unexpected laboratory abnormality, it is important to be sure that ionized calcium really is low and that hypocalcemia is not just the result of low protein-bound calcium. A rough correction for low albumin can be made by adding 0.8 mg/dL to the total serum calcium for every 1.0 g/dL of albumin lower than 4.0 g/dL.

Causes of Hypocalcemia.
The most common causes of hypocalcemia are PTH and vitamin D deficiency. Hypocalcemia due to PTH or vitamin D resistance or an abnormal calcium receptor protein does not occur often, but these disorders and hypocalcemia due to renal failure, severe hyperphosphatemia, or both illustrate major mechanisms of hormone action on calcium homeostasis.

Hypocalcemia Due to PTH Deficiency.
The most common cause of PTH deficiency is surgical damage or removal of the parathyroid glands during thyroid surgery, radical neck dissection, or extensive parathyroid surgery. Transient hypocalcemia for the first few days after removal of a parathyroid adenoma can occur due to postoperative edema or hemorrhage or "hungry bones" (patients with very active PTH-induced bone resorption rapidly

---

Causes of Hypocalcemia
PTH deficiency
   Surgical, hypomagnesemia, autoimmune, congenital
Vitamin D deficiency
PTH resistance
Vitamin D resistance
Abnormal calcium receptor protein
Renal failure (secondary hyperparathyroidism)
Severe hyperphosphatemia
Other
   Drug-induced, acute pancreatitis, acute rhabdomyolysis, transfusion of citrated blood

redeposit calcium and phosphorus in bone when the PTH-producing adenoma is removed). Prolonged postsurgical hypocalcemia indicates permanent damage.

Hypomagnesemia causes hypocalcemia because adequate magnesium is needed for both PTH synthesis and secretion.

Autoimmune hypoparathyroidism can be familial or sporadic and occurs alone or as part of a polyglandular deficiency syndrome. Polyglandular autoimmune hypoparathyroidism can also be associated with any of the following: vitiligo, adrenal insufficiency, alopecia, pernicious anemia, celiac disease, hypothyroidism, hypogonadism, type 1 diabetes mellitus, or mucocutaneous candidiasis.

Hypoparathyroidism in newborns due to congenital absence of the parathyroid glands is associated with other congenital anomalies in several syndromes. Isolated absence of the parathyroid glands is inherited as an X-linked or autosomal recessive disorder.

PTH deficiency is characterized by low PTH, low calcium, high phosphorus, and low $1,25(OH)_2D$ (see Table 7-8). Urine calcium is low. Treatment involves giving enough calcium and vitamin D supplements to keep plasma calcium in the low-normal range. Higher calcium levels are not desirable because without PTH to help retain urine calcium, patients are at risk for hypercalciuria and kidney stones. Calcium supplements are preferred to a diet high in dairy products because these also contain phosphorus.

Hypocalcemia Due to PTH Resistance (Pseudohypoparathyroidism [PHP]). Hypocalcemia occurs despite normal parathyroid activity if there is a defect in the parathyroid receptor, an abnormal G protein associated with the receptor, defective generation of cAMP, or failure anywhere in the subsequent cascade of phosphorylations. Calcium is low, but the PTH level is high because the parathyroid glands oversecrete PTH in an attempt to compensate. This situation is referred to as PHP. PHP is one of the causes of *secondary hyperparathyroidism*, so-called because the high PTH level is secondary to the hypocalcemia. Resistance to PTH results in high plasma phosphorus and low $1,25(OH)_2D$ (see Table 7-8). There are several clinical variants of PHP, depending on the site of the block. The classic test for PHP is the PTH infusion test. Patients with PHP do not have a normal increase in urinary cAMP and renal phosphorus excretion in response to PTH.

Patients with PHP type Ia have only 50% of the normal level of the $G_s\alpha$ protein, which responds to PTH receptor occupancy. They can have a similar deficiency in other glands, resulting in a diminished response to thyroid-stimulating hormone (TSH), follicle-stimulating hormone (FSH), and luteinizing hormone (LH) as well. These patients often have a distinct phenotype, which includes short stature, round faces, brachydactyly (short 4th and 5th metacarpals giving a knuckle-knuckle-dimple-dimple appearance to the hand), and subcutaneous ossification. This phenotype was first described by Fuller Albright, so PHP Ia is also called Albright's hereditary osteodystrophy (AHO).

Some patients have the physical characteristics of PHP Ia but have normal calcium and PTH levels and increases in urine cAMP and phosphorus in response to PTH infusion. They do not have PTH resistance. This variation is called pseudopseudohypoparathyroidism (PPHP) and can occur in families with members that have classic PHP. The cause of the abnormal phenotype in PPHP is not known.

The molecular defects causing the other variations of PHP are not known. The other variations do not have the abnormal phenotype.

The treatment of PHP is similar to the treatment for primary hypoparathyroidism.

Hypocalcemia Due to Vitamin D Deficiency. Vitamin D deficiency occurs because of defective supply or defective processing. Problems with obtaining enough vitamin D from the diet and adequate sunlight exposure have been discussed above. Malabsorption syndromes exacerbate any dietary deficiency. With severe liver and kidney disease, vitamin D cannot be hydroxylated to $25(OH)D$ and $1,25(OH)_2D$. Catabolism of vitamin D is accelerated by isoniazid, rifampin, and anticonvulsants such as phenytoin, which increase the activity of the liver P-450 enzyme system. Phenytoin also is thought to inhibit calcium absorption in the intestine.

Vitamin D deficiency in childhood results in *rickets*, which is characterized by the formation of disordered excess cartilage, poor bone formation at the epiphyseal growth plate, and poor mineralization of osteoid in cortical and trabecular bone. Infants

---

Major Causes of Vitamin D Deficiency
Diet low in vitamin D
Little sun exposure
Malabsorption of vitamin D
Severe liver disease
Renal failure
Increased catabolism

with rapidly growing bones develop widened cranial sutures, soft calvaria prone to deformity, bulging costochondral junctions (rachitic rosary on the anterior chest), wrist enlargement, and delayed eruption of teeth. Older children develop deformities due to pressure on weakened growth plates in weight-bearing bones that result in bowed legs (genu varum) or knock-knee (genu valgum) [Figure 7-5].

FIGURE 7-5
RICKETS IN THE RADIUS AND THE ULNA. The metaphyses are widened, irregular, and cupped. The bones in general are demineralized. (*Source:* Reprinted with permission from Klein GL: Nutritional rickets and osteomalacia. In *Primer on the Metabolic Bone Diseases and Disorders of Mineral Metabolism*, 3rd ed. Edited by Favus MJ. Philadelphia, PA: Lippincott-Raven, 1996, p 303.)

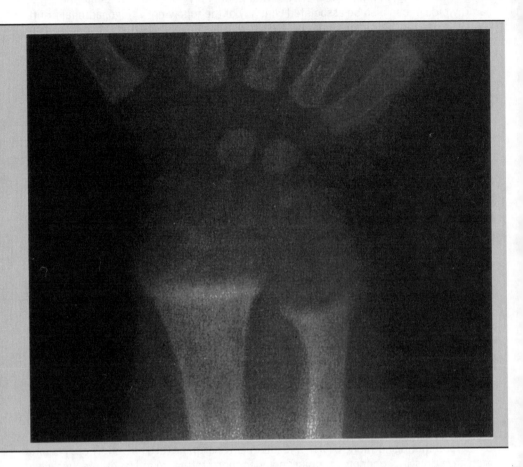

In adults whose epiphyseal growth plates have fused, severe vitamin D deficiency results in *osteomalacia*, a defect in bone mineralization. Bone biopsies show increased osteoid (unmineralized bone). The major clinical finding is diffuse bone pain. X-rays of the long bones may show thin radiolucent lines (Looser's lines) perpendicular to the cortex; these are not fractures. Both children and adults develop muscle weakness.

Laboratory findings (see Table 7-8) include a low calcium level and a high PTH level in response to the hypocalcemia (another example of secondary hyperparathyroidism). Calcium may be low-normal if the high PTH level causes enough bone resorption and renal calcium retention to compensate for the poor calcium absorption from the intestine. Phosphorus levels are low, partly due to decreased absorption from the intestine and partly due to the action of PTH on the kidney. Serum 25(OH)D levels are low. Conversion of 25(OH)D to 1,25(OH)$_2$D is increased in response to the high level of PTH, and 1,25(OH)$_2$D can remain in the normal range until the vitamin D deficiency is severe.

Treatment of vitamin D deficiency involves improving diet, increasing sunlight exposure, when possible, and supplementing with some form of vitamin D. Overtreatment results in hypercalciuria and hypercalcemia.

Hypocalcemia Due to Vitamin D Resistance. Rare genetic defects in vitamin D metabolism result in ineffective vitamin D action even though the supply of vitamin D is normal. Patients with severe defects present with childhood rickets; milder defects may result in osteomalacia later. Vitamin D–dependent rickets type I (VDDR-I) is an autosomal recessive disorder caused by defective renal 1α-hydroxylase.

Defective 1α-hydroxylase $\longrightarrow$ low $1,25(OH)_2D$ $\longrightarrow$ low calcium $\longrightarrow$ high PTH

Phosphorus is low due to decreased absorption from the intestine and PTH-induced renal excretion. Before $1,25(OH)_2D$ therapy was available, patients were treated with very large doses of vitamin D—hence the name "vitamin D–dependent" rickets. Very high doses of vitamin D result in very high levels of $25(OH)D$ or some other metabolite, which has some activity.

Vitamin D–dependent rickets type II (hereditary resistance to $1,25(OH)_2D$) is due to a defect in the $1,25(OH)_2D$ receptor or to a postreceptor defect so there is no response to $1,25(OH)_2D$.

Resistance to $1,25(OH)_2D$ $\longrightarrow$ low calcium $\longrightarrow$ high PTH $\longrightarrow$ high $1,25(OH)_2D$

The resulting hypocalcemia elicits a high level of PTH, which stimulates conversion of $25(OH)D$ to $1,25(OH)_2D$. Phosphorus levels are low as in VDDR-I. These patients also develop alopecia, indicating that $1,25(OH)_2D$ has some action on hair follicles. If the defect is mild, patients sometimes respond to vitamin D supplements. However, half the patients do not respond even to very high doses. These patients are treated with very high doses of calcium.

Hypocalcemia Due to Renal Failure (Secondary Hyperparathyroidism). In patients with severe kidney disease, there are several causes of the hypocalcemia that results in high PTH levels (secondary hyperparathyroidism). Loss of renal function results in loss of renal 1α-hydroxylase and inability to convert $25(OH)D$ to $1,25(OH)_2D$. Calcium absorption from the intestine is severely compromised. Patients with kidney failure are unable to excrete phosphorus, so phosphorus levels are high. Hyperphosphatemia lowers calcium levels directly (calcium + phosphorus $\rightarrow CaPO_4$). Hyperphosphatemia also suppresses 1α-hydroxylase.

Renal failure $\longrightarrow$ low $1,25(OH)_2D$ and high phosphorus $\longrightarrow$

low calcium $\longrightarrow$ high PTH

Prolonged renal failure results in significant, even severe, parathyroid hyperplasia. The high PTH levels increase osteoclastic resorption of bone, which releases both calcium and phosphorus. Since the phosphorus cannot be excreted, the hyperphosphatemia becomes even worse. Major bone resorption results in bone pain and fractures.

Medical treatment includes $1,25(OH)_2D$, calcium supplements, and phosphorus binders. If treatment is successful, parathyroid hyperplasia regresses. Prolonged hypocalcemia can cause progressive hyperplasia to the point that the parathyroid tissue appears autonomous. PTH production remains higher than normal, even if renal disease is corrected by renal transplant. If hypercalcemia develops also, the patients have developed tertiary hyperparathyroidism.

Hypocalcemia Due to an Abnormal Calcium Sensor (Hypercalciuric Hypocalcemia). Mutations in the calcium receptor protein on parathyroid and renal tubule cells can cause a gain in receptor function. These patients have low or low-normal PTH levels because the calcium receptor is oversensitive to extracellular calcium and PTH secretion is suppressed. They have hypocalcemia, hypercalciuria, and hypomagnesemia. These abnormalities are the opposite of those in families with FHH (see above) who have a decrease in calcium receptor function. Symptomatic patients should be given just enough vitamin D to raise the calcium to adequately suppress their symptoms. Asymptomatic patients should not be treated.

Hypocalcemia Due to Severe Hyperphosphatemia. Normally the product of the calcium $\times$ phosphorus concentrations is less than 60. If $[Ca] \times [P]$ is ≥ 70 after an oral or intravenous phosphorus load, $CaPO_4$ tends to precipitate in soft tissues. High phosphorus also suppresses renal 1α-hydroxylase, and the decrease in $1,25(OH)_2D$ also contributes to hypocalcemia.

Hyperphosphatemia severe enough to cause hypocalcemia occurs in renal failure or after chemotherapy or rhabdomyolysis, which cause massive cellular lysis with release of intracellular phosphorus.

Other Causes of Hypocalcemia. Drugs that effectively suppress osteoclasts and decrease calcium release from bone can cause hypocalcemia. Examples include bisphosphonates, fluoride, mithramycin (plicamycin), and high doses of parenteral calcitonin.

Transfusion with citrated blood or administration of contrast dyes that contain the calcium chelator EDTA can cause hypocalcemia.

Patients with pancreatitis can develop profound hypocalcemia, but the mechanisms are uncertain. Release of pancreatic lipase results in excessive release of free fatty acids, which bind calcium. These patients also have hypomagnesemia, which impairs PTH secretion and action.

Case Study: *Continued*	*Ms. A. R. developed classic symptoms and signs of hypocalcemia (perioral and peripheral tingling and Chvostek's sign). This was due to vitamin D deficiency. The high PTH level ruled out damage to her parathyroid glands during her earlier surgery as the cause. Her low vitamin D level was due to prolonged lack of exposure to sunlight plus phenytoin-induced catabolism of the vitamin D from her diet. Ms. A. R.'s bone and muscle pain and weakness suggested that she had developed osteomalacia.*

METABOLIC BONE DISEASE

Major Metabolic Bone Diseases
Osteoporosis—a disorder of excessive bone resorption
Osteomalacia—a disorder of bone formation
Paget's disease—a disorder of bone remodeling

The disorders referred to as metabolic bone diseases involve abnormal activity of packets of bone known as bone-forming units (BFUs). The normal balance between bone formation and bone resorption is upset, resulting either in loss of bone mass or formation of abnormal bone. The major metabolic bone diseases are osteoporosis, osteomalacia, and Paget's disease of bone.

BONE BALANCE AND BONE MASS

In young people, the main bone processes are modeling and growth. Growth factors, hormones, and exercise stimulate osteoblasts directly, and bone mass increases. Acquisition of bone mass is nearly complete by the end of adolescence, but another 5%–10% accumulates in the third decade of life when bone mass reaches its peak. Peak bone mass is largely genetically determined, although it is affected by many other factors including nutrition, activity, and illness. It is higher in men than in women and is higher in blacks than in whites or Asians.

After bone mass has reached its peak, the main process in adult BFUs is remodeling or repair of damaged bone. A hormonal or physical activation stimulus removes lining cells and exposes the bone surface (activation phase). This attracts osteoclasts that dig a resorption cavity (resorption phase). Eventually this process reverses, and a cement line is formed to cement together the old and new bone. Osteoblasts fill in the cavity with new matrix (osteoid), which is mineralized over a period of months (formation phase). Trapped osteoblasts become osteocytes. The whole sequence takes 3–6 months or more (Figure 7-6). In adults, bone resorption and bone formation are linked or coupled, and bone formation occurs only after bone resorption.

The extent of bone turnover depends on the *rate* of activation of BFUs and the *number* of BFUs activated. After age 30 or so, bone formation cannot keep up with bone resorption and a small amount of bone is lost with each cycle. Therefore, anything that activates BFUs and increases bone turnover is likely to contribute to bone loss. Trabecular bone, which turns over more rapidly than cortical bone, is more vulnerable.

PTH is one of many activators of BFUs. PTH interaction with its receptors on osteoblasts ultimately leads to release of cytokines from mononuclear cells. These cytokines activate osteoclasts and the BFU remodeling proceeds as shown in Figure 7-6. How PTH and other activators trigger release of cytokines such as interleukin-1 and interleukin-6 is unknown.

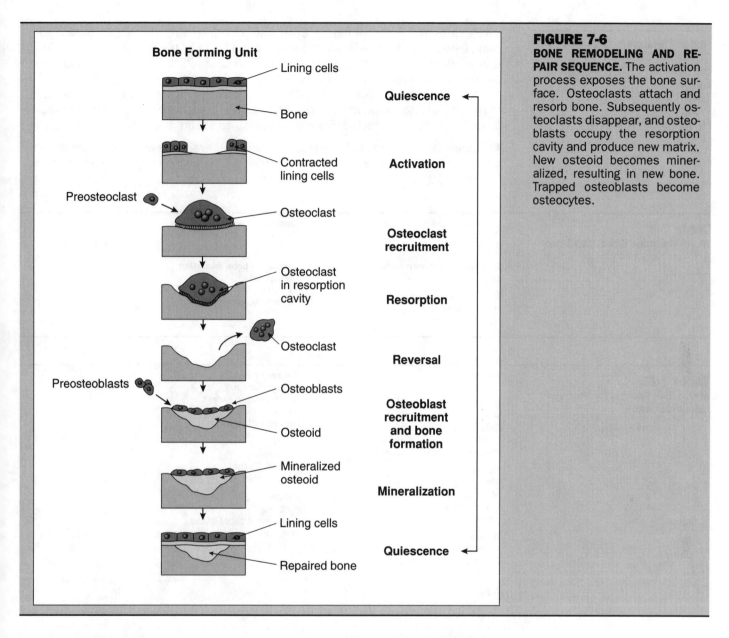

Bone Forming Unit

Lining cells

Bone

Quiescence

Contracted lining cells

Activation

Preosteoclast

Osteoclast

Osteoclast recruitment

Osteoclast in resorption cavity

Resorption

Osteoclast

Reversal

Preosteoblasts

Osteoblasts

Osteoid

Osteoblast recruitment and bone formation

Mineralized osteoid

Mineralization

Lining cells

Quiescence

Repaired bone

FIGURE 7-6
BONE REMODELING AND REPAIR SEQUENCE. The activation process exposes the bone surface. Osteoclasts attach and resorb bone. Subsequently osteoclasts disappear, and osteoblasts occupy the resorption cavity and produce new matrix. New osteoid becomes mineralized, resulting in new bone. Trapped osteoblasts become osteocytes.

In premenopausal women, estrogen acts as a brake on bone turnover. Estrogen is believed to inhibit release of cytokines, which activate osteoclasts. After menopause, the suppressive action of estrogen is gone, sensitivity to PTH increases, and osteoclast activity increases. This results in a high turnover state with deeper resorption cavities than usual. Osteoblast activity cannot keep up, bone trabeculae become eroded through, trabecular connections are lost, and complete repair is impossible. Women lose up to 25% of their trabecular bone and 10% of their cortical bone during the decade after menopause. Although the sensitivity to PTH is increased during this period, the excess calcium and phosphorus released from bone actually keep PTH and 25(OH)D activation by 1α-hydroxylase somewhat suppressed. Less calcium is absorbed from the gastrointestinal tract, and more calcium is lost in the urine. This prevents hypercalcemia but also accentuates total body loss of calcium.

Healthy men continue to produce testosterone until late in life, but if testosterone decreases, bone loss is comparable to that in postmenopausal women. Recent studies of two young adult men without functional estrogen receptors indicate that men also need estrogen action for normal bone maturation and repair.

After the first postmenopausal decade, the effects of estrogen deprivation diminish, and aging changes become dominant. Vitamin D activation and calcium absorption decrease with age. Plasma calcium decreases slightly, and PTH increases slightly (but

Major Regulators of Bone Mass
Genes
Hormones
Calcium
Exercise
Weight
Habits (alcohol, smoking)
Drugs

still remains in the normal range). Bone resorption increases to maintain plasma calcium. Osteoblasts become less and less active and fail to fill the resorption cavities. This may be due to failure of local growth factors. Slow loss of 25% of cortical and trabecular bone occurs with aging over a lifetime in both sexes.

Normal changes in bone mass with age are shown in Figure 7-7. Low bone mass is the major predictor of future fractures, and adults who start with a high peak bone mass at age 30 are better protected. Bone quality also matters, but this is difficult to measure.

Additional Determinants of Bone Mass. Although genes and age are major determinants of bone mass, many other factors also contribute. The major factors are listed in Tables 7-9 and 7-10.

Table 7-9
Major Hormone Effects on Bone

Increased bone resorption
Parathyroid hormone
Parathyroid hormone–related protein

Decreased bone formation
Glucocorticoids

Increased bone turnover
Hyperparathyroidism
Hyperthyroidism

Decreased bone resorption
Estrogen
Calcitonin

Increased bone formation
Testosterone
Growth hormone
Insulin-like growth factor 1

Table 7-10
Major Risk Factors for Osteoporotic Fractures

Aging

Genetic
White or Asian woman
Small peak bone mass
Low body mass index (kg/m^2)
Family history of osteoporosis

Nutritional
Malnutrition
Malabsorption
Low calcium intake
Low vitamin D

Diseases
Neoplasms affecting bone
Rheumatic diseases causing
    local bone loss

Other
Increased propensity to fall
    Poor vision
    Poor coordination
    Medications decreasing alertness
Poor bone quality
Previous osteoporotic fracture

Hormonal
Hypogonadism
Glucocorticoid excess
Hyperthyroidism
Hyperparathyroidism

Drugs
Heparin
Anticonvulsants
Cyclosporine

Habits
Smoking
Excessive alcohol intake
Low activity or immobilization

Major hormone effects on bone are summarized in Table 7-9. Hormone actions at the cellular level are complex. For example, PTH stimulates bone resorption, but small doses of PTH have an anabolic effect on trabecular bone. $1,25(OH)_2D$ increases bone formation by stimulating absorption of calcium and phosphorus, but large doses stimulate osteoclasts. Glucocorticoids suppress bone formation and also suppress calcium absorption from the intestine. Insulin-like growth factor-1 exerts local effects.

A high calcium intake during childhood and adolescence increases peak bone mass. In adults, a good calcium intake helps to overcome the decrease in efficiency of calcium absorption with aging.

Bone mass decreases or increases in response to unloading or loading. Bone is lost rapidly with immobilization, bed rest, and weightlessness (as in space satellite residence). Increased bone mass with habitual activity has been shown in children, adolescents, and young women. Trained athletes have higher bone mass. However, women who train to the level of amenorrhea have low bone mass due to loss of estrogen. The increased exercise does not compensate for this loss unless the loads on bone are extraordinary. In

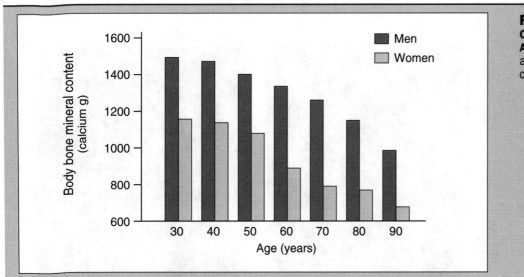

FIGURE 7-7
CHANGES IN BONE MASS WITH AGE. Changes in bone mass are indicated by total body calcium content.

nonathletes, controlled exercise trials have shown gains in bone mass of 1%–3%. Exercise also increases strength and coordination, which provide protection against falls.

Obese people have higher bone mass, partly due to the increased musculoskeletal effort of moving a heavier load. Also, adipose tissue contains aromatase, the enzyme that converts androgens to estrogens that are stored in fat. Obese postmenopausal women have higher estrogen stores.

Alcohol inhibits osteoblast activity. Smoking is associated with smaller bone mass. The mechanism is not certain, but smokers tend to be thinner.

Drugs can cause loss of bone by acting on bone directly (heparin, cyclosporine, glucocorticoids) or indirectly by increasing vitamin D catabolism (anticonvulsants) or decreasing calcium absorption (glucocorticoids).

OSTEOPOROSIS

Osteoporosis is defined as loss of bone mass *plus* accumulated microarchitectural damage resulting in enough bone fragility that fracture is likely with minimal trauma. Minimal trauma is defined as less trauma than that from a fall from a standing height. For women, the World Health Organization defines osteoporosis as a bone mass more than 2.5 SD below the young adult mean. Lesser degrees of bone loss are referred to as osteopenia. These are working definitions based on the increase in fracture risk at these levels of bone mass in epidemiologic studies. Such studies have not been done in men.

Osteoporotic bone is characterized by low bone mass, loss of horizontal trabeculae, and areas of microdamage (Figure 7-8), but composition of the remaining bone is normal. Patients with osteoporosis due to menopause and aging losses have normal calcium and phosphorus levels unless another illness prevents feedback control loops from operating normally.

Most fractures occur at sites containing trabecular bone, which turns over more rapidly and contains less calcium. The major sites of osteoporotic fractures, time of occurrence, and the lifetime risk for white women are shown in Table 7-11. Black women usually have a higher bone mass than white women and have far fewer fractures. Men are protected not only by larger peak bone mass but also by larger vertebral end plates. They also have more cortical bone, which is more highly mineralized and turns over slowly. Men rarely have wrist fractures. They have fewer vertebral fractures than women, and the fractures occur approximately 10 years later. Men have approximately half as many hip fractures as women.

Hip fractures are the most devastating in terms of pain, acute morbidity, long-term disability, mortality, and cost. Less than one-third of those who have a hip fracture have returned to their prefracture level of function 1 year later. Women at greatest risk for a hip fracture are women who have had a vertebral fracture, those whose mothers had a hip fracture, tall women (who have further to fall), and women who have a long hip axis (distance from the lateral surface of the trochanter to the inner surface of the pelvis along the axis of the femoral neck, measured on an x-ray).

Osteoporosis is loss of bone mass plus accumulated microarchitectural damage resulting in enough bone fragility that fracture is likely with minimal trauma.

FIGURE 7-8
SCANNING ELECTRON MICRO-
GRAPH OF TRABECULAR BONE
IN A HEALTHY YOUNG WOMAN
(A) AND A POSTMENOPAUSAL
WOMAN WITH OSTEOPORO-
SIS (B). In B, note the thinner
trabeculae and loss of horizontal trabecular connections.
(*Source:* Reprinted with permission from Dempster DW, et al: A
simple method for correlative
light and scanning electron microscopy of human iliac crest
bone biopsies. *J Bone Min Res*
1:19, 1986.)

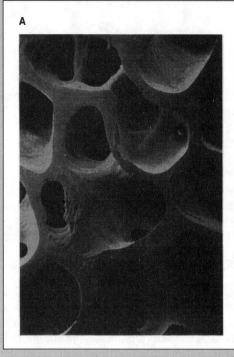
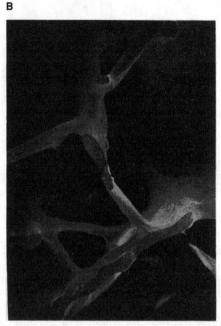

Table 7-11
Lifetime Osteoporotic Fracture
Risk[a]

FRACTURE SITE	USUAL AGE	PREVALENCE (BY AGE 80+)
Wrist	50+	24%
Spine	60+	33%
Hip	70+	15%

[a] Caucasian women in the United States.

Osteoporosis Evaluation
Risk factor assessment
Bone turnover assessment
  Tests of osteoclast activity
  Tests of osteoblast activity
Bone mineral density measure-
  ment
X-rays

Osteoporosis Evaluation. Risk factors for low bone mass (see Table 7-10) predict risk for fractures in populations better than in individuals. New biochemical markers of osteo-clast activity (pyridinolines and cross-linked N- and C-telopeptides measured in urine) measure breakdown products of type 1 collagen, the major protein of bone. Markers of osteoblast activity (propeptides of type 1 collagen, osteocalcin and bone-specific alka-line phosphatase) are osteoblast proteins. These are used primarily for research studies at this time since there is little longitudinal data in individual patients and day-to-day variation is large. Levels of osteoclast products change several months before levels of osteoblast products. Low levels of both formation and resorption markers indicate that bone turnover has been suppressed.

Bone mass (bone calcium/unit area) measured by *d*ual *e*nergy *x*-ray *a*bsorptiometry (DEXA) of the hip or spine currently is the best predictor of future fracture risk. It takes at least 1 year to measure significant changes. A DEXA scan should be obtained if the information will influence treatment. X-rays are much less sensitive and do not show changes in bone mass until one-third of bone has been lost.

Patients with osteoporosis should be evaluated for hyperparathyroidism, hyper-thyroidism, glucocorticoid excess, hypogonadism, and vitamin D deficiency, depending on the level of suspicion.

Osteoporosis Prevention. Prevention of bone loss is possible, but restoration after major bone loss is not. Pharmacologic treatments either suppress bone resorption by osteo-clasts (calcium, estrogen or an estrogen analog, calcitonin, bisphosphonates), increase bone formation by osteoblasts (testosterone, fluoride, low-dose PTH), or improve the calcium supply (calcium supplements, vitamin D).

Estrogen prevents osteoporotic fractures and has other beneficial effects (see Chap-ter 12), but progesterone must be added to prevent hyperstimulation of the endometrium unless the woman has had a hysterectomy. Concern about the effect of estrogen on breast cancer risk (controversial) and withdrawal bleeding limits patient acceptance of hormone replacement therapy. *Selective estrogen receptor modulators* (SERMs) interact with estrogen receptors and function as estrogen agonists in some tissues and antagonists in others, depending on their interaction with DNA and transcription factors. One of these compounds is raloxifene, which stabilizes bone mass and lowers low-density lipoprotein (LDL) cholesterol without stimulating the uterus or breast. The long-term effects of SERMs are not known. Calcitonin can be given as a nasal spray and has mild analgesic action in some patients. Bisphosphonates such as alendronate have an $RO_3P\text{-}C\text{-}PO_3R$ structure that binds tightly to hydroxyapatite and makes these drugs potent and long-lasting osteoclast inhibitors.

Significant suppression of osteoclast activity can result in hypocalcemia and secondary hyperparathyroidism. Patients treated with osteoclast inhibitors often need calcium supplements unless their dietary intake of calcium is high. Since $1,25(OH)_2D$ has complex actions on bone and often causes hypercalciuria, a physiologic dose of vitamin D such as 400 U/d usually is given when a supplement is required.

Since bone formation is coupled to bone resorption, any intervention that suppresses osteoclast activity eventually results in lower osteoblast activity, and bone mass reaches a plateau. Adding a stimulator of bone formation would be ideal. Slow-release fluoride, low-dose PTH, and anabolic steroids that do not have a virilizing effect are being tested in clinical trials. Testosterone is used to stimulate bone formation in hypogonadal males (Chapter 11).

Whatever the level of bone mass, it is important to decrease the risk of falling and to encourage exercise when this is possible.

OSTEOMALACIA

Osteomalacia is a disorder of bone mineralization resulting in accumulation of unmineralized osteoid, bone and muscle pain, weakness, and sometimes fractures. Osteomalacia and rickets caused by vitamin D deficiency are described above. Osteomalacia due to calcium deficiency is accompanied by osteopenia, because hypocalcemia elicits increased PTH, which increases bone resorption.

Osteomalacia also can be due to phosphorus deficiency. The inherited forms are due to a genetic defect in phosphorus transport in the renal tubule or to a humoral factor that stimulates renal phosphorus secretion. They are associated with a defect in the synthesis of $1,25(OH)_2D$. X-linked hypophosphatemia also is associated with defective osteoblast function. Patients are treated with oral phosphorus with $1,25(OH)_2D$ to increase calcium absorption.

Acquired hypophosphatemia can be due to very low phosphorus intake (unusual) or excessive binding of ingested phosphate by aluminum-containing antacids. More often, hypophosphatemia results from excessive renal phosphorus loss. Fanconi and other forms of renal tubular acidosis are associated with renal phosphorus wasting. Tumor-induced or oncogenic osteomalacia is characterized by phosphaturia, hypophosphatemia, and low $1,25(OH)_2D$. The tumors produce a humoral factor that affects phosphate resorption at the proximal renal tubule. The tumors are often small and very difficult to find, but bone healing occurs if the tumor can be removed.

Major features of osteoporosis and osteomalacia are compared in Table 7-12.

Osteoporosis Prevention
Decrease osteoclast action
  Calcium
  Estrogen
  Bisphosphonates
Stimulate osteoblast action
  Selective estrogen receptor
    modulators
  Testosterone
  Fluoride
  Calcitonin
Increase calcium supply
  Calcium
  Vitamin D
Exercise
Prevent Falls

Osteomalacia is a disorder of bone mineralization resulting in the accumulation of unmineralized osteoid, bone and muscle pain, and weakness.

Major Causes of Osteomalacia
Vitamin D deficiency
Calcium deficiency
Phosphorus deficiency

SYMPTOMS AND SIGNS	OSTEOPOROSIS	OSTEOMALACIA
Bone pain	Yes (with fractures)	Yes
Increased bone resorption	Yes	No
Decreased bone formation	Yes	Yes
Decreased bone mass	Yes	Yes
Bone composition normal	Yes	No (increased osteoid)
Muscle weakness	No	Yes
Serum calcium and phosphorus	Usually normal	Often low

Table 7-12
Manifestations of Osteoporosis and Osteomalacia

Case Study:
Continued

Ms. A. R. was treated for osteomalacia with high doses of calcium and vitamin D, and her bone and muscle pain and weakness resolved. Her calcium and vitamin D doses were decreased to more physiologic levels. Two years later, at the age of 67, Ms. A. R. developed sudden back pain while making her bed. Physical examination revealed loss of 1.5 inches in height from 2 years before and new tenderness over her mid-thoracic spine. Her calcium, albumin, phosphorus, 25(OH)D, and creatinine levels were normal. Spine x-rays revealed two thoracic vertebral fractures. A DEXA scan of her left hip showed low bone mass.

PAGET'S DISEASE OF BONE

Paget's disease is a disorder of bone remodeling. Giant multinucleated osteoclasts resorb bone. This is followed by compensatory but disorderly formation of woven bone by osteoblasts. Bone turnover is high, but resorption and formation are coupled, and plasma calcium and phosphorus usually are normal. Mineralization is normal. The result: local areas of enlarged, abnormally vascular, easily deformed bone that feel warm due to the increased blood flow. Paget's disease may affect one bone or several. The most common sites are the pelvis, femur, skull, tibia, and spine (Figure 7-9), but other bones also may be involved. X-rays show mixed areas of sclerosis and lucency.

Many patients are asymptomatic and are diagnosed when either an elevated alkaline phosphatase level (reflecting increased bone formation) or an abnormal x-ray is obtained during the workup for an unrelated problem. Pain can be due to the increased blood flow,

FIGURE 7-9
X-RAY OF A HUMERUS SHOWING TYPICAL CHANGES OF PAGET'S DISEASE OF BONE. In the distal half: thickened cortex, expansion, and mixed areas of lucency and sclerosis. (*Source:* Reprinted with permission from Siris ES: Paget's disease of bone. In *Primer on Metabolic Bone Diseases and Disorders of Mineral Metabolism*, 3rd ed. Edited by Flavus MJ. Philadelphia, PA: Lippincott-Raven, 1996, p 412.)

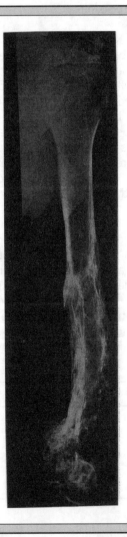

deformity, nearby nerve impingement, and degeneration of nearby joints if posture and gait are affected. Skull involvement can result in increased head size and deafness. Neoplastic degeneration occurs but is unusual (< 1%).

The cause of Paget's disease is unknown, though a virus is suspected, and there is a genetic component. Paget's disease is common in northern Europe, North America, Australia, and New Zealand. Treatment involves suppressing the osteoclasts, mostly with bisphosphonates or calcitonin (the same agents used to treat osteoporosis but at higher doses). It is unclear whether patients with mild disease (i.e., no symptoms and alkaline phosphatase < 1.5-2 × normal) should be treated to prevent progression.

Case Study:
Resolution

Ms. A. R. now has osteoporosis. She has had two vertebral fractures with minimal trauma. She no longer has symptoms or signs of osteomalacia, and her x-rays did not show Paget's disease. Her risk factors for osteoporosis include being a postmenopausal white woman with a family history of osteoporosis; previous high bone turnover due to hyperparathyroidism, low vitamin D, and modest calcium intake in the past; and a period of prolonged immobilization. It is unfortunate that her estrogen therapy was stopped after her accident. Estrogen was an excellent choice for her because estrogen helps prevent osteoclast resorption due to PTH.

Ms. A. R. was urged to continue her calcium and vitamin D supplements. She will increase her exercise, if possible, when her back pain lessens and will take extra precautions against falling. She is considering restarting estrogen and progesterone therapy. Bisphosphonate and calcitonin also are possible choices for her.

■ REVIEW QUESTIONS

Directions: For each of the following questions, choose the **one best** answer.

Questions 1 and 2

1. Sue R. is a 60-year-old woman who consults her physician because her mother has osteoporosis and has just fractured two vertebrae. Ms. R. has a history of exercise-induced asthma. She does not smoke and drinks an occasional glass of wine. She dislikes dairy products but drinks a glass of calcium-supplemented orange juice daily. She takes no medications and refuses estrogen therapy because her sister has breast cancer. The physical examination reveals a thin, healthy-appearing woman. When her bone mass is measured, it is found to be low. The physician would be most likely to recommend

   (A) thyroxine to suppress bone turnover
   (B) calcium to stimulate bone resorption
   (C) a bisphosphonate to suppress osteoclasts
   (D) fluoride to suppress osteoblast activity
   (E) calcitonin to stimulate osteoclasts

2. Two years later, Ms. R.'s asthma worsens, and she is started on chronic glucocorticoid therapy. The physician should be aware that glucocorticoids cause bone loss by

   (A) suppressing vitamin D activation
   (B) suppressing bone resorption
   (C) inhibiting bone formation
   (D) increasing calcium absorption from the intestine
   (E) increasing osteoblast proliferation

3. James T. is a 65-year-old man whose laboratory tests before knee replacement surgery reveal: calcium, 11.0 (normal: 8.5–10.5 mg/dL); phosphorus, 2.2 (normal: 2.3–4.5 mg/dL); and albumin and creatinine, normal. The urine calcium-to-creatinine ratio is low. Parathyroid hormone (PTH) is mildly increased. Mr. T. is unconcerned because he feels well except for knee pain, and both his son and granddaughter have high plasma calcium. They have no symptoms. The most likely cause of this man's hypercalcemia is

   (A) parathyroid hormone–related peptide (PTHrP)
   (B) primary hyperparathyroidism
   (C) secondary hyperparathyroidism
   (D) abnormal calcium sensor protein
   (E) vitamin D toxicity

4. An elderly man with a long smoking history is admitted to the hospital with complaints of weakness, fatigue, constipation, lethargy, and weight loss. Chest x-ray reveals a mass, which proves to be a squamous cell carcinoma. He also has high calcium and low phosphorus levels, which are most likely due to excess

   (A) endogenous $1,25(OH)_2D$
   (B) calcium-binding protein
   (C) parathyroid hormone (PTH)
   (D) calcitonin
   (E) parathyroid hormone–related peptide (PTHrP)

5. In clinic one afternoon a physician sees four patients with elevated PTH levels, but only one has hypercalcemia. Which patient is it most likely to be?

   (A) A 66-year-old man complaining of weakness, lethargy, and constipation; x-rays reveal osteoporosis and a kidney stone.
   (B) A 74-year-old woman who has a very limited diet and has been housebound because of a stroke. She complains of bone pain, and a bone biopsy reveals osteomalacia.
   (C) A 32-year-old man who has renal failure; he has not been treated with any medications.
   (D) A 27-year-old woman who is short, with a round face, and hand deformities. She is resistant to PTH and several other hormones.

Directions: The group of questions below consists of lettered choices followed by several numbered items. For each numbered item, select the appropriate lettered option with which it is most closely associated. Each lettered option may be used once, more than once, or not at all.

Questions 6–9

For each clinical scenario presented below, select the most likely laboratory test results. Assume that the albumin level is normal.

   (A) High calcium, high phosphorus (PO_4), low parathyroid hormone (PTH), high $1,25(OH)_2$ vitamin D
   (B) High calcium, low PO_4, high PTH, high $1,25(OH)_2D$
   (C) High calciuim, low PO_4, low PTH, normal $1,25(OH)_2D$
   (D) Low calcium, high PO_4, high PTH, low $1,25(OH)_2D$
   (E) Low calcium, high PO_4, low PTH, low $1,25(OH)_2D$
   (F) Low calcium, low PO_4, high PTH, low $1,25(OH)_2D$

6. An 82-year-old malnourished woman from a nursing home has bone pain and tenderness, muscle weakness, and tingling around her mouth. An iliac crest biopsy shows poorly mineralized osteoid (bone matrix).

7. A 45-year-old man recently underwent a near-total thyroidectomy for thyroid cancer. He complains of muscle spasms. His Chvostek's and Trousseau's signs are positive.

8. A lethargic 65-year-old woman has complained of fatigue, depression, weakness, and constipation for 15 years. She has been taking several over-the-counter vitamin preparations for years. Abdominal x-rays reveal three kidney stones, and her urine calcium is high. Her PTH level is low.

9. A 3-year-old girl has been confined indoors and is poorly nourished. She is weak, her legs are bowed, and during the physical examination, she cries when palpation exerts pressure on her bones.

▌ANSWERS AND EXPLANATIONS

1. The answer is C. Ms R. is a thin, postmenopausal woman with a family history of osteoporosis. She gets little exercise because of her asthma, and her dietary intake of calcium is low. Her bone mass is also low. Whether estrogen therapy significantly increases breast cancer risk is still unclear, but Ms. R. refuses estrogen. Thyroxine stimulates bone turnover, and excess thyroxine increases bone loss in postmenopausal women. Calcium suppresses PTH and suppresses bone resorption. Ms. R. should increase her calcium intake. Bisphosphonates and calcitonin suppress osteoclast activity and decrease bone resorption, which will diminish additional bone loss. Fluoride stimulates osteoblast activity.

2. The answer is C. Glucocorticoid therapy causes bone loss by inhibiting bone formation.

3. The answer is D. Mr. T. has familial hypocalciuric hypercalcemia (FHH), an autosomal dominant disorder caused by a defective calcium sensor protein. His parathyroid cells do not decrease PTH secretion until serum calcium is higher than normal. Most patients with FHH are asymptomatic except for newborns homozygous for the abnormal calcium sensor protein gene.

4. The answer is E. This man is most likely to have humoral hypercalcemia of malignancy due to tumor production of PTHrP. It is rare for a solid tissue malignancy to produce enough PTH to cause hypercalcemia. The diagnosis could be confirmed by measuring PTH, which should be suppressed by the hypercalcemia. (Measurement of PTHrP is more difficult and is less widely available.) Excess endogenous 1,25(OH)$_2$D is produced primarily by lymphomas and granulomatous diseases. Calcitonin is produced by medullary carcinoma of the thyroid, but patients with this malignancy are not hypercalcemic, perhaps due to downregulation of receptors in the face of such high concentrations of calcitonin.

5. The answer is A. The 66-year-old patient has classic symptoms and signs of longstanding primary hyperparathyroidism. The 74-year-old woman has osteomalacia. This most likely is due to vitamin D deficiency, which results in hypocalcemia and a compensatory increase in PTH. The 32-year-old man has renal failure resulting in hyperphosphatemia and low activation of vitamin 25(OH)D. These result in hypocalcemia, which elicits an increase in PTH. The 27-year-old woman has pseudohypoparathyroidism (the classic form also known as Albright's hereditary osteodystrophy). This patient is resistant to PTH because a defective G protein results in decreased formation of cAMP after PTH interacts with its receptor. Resistance to several hormones may be present if the defect in G protein is widespread.

6–9. The answers are: 6-F, 7-E, 8-A, 9-F. The 82-year-old woman has classic signs of hypocalcemia and osteomalacia due to 1,25(OH)$_2$D deficiency. She has been confined indoors, and her diet is poor. Decreased calcium absorption results in high PTH. Phosphorus is low, partly due to low absorption and partly due to the action of PTH on the kidneys.

The 45-year-old man has symptoms and signs of hypocalcemia, which are most likely due to inadvertent destruction of the parathyroid glands during thyroid surgery. Low PTH results in hypocalcemia and hyperphosphatemia. The hypocalcemia is partly due to decreased bone resorption and decreased renal calcium retention and partly due to low 1α-hydroxylase activity and decreased activation of vitamin D in the absence of normal PTH.

The clinical picture of the 65-year-old woman is most likely the result of vitamin D excess due to years of taking multiple vitamin pills containing vitamin D. Both phosphorus and calcium would be high, and PTH would be suppressed by the hypercalcemia. The long history of symptoms makes hypercalcemia due to malignancy unlikely.

The 3-year-old girl represents the classic picture of rickets due to vitamin D deficiency in childhood.

■ REFERENCES

Adami S, Rossini M: Hypercalcemia of malignancy: pathophysiology and treatment. *Bone* 13:S51–S55, 1992.

Audran M, Kumar R: The physiology and pathophysiology of vitamin D. *Mayo Clin Proc* 60:851–866, 1985.

Consensus Development Conference Panel: Diagnosis and management of asymptomatic primary hyperparathyroidism: consensus development conference statement. *Ann Intern Med* 114:593–597, 1991.

Favus MJ (ed): *Primer on the Metabolic Bone Diseases and Disorders of Mineral Metabolism*, 3rd ed. Philadelphia, PA: Lippincott-Raven, 1996.

Fuleihan GE-H: Tissue-specific estrogens—the promise for the future. *N Engl J Med* 337(23):1686–1687, 1997.

Heaney RP: Nutritional factors in osteoporosis. *Ann Rev Nutr* 13:287–316, 1993.

Holick MF: Vitamin D—new horizons for the 21st century. *Am J Clin Nutr* 60:619–630, 1994.

Levine MA, Downs RW, Moses AM, et al: Resistance to multiple hormones in patients with pseudohypoparathyroidism. *Am J Med* 74:545–556, 1983.

Pearce SHS, Brown EM: Calcium-sensing receptor mutations: insights into a structurally and functionally novel receptor. *J Clin Endocrinol Metab* 81:1309–1311, 1996.

Riggs BL, Melton LJ: Involutional osteoporosis. *N Engl J Med* 314:1676–1686, 1986.

Silverberg SJ, Bilezikian JP: Evaluation and management of primary hyperparathyroidism. *J Clin Endocrinol Metab* 81:2046–2040, 1996.

Chapter 8

PANCREATIC ISLET HORMONES, DIABETES MELLITUS, AND HYPOGLYCEMIA

Elizabeth R. Seaquist, M.D.

▌CHAPTER OUTLINE

Case Study:
Introduction

Mary Anderson is a 21-year-old college student who presented to the College Health Service because of frequent urination during the last week. She had been drinking more fluids and feeling hungrier than usual. Despite her good appetite, she had lost approximately 10 lbs this semester. She had always been healthy and denied taking any medication. Her grandmother recently was told she had diabetes.

On physical examination, she appeared well. Her height was 5'5", and weight was 120 lbs. Her blood pressure was 110/75 mm Hg, her pulse was 76 beats/min, and neither changed when she moved from a supine to standing position. Her general examination was unremarkable.

Laboratory data revealed the following: glucose, 320 mg/dL (normal: 70–110 mg/dL); sodium, 135 mEq/L (normal); potassium, 3.9 mEq/L (normal); bicarbonate, 22 mEq/L (normal: 23–29 mEq/L); creatinine, 0.8 mg/dL (normal); and urinalysis, 4+ glucose (normal: 0 glucose). Blood for an insulin level was sent to an outside laboratory. The level was less than 2 μU/mL (low).

▌INTRODUCTION

REGULATION OF BLOOD GLUCOSE CONCENTRATION

Normal blood glucose concentrations are maintained by a balance between glucose coming into and exiting the blood space. Hormones from the pancreatic islets are of primary importance in maintaining this balance (Figure 8-1).

FIGURE 8-1
REGULATION OF BLOOD GLU-COSE CONCENTRATION.

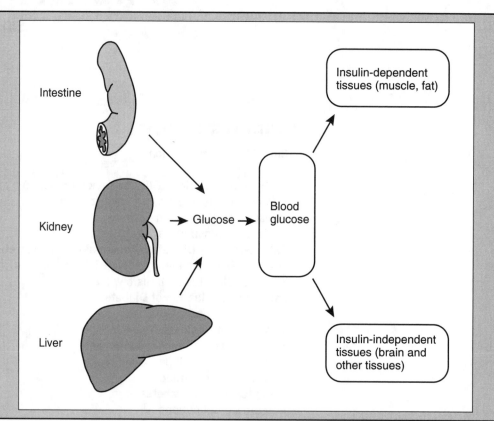

PANCREATIC ISLET STRUCTURE AND HORMONES

The endocrine pancreas consists of the islets that are dispersed throughout the exocrine pancreas. Four different hormonal products are secreted from four different cell types in the islet, as shown in Figure 8-2.

FIGURE 8-2
STRUCTURE OF THE PANCRE-ATIC ISLET.

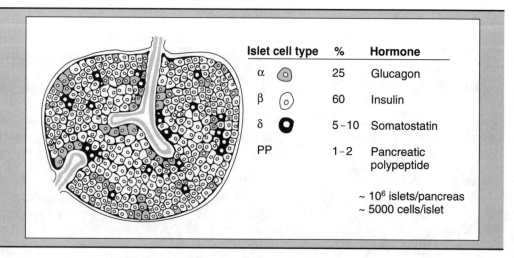

Islet cell type		%	Hormone
α		25	Glucagon
β		60	Insulin
δ		5–10	Somatostatin
PP		1–2	Pancreatic polypeptide

~ 10^6 islets/pancreas
~ 5000 cells/islet

Insulin is generated from its precursor proinsulin. In the secretory granule, proinsulin is cleaved into the 51–amino acid insulin peptide and the 31–amino acid C-peptide (for connecting peptide). They are cosecreted in an equimolar ratio. C-peptide can be used as an indicator of endogenous insulin secretion (Figure 8-3).

Major Islet Cell Hormones
Insulin
Glucagon
Somatostatin

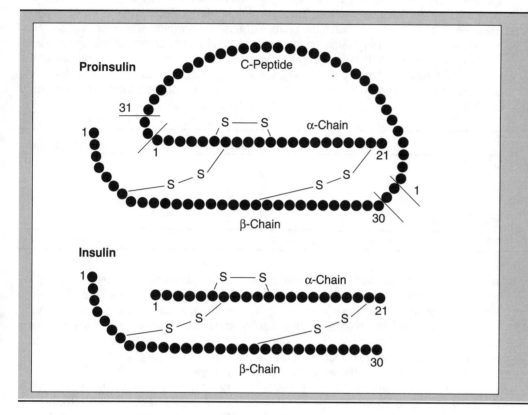

FIGURE 8-3
STRUCTURE OF PROINSULIN AND INSULIN. Proinsulin is cleaved into insulin and C-peptide in the secretory granule. Insulin is composed of α- and β-chains that are joined by two sulfhydryl bridges. Each *dot* represents an amino acid. *Slashes* indicate points of cleavage. *Numbers* refer to the respective position of the amino acid on the α- and β-chains and C-peptide. The final α- and β-chains contain 21 and 30 amino acids.

The regulation of islet hormone secretion is complex. Because of the order in which islet cells are perfused, the upstream hormone serves to modulate the function of the downstream cell. Perfusion goes from the core to the mantle of the islet such that the beta cell has a paracrine effect on the alpha and the delta cells, and the alpha cell has a paracrine effect on the delta cell.

Pancreatic islets are richly innervated. Parasympathetic nerves travel via the vagus nerve and may play a role in the cephalic phase of insulin release that occurs at the sight and smell of food. The sympathetic nerves have a role in the acute response to stress in which insulin secretion is inhibited and glucagon secretion is stimulated. In addition, many neuropeptides, including vasoactive intestinal peptide (VIP), cholecystokinin (CCK), galanin, and neuropeptide Y are found within islet nerve terminals (Table 8-1).

INSULIN SECRETION (BETA CELL)		GLUCAGON SECRETION (ALPHA CELL)	
Stimulators	**Inhibitors**	**Stimulators**	**Inhibitors**
Glucose	Somatostatin	Arginine	Somatostatin
Arginine	Epinephrine	Hypoglycemia	Glucose
Leucine			Insulin
Secretin and other intestinal hormones			
Acetylcholine			
Glucagon			

Table 8-1
Modulators of Insulin and Glucagon Secretion

INSULIN AND GLUCAGON ACTIONS

Insulin and glucagon oppose each other in regulating glucose metabolism (Table 8-2). Insulin acts to move glucose into insulin-sensitive tissues, such as muscle and fat, and enhances the storage of fuels. Insulin promotes the storage of glucose as glycogen by increasing the rate of glycogen formation and decreasing the rate of glycogenolysis in both the liver and skeletal muscle. Through its inhibitory effects on both lipolysis and proteolysis, insulin also promotes the storage of fats and proteins. Glucagon opposes all of these actions of insulin. Glucagon increases blood glucose concentrations by increasing gluconeogenesis and by increasing glycogenolysis in both the liver and skeletal muscle. By promoting both lipolysis and proteolysis, glucagon also increases the delivery of glucose precursors to the gluconeogenic pathway. Somatostatin inhibits the secretion of both insulin and glucagon and reduces the effects of these hormones.

Table 8-2
Metabolic Actions of Insulin and Glucagon

	INSULIN	**GLUCAGON**
Lipolysis	↓	↑
Ketogenesis	↓	↑
Gluconeogenesis	↓	↑
Glycogenesis	↑	↓
Glycogenolysis	↓	↑
Glycemia	↓	↑

Note. ↑ = increased; ↓ = decreased.

Under healthy conditions, the pancreatic islet secretes a small amount of insulin throughout the day to maintain a normal plasma glucose concentration. This basal level of insulin secretion is particularly important in regulating the rates of gluconeogenesis and glycogenolysis in the liver and kidney. In response to eating, insulin secretion is increased to prevent excessive postprandial glucose excursions. The amount of insulin secreted by the endocrine pancreas to maintain normal glucose tolerance is tightly regulated by the arterial glucose concentration; thus, in healthy individuals, the range of glycemia is not large.

The actions of both insulin and glucagon on target cells are mediated by cell surface receptors that bind specifically to each hormone. The insulin receptor is a tetrameric structure consisting of two α-subunits (M_r = 135,000) and two β-subunits (M_r = 95,000) joined together by disulfide bonds. The α-subunits are extracellular in location and contain the insulin-binding site, which is rich in cysteine residues. The β-subunits span the plasma membrane and anchor the receptor to the cell. Single cysteine residues are believed to be important in the formation of the α_2-β_2 complex. The β-subunits contain specific tyrosine residues that are autophosphorylated by the receptor when insulin binds to the α-subunit. This autophosphorylation turns the receptor into a tyrosine kinase, which phosphorylates other cellular proteins, thereby mediating the effects of insulin on cellular metabolism (Figure 8-4).

The glucagon receptor is a G-protein–linked receptor. Like other receptors in this family, the glucagon receptor has seven transmembrane-spanning domains that couple glucagon binding to adenylate cyclase through G-protein effectors.

GLUCOSE TRANSPORTERS

Glucose movement from the blood into tissue requires the action of a glucose transporter (GLUT). GLUTs are membrane-associated glycoproteins with 12 transmembrane domains, a cytoplasmic NH_2 terminus and COOH terminus, and a large extracellular loop. Five glucose transporters have been identified (Table 8-3). Insulin regulates the action of GLUT-4. Following insulin binding to its receptor, GLUT-4 is translocated to the cell membrane to facilitate glucose transport.

Table 8-3
Location of Glucose Transporters

GLUCOSE TRANSPORTER	LOCATION
GLUT-1	Ubiquitous and also placenta
GLUT-2	Beta cell, liver, kidney, and intestine
GLUT-3	Ubiquitous
GLUT-4	Muscle and fat
GLUT-5	Jejunum

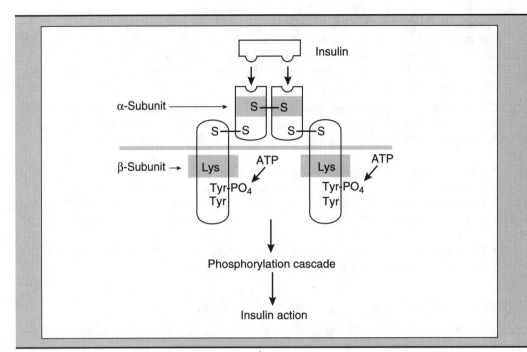

FIGURE 8-4
INSULIN INTERACTION WITH THE INSULIN RECEPTOR. Insulin interaction with its receptor results in phosphorylation of the receptor. This initiates a series of phosphorylations, which results in insulin action. Lys = lysine; Tyr = tyrosine; ATP = adenosine triphosphate; Tyr-PO_4 = tyrosine phosphate.

PATHOGENESIS OF DIABETES: ABNORMAL INSULIN SECRETION AND RESISTANCE

To maintain normal glucose tolerance, an individual must have both normal insulin secretion and normal sensitivity to insulin. Absolute insulin deficiency or abnormalities in both insulin secretion and insulin action can lead to diabetes. Diabetes can be either primary or secondary to other diseases such as exocrine pancreas disease, drugs, hormonal disorders such as acromegaly or glucagonoma, or genetic syndromes. Primary diabetes is classified as type 1 or type 2 diabetes mellitus, depending upon the pathogenesis.

Diabetes mellitus is a disorder of glucose metabolism resulting in hyperglycemia as a result of absolute insulin deficiency or abnormalities in insulin secretion and insulin action.

TYPE 1 DIABETES MELLITUS (TYPE 1 DM)

This form of diabetes was formerly known as juvenile onset diabetes, ketosis-prone diabetes, or insulin-dependent diabetes mellitus (IDDM).

Pathophysiology. Type 1 DM is caused by an absolute deficiency of insulin. It occurs because of autoimmune destruction of the pancreatic beta cells. It is believed to arise in genetically susceptible individuals who are exposed to an environmental factor that initiates the autoimmune response. The nature of this environmental factor is unknown, but it is hypothesized to be a viral infection, an environmental toxin, or a dietary component. Once the triggering event occurs, beta-cell destruction ensues, and there is progressive loss of the beta cells over years. The rate at which this destruction occurs is variable, but beta-cell attrition is believed to be more rapid in persons who are diagnosed in childhood. Overt diabetes does not appear until approximately 90% of the beta cells are destroyed.

Autoimmune destruction of pancreatic beta cells sometimes can be detected in children by measurement of circulating islet-cell antibodies. Between 50%–85% of children with type 1 DM have antibodies to islet cells (ICA, islet-cell antibodies) present in their serum at the time of diagnosis, and some children also have antibodies to insulin. These antibodies are not directed against the antigen that incites the autoimmune process but are antibodies generated in response to the destruction of the beta cell. Adults do not usually have detectable concentrations of these antibodies in the serum at the time of diagnosis, perhaps because the onset of the autoimmune destruction of their beta cells occurred years earlier and the rate of beta cell destruction was so slow that antibody production disappeared.

In contrast to ICA, antibodies to the enzyme glutamic acid decarboxylase (GAD) are thought to be important in inciting the autoimmune destruction of beta cells. Anti-GAD antibodies often are detected in children and adults at the time diabetes is diagnosed.

Major Classes of Diabetes
Primary diabetes
  Type 1 DM
  Type 2 DM
Secondary diabetes
  Due to pancreatic destruction
  Due to hormonal diseases
  Due to genetic syndromes

Signs of Hyperglycemia
Excessive urination (polyuria)
Excessive thirst (polydipsia)
Excessive eating (polyphagia)
Weight loss

Prevalence. In the United States, approximately 0.3% of the population develop type 1 DM by 20 years of age. The worldwide prevalence varies significantly. The highest prevalence is found in Finland, where two to three times as many people develop type 1 DM as in the United States. Japan has a rate that is about one-tenth that of the rate in the United States. Type 1 DM is rare in African Americans, Hispanics, and Native Americans.

Clinical Features. The peak age of onset of type 1 DM occurs between the ages of 10 and 16 and coincides with puberty. A second peak of onset occurs in the late 30s and early 40s. Patients with type 1 DM are usually lean. Presenting symptoms include:

- Excessive urination (*polyuria*), which occurs because of glucosuria.
- Excessive thirst (*polydipsia*), which occurs in response to dehydration.
- Excessive hunger (*polyphagia*), which occurs because of persistent loss of calories as a result of glucosuria and the possible effects of diabetes on satiety signals in the brain.
- Unexplained weight loss, which occurs because of the inability to eat enough calories to compensate for loss of glucose in the urine.

TYPE 2 DIABETES MELLITUS (TYPE 2 DM)

This form of diabetes was formerly known as adult onset diabetes or non–insulin-dependent diabetes (NIDDM).

Pathophysiology. Type 2 DM occurs because of abnormalities in *both* insulin secretion and insulin action, as shown in Figure 8-5. Which defect comes first has long been the subject of debate, but current research suggests that different populations may start with different primary defects. Some populations may have a primary defect in insulin

FIGURE 8-5
MULTIPLIER HYPOTHESIS. Both defective glucose-induced insulin secretion and defective tissue response to circulating insulin are required for type 2 diabetes mellitus (type 2 DM) to manifest itself. These two defects in concert lead to increased liver glucose production, decreased cellular glucose uptake, and hyperglycemia. Hyperglycemia then leads to glucose desensitization of the beta cell. This leads to further impairment of beta-cell function. Hyperglycemia is also associated with decreased glucose transport, basal hyperinsulinemia, decreased insulin binding, and postreceptor defects—all of which promote insulin resistance. Progressive impairment in insulin secretion and insulin sensitivity ultimately produce the syndrome of type 2 DM. (*Source:* Reprinted with permission from: Robertson RP: Defective insulin secretion in NIDDM: integral part of a multiplier hypothesis. *J Cell Biochem* 48: 228, 1992.)

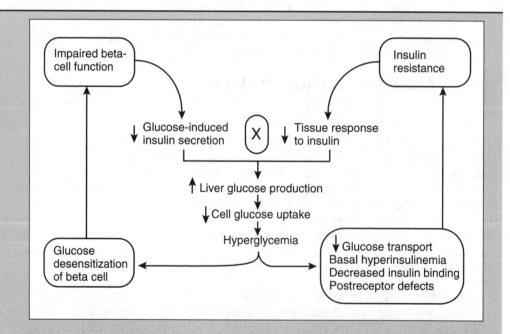

secretion, which can lead to hyperglycemia when coupled with insulin resistance. Others may have a primary defect in insulin resistance but will not develop hyperglycemia until their beta cells become unable to secrete enough insulin to maintain normal blood glucose concentrations. In either case, the result is that glucose production from the liver increases, and glucose uptake into tissues decreases. The hyperglycemia that ensues exacerbates the problem by leading to further impairment of beta-cell function and insulin action.

One variant of type 2 DM called maturity onset diabetes of the young (MODY) is due to a mutation in the enzyme glucokinase. This leads to abnormal glucose sensing by the beta cell and impaired insulin secretion. Insulin secretory abnormalities in type 2 DM are specific to glucose-stimulated insulin secretion. Insulin secretion in response to other stimuli is normal.

Type 2 DM has a strong genetic component, but its development is influenced by environmental factors such as obesity and lack of exercise, which increase insulin resistance. Insulin resistance also can arise because of a defect in one or more areas of insulin action.

Causes of insulin resistance include the following:

- *Prereceptor defects.* These are rare problems due to either an abnormal insulin molecule or antibodies to insulin that prevent it from binding to its receptor.
- *Receptor defects.* These rare abnormalities include syndromes of severe insulin resistance where the number of receptors is decreased, unusual autoimmune disorders in which antibodies directed against the insulin receptor prevent hormone binding and subsequent action, and mutations in the receptor that alter the affinity for insulin.
- *Postreceptor defects.* These abnormalities include mutations in the insulin receptor gene that prevent the receptor from effectively participating in insulin signal transduction or abnormalities of any of the intracellular messengers mediating the effects of insulin in the cell.

Causes of Insulin Resistance
Prereceptor defects
  Abnormal insulin
  Anti-insulin antibodies
Insulin receptor defects
  Decreased receptor number
  Abnormal receptors
  Antibodies to receptor
Postreceptor defects

Prevalence. In the United States, 6%–10% of the population develop type 2 DM. The prevalence rate is higher in African Americans, Hispanics, and Native Americans.

Clinical Features. Most patients with type 2 DM present over the age of 40 years. Some families have an unusual autosomal dominant form of type 2 DM called MODY that presents in childhood. Most patients with type 2 DM are obese and have a strong family history of the disease.

Approximately 50% of Americans with type 2 DM do not know they have the disease, either because their hyperglycemia is not severe enough to cause symptoms or because they do not recognize the symptoms of hyperglycemia. The diagnosis often is made in asymptomatic individuals when they are being evaluated for another problem. Patients with type 2 DM can present with the same symptoms as patients with type 1 DM (Table 8-4) if they are sufficiently hyperglycemic.

	TYPE 1 DM	TYPE 2 DM
Synonyms	IDDM, juvenile-onset diabetes	NIDDM, adult-onset diabetes
Age of onset	Usually < 30 years	Usually > 40 years
Ketosis	Common	Rare
Body weight	Nonobese	Obese (80%)
Prevalence	0.5%	6%–10%
Genetics	HLA-associated, 40%–50% concordance rate in twins	Non–HLA-associated, 95%–100% concordance rate in twins
Circulating islet cell antibodies	50%–85%	< 10%
Treatment with insulin	Necessary for survival	Not necessary for survival
Complications	Frequent	Frequent

Table 8-4
Comparison of Type 1 Diabetes Mellitus (Type 1 DM) and Type 2 Diabetes Mellitus (Type 2 DM)

■ LABORATORY EVALUATION OF DIABETES

The hallmark of diabetes is hyperglycemia. The Expert Committee on the Diagnosis and Classification of Diabetes Mellitus has formulated the diagnostic criteria for diabetes mellitus listed in Table 8-5. Symptomatic patients who present with blood glucose concentrations greater than 200 mg/dL or patients who display ketonuria and clearly have type 1 DM usually require no further evaluation to make the diagnosis of diabetes.

Table 8-5
Diagnostic Criteria for Diabetes

TEST	DIABETES MELLITUS	IMPAIRED GLUCOSE TOLERANCE
Fasting glucose (on two or more occasions)	≥ 126 mg/dL (7.0 mM)	110–125 mg/dL (6.1–6.9 mM)
OGTT (2-hr plasma glucose)	≥ 200 mg/dL (11.1 mM)	140–199 mg/dL (7.8–11.0 mM)

Note. OGTT = oral glucose tolerance test.

Asymptomatic patients with blood glucose concentrations greater than 200 mg/dL or symptomatic patients with random blood glucose concentrations less than 200 mg/dL (11.1 mM) should have their glucose concentrations measured in the fasting state. If the fasting plasma glucose concentration is greater than or equal to 126 mg/dL (7.0 mM) on two or more occasions, the diagnosis of diabetes is made. However, if they have fasting glucose concentrations less than 126 mg/dL, they may have diabetes, impaired glucose tolerance, or be normal. Such patients may not need to undergo additional diagnostic testing if the initial recommendations for weight loss and increased exercise would be the same whether or not they meet the official diagnostic criteria for diabetes. When an official diagnosis must be made, an oral glucose tolerance test should be performed in which 75 g of glucose are ingested at time zero and blood samples for measurement of plasma glucose are obtained at 2 hours. Table 8-5 lists the blood glucose responses to this test required for the designation of diabetes or impaired glucose tolerance. Individuals with impaired glucose tolerance do not always develop diabetes, but many do. This is more likely if they are obese.

In clinical practice, laboratory evaluation is often enhanced by the measurement of glycosylated hemoglobin. Glucose contains a carbonyl group that can react with a N-terminal amino group of a protein such as hemoglobin. This reaction is called glycation or glycosylation. The amount of hemoglobin glycosylated is directly related to the degree of hyperglycemia. Hemoglobin A_{1c} (HbA_{1c}) is the largest subfraction of hemoglobin, and glycosylation of this subfraction is measured most frequently. Since the life span of a red blood cell is approximately 90 days, the percentage of glycosylated hemoglobin (or glycosylated HbA_{1c}) provides information about the level of glycemia for the past 3 months. Glycosylated hemoglobin measurements are not part of the official diagnostic criteria for diabetes, but these values correlate well with fasting glucose values, and a high glycosylated hemoglobin level is used as a marker for diabetes.

Case Study:
Continued

Mary Anderson presented at the college health service with classic symptoms of hyperglycemia. Her laboratory data confirmed that she was hyperglycemic without any other electrolyte abnormalities. Her blood insulin level was inappropriately low for her serum glucose, indicating an insulin-deficiency state. This, her young age, lean weight, and lack of a strong family history for type 2 DM all support the diagnosis of type 1 DM. Ms. Anderson was placed on insulin therapy and encouraged to receive ongoing care with her diabetes care team. For the next 2 years, she managed her diabetes very well.

■ TREATMENT OF DIABETES

The goal of diabetes therapy is twofold: (1) to correct the symptoms of diabetes, and (2) to normalize plasma glucose concentration as much as possible to prevent the long-term complications of diabetes. When designing a treatment program, it is useful to consider therapies that correct the underlying pathophysiologic defect that led to diabetes in the first place. Since type 1 DM develops because of insulin deficiency that results from beta-cell destruction, the appropriate therapy for type 1 DM patients is insulin replacement.

Patients with type 2 DM have defects both in insulin secretion and insulin action. Therapy for these individuals should be directed to overcome these metabolic abnormalities. The specific strategies used to meet the goals of therapy depend on the type of diabetes present.

MANAGEMENT OF TYPE 1 DM

Type 1 DM requires that patients take insulin to sustain life. Patients with this disorder have an absolute insulin deficiency, and therapies are designed to replace insulin in as physiologic a way as possible. To replicate the normal pattern of insulin secretion in a person with type 1 DM, insulin must be present throughout the day at a level sufficient to maintain normal glycemia and must be increased after meals to prevent hyperglycemia. Ideally, the person administering exogenous insulin should know the insulin dose that maintains normal plasma glucose concentrations under a variety of circumstances. Unfortunately, determining the correct dose of insulin necessary to meet the metabolic needs of the moment and estimating the actual pharmacokinetics of the available insulin preparations are very difficult. Many patients with type 1 DM find it impossible to achieve consistent normoglycemia.

The insulin preparations commonly used for the treatment of diabetes include the short-acting lispro and regular insulins and the intermediate-acting neutral protamine Hagedorn (NPH), Lente, and Ultralente insulins. As shown in Table 8-6, all of these insulins except lispro have a lag time between the time of injection and the time at which they begin to affect blood glucose concentrations. They have different times of peak effect and predicted duration of action. Depending on the schedule and preferences of a given patient, these insulins can be used alone or in combination, as shown in Figure 8-6.

Table 8-6
Pharmacokinetics of Insulin Action

INSULIN	ONSET OF ACTION (hr)	PEAK ACTION (hr)	AVERAGE DURATION OF ACTION (hr)	MAXIMUM DURATION (hr)
Regular	0.5–1.0	2–3	3–6	4–8
Lispro	Immediate	1–2	2–4	4
NPH	2–4	4–10	10–16	14–18
Lente	3–4	4–12	12–18	16–20
Ultralente	6–10	None	18–20	18–24

Note. NPH = neutral protamine Hagedorn; hr = hours after insulin injection.

In designing treatment strategies for patients with type 1 DM, it is essential to remember that each blood glucose concentration is the result of three variables: the food eaten and absorbed, the exercise performed (exercise increases sensitivity to insulin), and the insulin taken in the hours before measurement. To achieve normoglycemia in type 1 DM, a schedule with consistent times for insulin injection, meals, and exercise, in which the carbohydrate content of the meals and duration and intensity of exercise also remain stable, is recommended. If one of these three variables changes, the other two must be adjusted if normoglycemia is to be maintained.

MANAGEMENT OF TYPE 2 DM

Type 2 DM results from defects in both insulin secretion and insulin action. Therefore, treatments are designed both to improve insulin secretion and to overcome insulin resistance. Most clinicians follow a stepped approach to treating type 2 DM. Diet and exercise are generally the first line of therapy used unless patients are very symptomatic or hyperglycemic. If the patient is obese, as most persons with type 2 DM are, the primary goal of diet therapy should be calorie reduction to achieve weight loss. Weight loss decreases insulin resistance.

If adequate glycemic control cannot be obtained through changes in diet and exercise alone, pharmacologic therapy is added. Blood glucose lowering drugs act by increasing insulin secretion, lowering hepatic glucose output, slowing the rate of starch digestion or by increasing the efficiency of glucose uptake by muscle (decreasing insulin resistance). Oral hypoglycemic agents usually are tried first, but insulin also can be given.

FIGURE 8-6
INSULIN DOSING REGIMEN. Three insulin dosing regimens are shown. The *top panel* depicts the expected insulin effect derived from a twice daily injection schedule, the *middle panel* depicts a schedule with three injections each day, and the *bottom panel* reflects a more vigorous four-injection regimen. The short-acting insulin R is used to prevent postprandial hyperglycemia, and the intermediate-acting insulin (neutral protamaine Hagedorn [NPH] or Ultralente [UL]) provides more basal coverage. *Shaded areas* indicate action times of regular insulin. R = regular; NPH/R = a mixture of NPH and regular insulin.

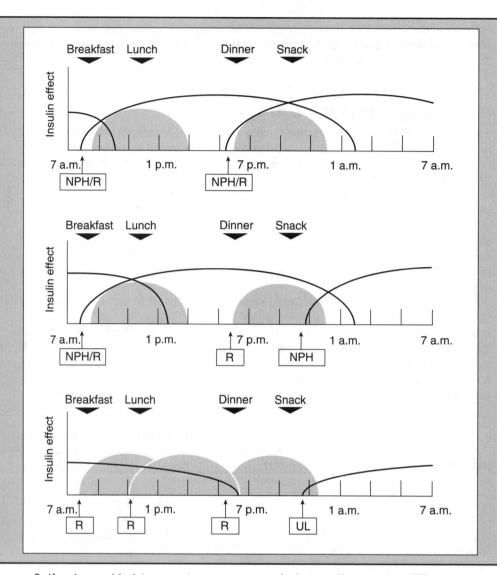

Locations for Control of Hyperglycemia
Control glucose entry from intestine
Control liver glucose output
Control muscle glucose uptake
Augment pancreatic insulin secretion

Sulfonylureas bind to receptors on pancreatic beta cells, causing ATP-dependent potassium channels to close and calcium channels to open. Intracellular calcium increases and glucose-induced insulin secretion increases. Biguanides reduce liver glucose production; the mechanism is uncertain. Starch blockers inhibit α-glucosidase and sucrase, which are intestinal enzymes that digest starch and sucrose (table sugar). Therefore, glucose is absorbed more slowly. Thiazolidenediones increase cell responsiveness to insulin by binding to nuclear receptors that regulate transcription of insulin-responsive genes. The actions of these drugs, their expected effects on blood glucose, and their side effects are shown in Table 8-7. Rapaglinide is a new short-acting stimulator of insulin secretion that restores postmeal glucose concentrations toward normal when given with meals. Several other new classes of hypoglycemic agents are being investigated.

Over the course of time, most patients with type 2 DM find that the original oral medication used to treat their diabetes is no longer enough. To prevent hyperglycemia, oral medications with different mechanisms of action can be combined, or insulin can be added. Eventually it may be necessary to give combinations of insulins or to give insulin several times daily. Patients with type 2 DM do not require insulin to maintain life, but insulin therapy may be necessary to control hyperglycemia.

Case Study:
Continued

Two years after her diagnosis of diabetes, Mary Anderson developed a severe gastroenteritis that resulted in nausea and vomiting. She was unable to eat, and her fluid intake also was decreased. She reduced her insulin doses substantially because she thought this would help her avoid hypoglycemia during her illness-imposed fast. However, her blood glucose became very high, and she presented to the emergency room feeling lightheaded and weak. In the emergency room, she was found to have orthostatic changes in her blood pressure and pulse, but the rest of her examination was normal. Laboratory data included a serum sodium of 129 mEq/L (normal: 138–147 mEq/L), potassium of 4.0 mEq/L (normal), bicarbonate of 15 mEq/L (normal: 23–29 mEq/L), glucose of 540 mg/dL (normal: 70–110 mg/dL), a blood urea nitrogen (BUN) of 30 mg/dL (normal: 10–20 mg/dL), a creatinine of 2.2 mg/dL (normal: 0.6–1.2 mg/dL), and a pH of 7.2 (normal: 7.4). Serum ketones were high, and ketonuria was present.

Case Study:
Continued

Table 8-7
Major Drugs for the Treatment of Type 2 DM

DRUGS	SITES OF ACTION	ACTIONS	EFFECTS ON GLYCEMIA FPG (mg/dL)	EFFECTS ON GLYCEMIA HbA$_{1c}$ (%)	SIDE EFFECTS
Sulfonylureas Glyburide Glipizide Glimepiride Tolazamide	Pancreas	Increase insulin secretion	↓	↓ 1.0–1.5	Hypoglycemia, weight gain
Biguanides Metformin	Liver	Decrease hepatic glucose production	↓ 50–60	↓ 1.0–1.5	Anorexia, diarrhea and lactic acidosis in susceptible individuals
Inhibitors of starch digestion Acarbose Miglitol	Intestine	Delay starch and sucrose digestion, delay glucose absorption	↓ PP–PG	↓ 0.5–1.0	Flatulence, diarrhea, abdominal pain
Thiazolidenediones Troglitazone	Muscle and liver	Increase muscle glucose uptake, decrease liver glucose output	↓ 20–50	↓ 0.6–1.0	Increased plasma volume, liver toxicity

Note. FPG = fasting plasma glucose; PP-PG = postprandial plasma glucose; HbA$_{1c}$ = hemoglobin A$_{1c}$; ↓ = decreased; ↑ = increased.

COMPLICATIONS OF DIABETES

ACUTE COMPLICATIONS

The acute complications of diabetes are due to the immediate effects of hyperglycemia on fluid and electrolyte balance. Because of the osmotic diuresis that ensues during hyperglycemia, dehydration occurs in patients who are unable to maintain sufficient water intake. Excessive and prolonged hyperglycemia can lead to life-threatening illness in patients with both type 1 DM and type 2 DM. However, the pathophysiology depends on the type of diabetes present.

Acute Complications of Diabetes
Dehydration
Diabetic ketoacidosis
Hyperosmolar coma

Type 1 DM. Hyperglycemia in a patient with type 1 DM indicates insulin deficiency and carries the risk of ketoacidosis. Diabetic ketoacidosis (DKA) is characterized by extreme hyperglycemia (generally > 300 mg/dL), an increased anion gap, metabolic acidosis (usually pH < 7.3), and an increase in the concentrations of total blood ketones (usually > 5 mM). In the setting of absolute insulin deficiency, glucagon action on adipose tissue and the liver are unopposed. Consequently, lipolysis is unrestrained, and free fatty acids accumulate in the blood. These free fatty acids are transported to the liver where they provide energy for gluconeogenesis. Excess free fatty acids, which cannot be completely oxidized, are converted by the liver to ketones: acetone, acetoacetate and β-hydroxybutyrate. These appear in the blood as organic acids and are excreted in the urine, producing ketonuria. Proteolysis is increased in the absence of insulin, and the amino acids provide substrate for gluconeogenesis. Hepatic glucose output increases, since glucagon stimulates both gluconeogenesis and glycogenolysis. Glucose utilization decreases, because without insulin glucose uptake by skeletal muscle is decreased. Persistent hyperglycemia causes an osmotic diuresis, which leads to extreme dehydration inadequate renal function, and growing acidosis. These relationships are outlined in Figure 8-7.

FIGURE 8-7
METABOLIC CONSEQUENCES OF SEVERE INSULIN DEFICIENCY (DIABETIC KETOACIDOSIS). In the setting of severe insulin deficiency the ratio of glucagon to insulin is shifted in favor of glucagon, resulting in lipolysis and ketogenesis. Lipolysis contributes fuel (free fatty acids), and increased proteolysis contributes amino acids to the liver for gluconeogenesis, which is stimulated by glucagon. Glucagon also stimulates glycogenolysis. Liver glucose production increases. Glucose uptake by muscle is markedly decreased. Acidosis and renal insufficiency occur in response to rising blood concentrations of ketones and glucose. If insulin deficiency is left untreated, diabetic keto-acidosis occurs.

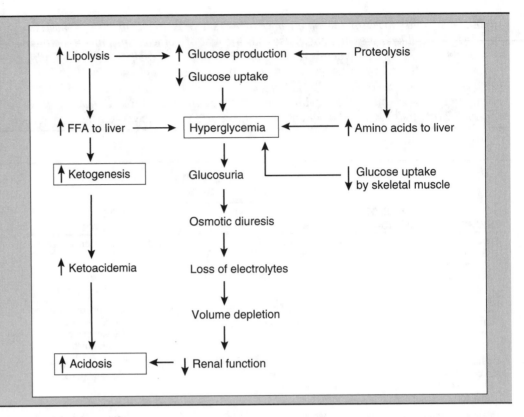

The presence of acetone may impart a fruity odor to patients' breath. In addition to hyperglycemia, glucosuria, ketonemia and ketonuria, patients present with low bicarbonate as a result of the acidosis and elevated blood urea nitrogen and creatinine as a result of dehydration. Total body potassium and phosphorus are depleted by gastrointestinal loss because DKA frequently is accompanied by nausea and vomiting and by diuresis and acidosis. However, serum levels may be normal or elevated because of shifts to the extracellular space in the presence of acidosis. Serum sodium may be low because plasma volume is expanded by the excess glucose.

Case Study:
Continued

Two years after her diagnosis, Ms. Anderson presented with diabetic ketoacidosis, which developed as a result of inadequate insulin dosing in the setting of an acute illness. This illustrates the importance of educating patients in how to adjust their diabetes therapy under a variety of circumstances. When she presented with her DKA, Ms. Anderson was significantly dehydrated, as demonstrated by her orthostatic hypotension and elevated BUN and creatinine levels. She was treated with intravenous fluids and insulin and was taught appropriate sick-day management techniques. She made a quick and complete recovery.

The treatment of DKA requires that insulin be administered to correct the insulin deficient state and to overcome the excess glucagon effect. Insulin decreases lipolysis, proteolysis, and ketone body formation and increases glucose uptake into fat and muscle. The dehydration and electrolyte abnormalities associated with DKA must be corrected by the administration of intravenous fluids. It is essential to determine and treat whatever caused the severe metabolic decompensation. Illness, with its attendant rise in the insulin-opposing hormones cortisol and epinephrine, is a common cause of DKA. Undetected myocardial ischemia, pregnancy, or poor compliance with the diabetes care regimen also may be responsible.

Type 2 DM. Hyperglycemia in a patient with type 2 DM can lead to hyperosmolar coma. Insulin deficiency is not absolute, so significant ketosis and severe acidosis (DKA) usually do not occur. However, these patients can develop hyperglycemia and dehydration that are much more severe than that seen in patients with DKA. Hyperosmolar coma is characterized by an increase in blood glucose to greater than 600 mg/dL, profound dehydration due to the hyperglycemia, and increased serum osmolality to greater than 320 mOsm/kg. Bicarbonate remains greater than 15 mEq/L (normal: 23–29 mEq/L), pH remains greater than 7.3 (normal: 7.4), and severe ketosis is absent. This syndrome usually occurs in elderly patients and may be precipitated by illness or drugs. Therapy depends on detection and treatment of the underlying cause of the disorder, aggressive hydration, and replacement of electrolyte deficiencies. Hyperglycemia improves with hydration alone, since increased plasma volume increases renal blood flow and allows excess glucose to be excreted in the urine. However, insulin is usually included in the treatment program.

Case Study:
Continued

Fifteen years later, Ms. Anderson returned to her physician's office for help in managing her diabetes. During the previous week, she had experienced a severe hypoglycemic reaction while working at home alone in the afternoon. When her family came home for dinner, they found her unconscious on the floor. The paramedics were called and found her blood glucose to be 20 mg/dL (normal: 70–110 mg/dL). After receiving an intravenous injection of glucose, she regained consciousness. Although this was the first time she had ever needed the help of paramedics to treat an insulin reaction, she had had difficulty in detecting low blood sugars recently. On several occasions over the last few months she had not been aware that she was hypoglycemic until a family member noted that she was confused. With some difficulty, they were able to get her to drink a glass of juice and help her restore her blood sugar to normal. Ms. Anderson also said that she was often surprised to find her fasting blood sugars around 40 mg/dL because she had no symptoms of hypoglycemia.

On physical examination, her blood pressure was 150/95 mm Hg with a heart rate of 96 beats/min. Her funduscopic examination was significant for dot hemorrhages and hard exudates in both eyes. Her neurologic examination revealed absent deep tendon reflexes in her legs and markedly decreased sensation in a stocking distribution to mid calf bilaterally. Examination of her feet revealed normal pulses and mild edema. The rest of her examination was unremarkable.

Her laboratory data were significant for a glycosylated hemoglobin of 7.8% (normal: 4.5%–6.0%), a glucose level of 240 mg/dL (normal: 70–110 mg/dL), a creatinine level of 2.5 mg/dL (normal: 0.6–1.2 mg/dL), and 4 + protein on her urinalysis (normal: 0 protein).

CHRONIC COMPLICATIONS

Chronic complications of diabetes arise when tissues that are freely permeable to glucose are exposed to chronic hyperglycemia. These complications of diabetes mellitus can be categorized as microvascular or macrovascular complications, as shown in Figure 8-8.

All of these complications can occur in patients with both type 1 DM and type 2 DM, but all patients with diabetes do not develop complications. Other factors, such as

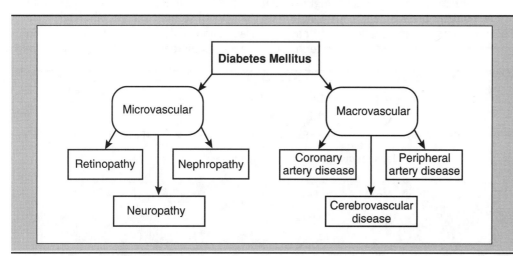

FIGURE 8-8
CHRONIC COMPLICATIONS OF DI-ABETES MELLITUS. The chronic complications of diabetes are classified according to the size of the blood vessel affected by the disease. In microvascular complications, small arterioles and capillaries are altered by hyperglycemia, whereas in macrovascular complications, the affected blood vessels are large arteries. Microvascular complications are unique to diabetes, but macrovascular complications occur in the nondiabetic population.

genetic susceptibility, also play a role. Nonetheless, reduction of hyperglycemia is effective in preventing the development and progression of the long-term complications of diabetes. In the Diabetes Control and Complications Trial, a prospective randomized study in which patients with type 1 DM were randomized to receive either standard therapy or intensive therapy for more than 5 years, the group that received intensive therapy significantly reduced their risk of developing all of the microvascular complications of diabetes.

Why chronic hyperglycemia results in long-term complications is uncertain. One hypothesis is that tissue proteins are nonenzymically *glycated* or *glycosylated* by glucose in direct proportion to the ambient glycemia (Figure 8-9). The products are ultimately converted into highly reactive carbonyl compounds and reactive oxidative species that can cause proteins to become abnormally cross-linked to each other. This alters both protein structure and function. Because these advanced glycation end products (AGEs) can be very long-lived, and because they can continue to react with proteins even after blood glucose concentrations are normalized, hyperglycemia may have lasting effects on the integrity of tissue proteins. This may be particularly true in the extracellular matrix where AGE-modified proteins alter both matrix–matrix and matrix–cell interactions. Increased cross-linking of lens proteins leads to lens opacities (cataracts). Intracellular proteins such as basic fibroblast growth factor can also be AGE-modified and lead to changes in cellular mitogenic activity. Specific receptors for AGEs have been identified on many cell types, including monocytes, macrophages, glomerular mesangium, and endothelium. Binding of AGEs to these receptors can result in altered rates of gene transcription, leading to increased cytokine production and generation of oxygen free radicals, which also are highly reactive.

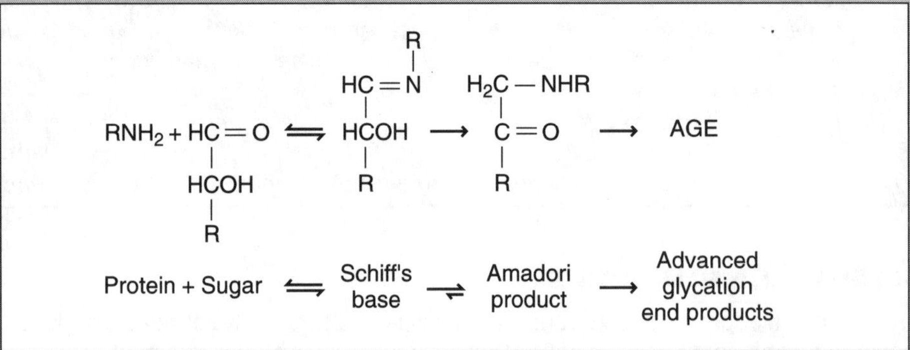

Chronic Complications of Diabetes

Microvascular complications (affect arterioles and capillaries)
Nephropathy
Neuropathy
Retinopathy
Macrovascular complications (affect larger vessels)
Myocardial infarctions
Strokes
Ischemic ulcers
Amputations

FIGURE 8-9
FORMATION OF ADVANCED GLYCATION END PRODUCTS (AGEs). Formation of AGEs begins with reversible interactions between a protein amino group (RNH$_2$) and a sugar molecule containing a reactive aldehyde group (HC = O) to form a glycated protein (Schiff's base). Further rearrangement of the glycated protein leads to the irreversible production of AGEs.

$$RNH_2 + HC=O \rightleftharpoons \underset{\overset{|}{HCOH}}{\overset{R}{|}} HCOH \longrightarrow \underset{\overset{|}{R}}{\overset{HC=N}{|}} HCOH \longrightarrow \underset{\overset{|}{R}}{\overset{H_2C-NHR}{|}} C=O \longrightarrow AGE$$

Protein + Sugar $\rightleftharpoons$ Schiff's base $\rightleftharpoons$ Amadori product $\longrightarrow$ Advanced glycation end products

Chronic hyperglycemia also increases flux through the polyol pathway. This results in increased accumulation of intracellular sorbitol, a sugar alcohol made from glucose by the enzyme aldose reductase (Figure 8-10). Sorbitol accumulation increases intracellular osmotic pressure and causes fluid retention. When sorbitol accumulation occurs in the lens, fluid accumulation can cause blurred vision. This resolves after a period of improved glucose control. Long-term consequences of increased flux through the polyol

FIGURE 8-10
FLUX THROUGH THE POLYOL PATHWAY. Aldose reductase converts D-glucose to sorbitol. The rate of this reaction is dependent on the cellular concentration of glucose. NAD = nicotinamide adenine dinucleotide; NADH = the reduced form of NAD; NADP = nicotinamide adenine dinucleotide phosphate; NADPH = the reduced form of NADP.

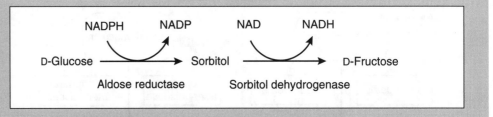

pathway could occur by two mechanisms. (1) Sorbitol accumulation impairs sodium (Na+)–potassium (K+) adenosine triphosphatase (Na+–K+-ATPase) activity, leading to decreased adenosine triphosphate (ATP) concentrations and cell death. (2) Increased sorbitol formation consumes NADPH (the reduced form of nicotinamide-adenine dinucleotide phosphate), which is used for synthesis of the vasodilator nitric oxide. Decreased nitric oxide could lead to reduced blood flow and ischemia in tissues, including nerves and the retina.

Abnormalities in vascular endothelium and platelets and defects in cells supporting capillaries, such as retinal pericytes or glomerular mesangial cells, have been implicated in the development of the complications of diabetes. An imbalance in insulin intracellular signaling also might contribute to the development of complications. Insulin responsive tissues may be more sensitive to the effects of insulin on cellular proliferation than on glucose transport. Consequently, the amount of insulin required to overcome the defect in glucose transport and correct hyperglycemia might also stimulate abnormal cell growth. Given the number of theories that have been proposed to explain the pathogenesis of diabetes complications, it is likely that more than one mechanism is involved.

Diabetic Nephropathy. Diabetic nephropathy occurs in 20%–40% of patients after 5–10 years of diabetes. Thickening of capillary basement membranes and the mesangium of the glomeruli results in glomerular sclerosis and renal insufficiency. The onset of nephropathy is heralded by the appearance of albumin in the urine. Because early treatment of diabetic nephropathy slows the rate of progression, all patients with diabetes should be screened for the presence of albumin in their urine. Screening is performed by measuring the amount of albumin in a timed collection of urine. Based on this screening test, patients can be categorized as having either normal renal function, microalbuminuria (30–300 mg albumin/d or 30–300 mg albumin/g creatinine), or proteinuria (> 300 mg albumin/d or > 300 mg albumin/g creatinine). Once the stage of proteinuria (macroalbuminuria) is reached, the glomerular filtration rate begins to fall. Patients with type 1 DM develop hypertension at this time. Progression of hypertension and azotemia results in end-stage renal disease after 15–25 years of diabetes in 20%–30% of patients. Progression of diabetic nephropathy is strongly associated with acceleration and earlier death from atherosclerosis. The mechanisms other than hypertension are not certain.

Pathogenesis of nephropathy is the same in patients with type 2 DM, but these patients often are older and the course is complicated by hypertension and atherosclerosis, which were already present when the diagnosis of diabetes was made.

Development and progression of microalbuminuria and proteinuria can be prevented or delayed by good control of glycemia and hypertension. Treatment with an angiotensin-converting enzyme inhibitor has been shown to slow the rate of progression toward end-stage renal disease.

Diabetic Neuropathy. The manifestations of diabetic neuropathy are protean. Patients can develop neurologic complications at any time after diagnosis, and more than one type of neuropathy may appear in the same patient. The number of diabetic patients who develop neuropathy is difficult to determine, since abnormalities on testing are not always associated with symptoms. However, most diabetic patients experience some neurologic complication at some point in their lives. The major types of neuropathy are listed in Table 8-8.

Diabetic Retinopathy. Some degree of retinopathy occurs in more than 90% of patients with diabetes, but vision-threatening complications occur in less than 30%. Patients usually have had diabetes for 5 years before the first signs of retinopathy become apparent, but new eye problems can develop at any time. Retinopathy occurs in predictable stages, as listed below.

Background or nonproliferative retinopathy
- Dot and blot hemorrhages as a result of the escape of erythrocytes from microaneurysms
- Hard exudates as a result of extravasation of serous fluid from capillaries into retina

Preproliferative retinopathy
• Cotton wool spots as a result of retina ischemia and infarction in the nerve layer

Proliferative retinopathy
  • Neovascularization. Fragile new vessels develop in response to ischemia

Table 8-8
Diabetic Neuropathies

NEUROPATHY	SYMPTOMS	PHYSICAL SIGNS	TREATMENT
Distal symmetric sensorimotor neuropathy	Paresthesia or pain in stocking/glove distribution	Decreased reflexes, decreased sensation, muscle wasting	Foot care education, pain management
Autonomic neuropathy Cardiac	Lightheadedness	Orthostatic hypotension and resting tachycardia	Fludrocortisone, compression stockings
Gastrointestinal	Early satiety, nausea, vomiting, constipation, diarrhea		Prokinetic agents such as metoclopramide and cisapride
Genitourinary	Impotence, retrograde ejaculation		Penile or urethral injections with papaverine, phentolamine, prostaglandin E_2 or vacuum device or implantable prothesis
Amyotrophy	Severe pain, weakness, weight loss	Muscle weakness, cachexia	Supportive care Self-limited
Mononeuritis multiplex	Weakness or loss of sensation in distribution of single nerve, often cranial nerves III–VI	Muscle weakness or decreased sensation in the distribution of a single nerve	Self-limited

Vision loss from diabetic retinopathy occurs because of hemorrhage of the fragile new blood vessels into the vitreal cavity. The accumulation of blood can obscure vision, but it is the subsequent fibroproliferative changes in the clot that result in retinal detachment and permanent vision loss. Early detection of preproliferative and proliferative retinopathy allows treatment with photocoagulation. This eliminates the neovascularization and decreases the stimulus to additional proliferation. Because patients are asymptomatic until serious vision loss occurs, they must be screened for the development of retinopathy by an ophthalmologist each year.

Macrovascular Complications. Patients with diabetes experience cardiovascular disease more frequently and at an earlier age than people without diabetes, and the outcome is more severe. All of the major blood vessels are affected, and atherosclerosis also extends to the vessels in the feet. Women with diabetes do not have the protection from the development of coronary heart disease before menopause that women without diabetes have. Diabetes synergizes with other risk factors for coronary heart disease. For example, both diabetes and smoking increase the risk for a myocardial infarction threefold, but the combination of diabetes and smoking increases the risk thirteenfold. A thrombembolic stroke is two to three times more likely to occur in patients with diabetes, the incidence of peripheral vascular disease is four times greater, gangrene is fifteen times more common, and the amputation rate is two to four times greater.

The reason for the increased severity of atherosclerosis is not known, but several abnormalities contributing to atherosclerosis and thrombosis have been implicated. These include endothelial dysfunction; increased fibrinogen; increased platelet aggregation; small dense lipoproteins, which are readily taken up into vessel walls; increased glycosylated and oxidized LDLs (low-density lipoproteins); and increased stiffness of blood vessels resulting from abnormal cross-linking of glycated proteins.

Impaired glucose tolerance and type 2 DM often develop in patients who already have the insulin resistance syndrome, sometimes called syndrome X or the deadly quartet: central obesity, hyperinsulinemia, hypertension, and dyslipidemia (hypertriglyceridemia and low high-density lipoprotein [HDL] cholesterol). The insulin resistance syndrome is strongly associated with the development of coronary heart disease.

Macrovascular disease is the most common cause of death in all patients with diabetes mellitus. For this reason, management of cardiovascular risk factors is of particular importance in the diabetic patient, and hypertension and hyperlipidemia warrant particularly aggressive treatment.

Some complications of diabetes can be attributed to the presence of both microvascular and macrovascular disease. Foot ulcers that fail to heal and ultimately lead to amputation are usually due to neuropathy and insufficient blood flow to the feet because of atherosclerosis. In patients with peripheral neuropathy, injury to the feet is common because they do not detect pain with foot trauma. These injuries are often left untreated because the patient is unaware of their presence. Infection sets in, and the wound increases in size. To heal such an injury, sufficient tissue oxygenation must be present. When atherosclerosis is present in the arteries of the affected leg, sufficient oxygen is not available, and the ulcer heals slowly, if at all.

Impotence is another complication that usually is due to a combination of microvascular and macrovascular disease. To achieve and sustain an erection, a man must have normal neural connections and sufficient delivery of arterial blood to the corpora cavernosa to develop tumescence. Men with diabetic neuropathy and diffuse atherosclerosis in the pelvic arteries can become impotent because of neurologic dysfunction and inadequate blood flow.

HYPOGLYCEMIA

Hypoglycemia refers to a lower-than-normal blood glucose level. Hypoglycemia is dangerous because glucose is the primary fuel of the brain. Symptoms of hypoglycemia usually begin when the plasma glucose concentration falls to 45–50 mg/dL (normal: 70–110 mg/dL) and can be divided into two categories:

1. Adrenergic symptoms are due to excessive secretion of epinephrine in response to hypoglycemia and consist of sweating, tremor, tachycardia, anxiety, and hunger.
2. Neuroglycopenic symptoms are due to dysfunction of the central nervous system (CNS) due to hypoglycemia and consist of dizziness, headache, clouding of vision, blunted mental activity, loss of fine motor skill, confusion, abnormal behavior, convulsions, and loss of consciousness.

Hypoglycemia occurs most frequently in patients with type 1 DM and is usually due to difficulty in matching exogenous insulin injections with anticipated blood glucose levels. Hypoglycemia is a particularly serious problem for patients attempting to normalize their blood glucose concentrations using intensive insulin regimens. In fact, the intensively treated group in the Diabetes Control and Complications Trial had a 2–3 times greater risk of developing hypoglycemia than the control group receiving standard treatment. The risk of hypoglycemia often limits how successfully blood glucose concentrations can be normalized in patients with diabetes.

Early in the course of type 1 DM, recovery from hypoglycemia is brought about by glucagon release from pancreatic islet alpha cells. Glucagon stimulates glycogenolysis in the liver, which causes hepatic release of glucose and restoration of normoglycemia. Epinephrine release from the adrenal medulla provides a secondary defense, because epinephrine is released if glucose drops further. Epinephrine also stimulates glycogenolysis. Cortisol and growth hormone are important in recovery from prolonged hypoglycemia, but they contribute little to restoring normoglycemia in the acute setting.

In patients with long-standing diabetes, glucagon responsiveness to hypoglycemia is lost, and epinephrine responsiveness is attenuated. In this situation, ingestion or injection of glucose is mandatory for recovery from hypoglycemia.

Hormones Counter-regulating Hypoglycemia
Glucagon
Epinephrine
Growth hormone
Cortisol

HYPOGLYCEMIC UNAWARENESS

Patients who have achieved near-normal blood glucose concentrations by intensive insulin therapy may no longer have warning symptoms of hypoglycemia that prompt them to eat when their blood glucose concentration is very low. They may even go directly into an altered mental state as their blood glucose falls, without any warning symptoms at all. This is known as "hypoglycemic unawareness." The cause is uncertain but may relate to alterations in the delivery of glucose to the brain in well-controlled diabetic patients. Hypoglycemic unawareness is different from loss of epinephrine-induced symptoms because of autonomic neuropathy. In patients with hypoglycemic unawareness, the symptomatic response to hypoglycemia can be restored if they allow their blood glucose concentrations to be somewhat higher for several weeks.

Hypoglycemic unawareness usually occurs in patients with type 1 DM who have had diabetes for a long time. They may have a mixture of hypoglycemic unawareness and defective epinephrine secretion. Hypoglycemic unawareness also can occur in patients with insulin-secreting tumors. In this case, the syndrome disappears if the tumor is removed.

HYPOGLYCEMIA UNRELATED TO DIABETES

Hypoglycemia also can occur in people who do not have diabetes. Determining whether the insulin concentration is high or low can help to diagnose the cause of hypoglycemia. High insulin concentrations occur because of excessive release of insulin from the pancreas or because of the surreptitious administration of exogenous insulin. Measurement of the serum C-peptide concentration differentiates between endogenous or exogenous hyperinsulinemia because C-peptide is cosecreted in equimolar amounts with endogenous insulin. When insulin secretion is excessive, C-peptide levels are elevated in proportion to the insulin concentration. In the presence of exogenous insulin, C-peptide concentrations are low because secretion of both C-peptide and endogenous insulin is suppressed. Causes of hypoglycemia associated with excessive insulin secretion include insulin-producing tumors and the use of drugs like sulfonylureas, pentamidine, quinine, or monoamine oxidase inhibitors, which stimulate insulin release. Patients with very rapid gastric emptying following gastric surgery may also develop hypoglycemia with high insulin levels. In these patients with alimentary hypoglycemia, the rapid absorption of food provides a strong stimulus for insulin secretion. Since insulin secretion lags behind absorption, hyperinsulinemia persists after the disappearance of nutrients from the gastrointestinal tract, and hypoglycemia occurs.

Hypoglycemia can also occur in the setting of low insulin concentrations. When gluconeogenesis is decreased, as occurs with alcohol excess, liver failure, malnutrition, or growth hormone or cortisol deficiency, hypoglycemia can occur with fasting. Large mesenchymal tumors that produce insulin-like growth factors also can lead to low insulin hypoglycemia.

Case Study:
Resolution

Fifteen years after her diagnosis of diabetes, Ms. Anderson presented with hypoglycemic unawareness. Her clinical course suggested that she no longer had hypoglycemia-induced glucagon or catecholamine secretion. She was instructed on how to avoid hypoglycemia by more consistent timing of her medications, snacks, and exercise and by adjusting her insulin doses, and family members were taught how to give glucagon in an emergency situation.

Ms. Anderson also displayed physical findings consistent with diabetic retinopathy and peripheral diabetic neuropathy. The presence of edema, proteinuria, and an elevated creatinine level indicated that she also had diabetic nephropathy. She was referred to an ophthalmologist for careful evaluation. She was given intensive instruction in appropriate foot care techniques and was given antihypertensive therapy with an ACE inhibitor, which has been shown to retard progression of diabetic nephropathy.

■ REVIEW QUESTIONS

Directions: For each of the following questions, choose the **one best** answer.

Questions 1 and 2

A 58-year-old man comes to the physician's office complaining of recent onset of fatigue, a 20-lb weight loss, and the need to urinate two or three times each night. He is 6′ tall and weighs 275 lbs. His blood pressure is 135/88 mm Hg and does not change with movement from a supine to upright position. He has no other abnormalities. Laboratory data reveal a fasting glucose of 270 mg/dL. Urinalysis reveals high urine glucose but no ketones.

1. What is the most likely cause of this man's symptoms?

    (A) Type 1 diabetes mellitus (type 1 DM)
    (B) Type 2 diabetes mellitus (type 2 DM)
    (C) Diabetes insipidus
    (D) Urinary tract infection

2. Further investigation of this patient would be most likely to reveal

    (A) increased insulin resistance
    (B) severe beta-cell depletion
    (C) evidence of other autoimmune disorders
    (D) propensity to develop ketoacidosis

3. A 45-year-old man has had type 2 diabetes mellitus for 5 years. He has been following a weight-reduction diet and has increased his exercise. He is interested in minimizing his risk of developing the long-term complications of diabetes. Which of the following is most likely to be the best long-term strategy to help him achieve his goal?

    (A) Monitoring his blood pressure annually and examining his fundi every 5 years.
    (B) Maintaining his blood glucose level as close to normal as possible
    (C) Avoiding all alcohol consumption
    (D) Exercising at least three times a week and examining his feet every six months
    (E) Increasing his rate of starch digestion and his fasting hepatic glucose output to avoid hypoglycemia

4. A 37-year-old man with a 22-year history of type 1 diabetes mellitus comes into the physician's office with his wife for marital counseling. The wife feels that her husband has had a personality change. If she offers him something to eat when she thinks he is having an insulin reaction, he becomes belligerent. This behavior is in marked contrast to his former even-tempered manner. He says that he used to become sweaty and shaky during insulin reactions, but during the last year he has had no symptoms when his blood sugar levels are low. What is the most likely cause of his mood swings and personality change?

    (A) After 22 years of diabetes, he is frustrated when others tell him what to do
    (B) He has increased cortisol and growth hormone secretion in response to hypoglycemia
    (C) He has lost his ability to secrete catecholamines in response to hypoglycemia
    (D) He has increased secretion of glucagon in response to hypoglycemia

Directions: The group of questions below consists of lettered choices followed by several numbered items. For each numbered item, select the appropriate lettered option with which it is most closely associated. Each lettered option may be used once, more than once, or not at all.

Questions 5–8

For each case history that follows, select the diagnosis that is most appropriate.

- **(A)** Type 1 diabetes mellitus (type 1 DM)
- **(B)** Type 2 diabetes mellitus (type 2 DM)
- **(C)** Hypoglycemic unrelated to diabetes
- **(D)** Hypoglycemic unawareness

5. A 30-year-old Native American man is found to have glucose in his urine during a physical examination. He had slightly high blood glucose concentrations 2 years ago but was never told that he had diabetes. He feels well. Both of his parents, his two older brothers, and several aunts and uncles have diabetes. All are taking pills to control their blood sugar. On physical examination, he weighs 280 lbs, and his height is 5′9″. His laboratory data include a fasting blood glucose concentration of 160 mg/dL (normal: 70–110 mg/dL), a glycosylated hemoglobin of 10.0% (normal: 4.5%–6.0%), and a urinalysis remarkable only for the presence of glucose.

6. A 25-year-old woman comes to the physician's office because of a 2-week history of polyuria and polydipsia. She reports feeling ravenously hungry and asks if she can finish her lunch while she talks to you. In the last month she has eaten more than usual but has lost 10 lbs. All of her family members are well. On physical examination, she is 5′4″ tall and weighs 120 lbs. Her blood glucose concentration was 280 mg/dL. Other laboratory data include a C-peptide concentration of 50 pg/mL (normal: 500–2500 pg/mL).

7. A 12-year-old boy is brought to the emergency room by his parents because he had become increasingly lethargic over the last 4 hours. He stayed home from school in the morning because of abdominal pain and lightheadedness. These symptoms persisted all day. His mother reports that he has been getting up twice each night to urinate for the last few days, and she thinks he has lost weight. On physical examination, his supine blood pressure is 100/60 mm Hg, and his supine heart rate is 90 beats/min. His upright blood pressure is 80/45 mm Hg, and his upright heart rate is 130 beats/min. His laboratory data include a blood glucose concentration of 450 mg/dL (normal fasting concentration: 70–110 mg/dL), an arterial pH of 7.1 (normal: 7.35–7.45), and a urinalysis remarkable for the presence of glucose and ketones.

8. A 65-year-old woman comes to the physician's office because she feels tired all the time. She attributes this to extra work at home caring for her father who was recently discharged from the hospital following amputation of his foot. On physical examination, she is 5′7″ and weighs 250 lbs. Laboratory data reveal a blood glucose concentration of 250 mg/dL (normal fasting concentration: 70–110 mg/dL), a glycosylated hemoglobin of 10.2% (normal: 4.2%–6.0%), and a C-peptide concentration of 2500 pg/mL (normal: 500–2500 pg/mL).

Questions 9–13

For each of the patients with diabetes mellitus described below, select the complication that is most likely to be present.

(A) Diabetic retinopathy
(B) Peripheral vascular disease
(C) Diabetic nephropathy
(D) Diabetic neuropathy

9. A 34-year-old woman who is a day-care worker has a 30-year history of type 1 diabetes mellitus. She comes into the clinic complaining of bloating after she eats and intermittent nausea and vomiting. She also feels lightheaded if she rises quickly after reading stories to her students on the floor. On physical examination, her supine blood pressure is 180/95 mm Hg with a pulse of 110 beats/min, and her upright blood pressure is 90/50 mm Hg with a pulse of 110 beats/min. Her neurologic examination demonstrates absent deep tendon reflexes and loss of light touch sensation in her feet. The remainder of her examination is unremarkable.

10. A 72-year-old retired electrician comes into the clinic complaining that his feet feel like someone is giving him electric shocks at night when he is trying to sleep. He has had type 2 diabetes for 7 years. His examination is significant for absent vibration and pinprick sensation in his feet and lower legs. His dorsalis pedis pulses are palpable.

11. A 23-year-old librarian who developed type 1 diabetes mellitus at age 11 comes to the physician's office for a routine visit. He has no complaints and reports that his blood glucose values measured at home range from 80–250 mg/dL. His blood pressure is 140/88 mm Hg. Examination of his fundi reveals several hard exudates, some arterioventricular nicking, and several microaneurysms, although his visual acuity is normal at 20/20. His urinalysis is unremarkable.

12. A 28-year-old medical student who developed type 1 diabetes mellitus at age 11 comes to the physician's office for a routine visit. She has no complaints and reports that her blood glucose values measured at home range from 80–250 mg/dL. Her blood pressure is 145/94 mm Hg. Her visual acuity is 20/20. Her 24-hour urinary albumin excretion rate is 300 mg/day.

13. A 58-year-old basketball coach with a 10-year history of type 2 diabetes presents because of a sore on his foot that developed 2 weeks ago. It is not painful, but his leg often aches by the end of basketball practice. The physician finds an ulcer on his second right toe that is 0.5 × 0.5 cm in size. His right foot is cooler than his left foot, and the pulses on the right are weaker than on the left. On neurologic examination, his deep tendon reflexes are present in all limbs, and his sensation to light touch appears normal.

■ ANSWERS AND EXPLANATIONS

1. The answer is B. The 58-year-old man described in the question is likely to have type 2 DM because he is an overweight adult with increased serum glucose in the absence of ketonuria. His age, size, and lack of ketonuria make type 1 DM unlikely. Diabetes insipidus results from an inadequate quantity or inadequate effect of antidiuretic hormone (see Chapter 3). It causes dehydration due to the inability to concentrate urine, but it does not cause glucosuria. A simple urinary tract infection may cause polyuria but should not cause weight loss or glucosuria.

2. The answer is A. Patients with type 2 diabetes mellitus (type 2 DM) have insulin resistance. Their beta-cell capacity for insulin secretion is sufficient to prevent keto-acidosis but is not sufficient to prevent hyperglycemia. Type 2 DM is not an autoimmune disorder and is not HLA-associated.

3. The answer is B. Normalizing glucose concentrations has been shown to slow the rate of development and perhaps prevent the microvascular complications of diabetes. Blood pressure control is also important in slowing the rate of development of retinopathy, nephropathy, and the macrovascular complications of diabetes. Annual monitoring of blood pressure may not be enough and fundus examinations should be done annually. Modest alcohol consumption is not necessarily contraindicated, but the calories and any accompanying carbohydrate must be taken into account. Regular exercise is excellent but may have to be modified if the patient develops significant retinopathy, neuropathy, or coronary or peripheral vascular disease. Patients who develop peripheral neuropathy or have impaired blood flow to their feet should examine their feet daily. Increasing his rate of starch digestion and his hepatic glucose output on an ongoing basis would increase his hyperglycemia. These measures are used if hypoglycemia already has occurred.

4. The answer is C. The patient is no longer able to recognize hypoglycemia before he develops neuroglycopenic symptoms because his ability to secrete catecholamines in response to hypoglycemia is gone or severely impaired. He also is unable to secrete glucagon in response to hypoglycemia. Increased cortisol and growth hormone are appropriate responses to hypoglycemia and would not cause his symptoms. Frustration would not account for his loss of adrenergic symptoms and signs in response to hypoglycemia.

5–8. The answers are: 5-B, 6-A, 7-A, 8-B. The 25-year-old Native American illustrates a classic presentation of type 2 DM, which is very prevalent among Native American populations. Patients with type 2 DM are often asymptomatic, and their diabetes is often discovered as part of another investigation. Obesity and a family history of type 2 DM are common in patients with type 2 DM.

The 25-year-old woman has classic symptoms of severe hyperglycemia. Low C-peptide indicates insulin deficiency consistent with type 1 DM. Weight loss, polyphagia, polyuria, and polydipsia all occur with hyperglycemia.

The 12-year-old boy has severe type 1 DM and is presenting with diabetic keto-acidosis. The presence of ketones indicates that he needs insulin. His orthostatic blood pressure changes and lightheadedness indicate that he has severe volume depletion.

High glucose in the face of considerable insulin secretion (as indicated by the high normal level of C-peptide in the 65-year-old woman) illustrates the insulin resistance seen with type 2 DM. Her obesity makes her insulin resistant. Hyperglycemia may present as fatigue.

9–13. The answers are: 9-D, 10-D, 11-A, 12-C, 13-B. The 34-year-old day-care worker has signs and symptoms of autonomic neuropathy (bloating, nausea, vomiting, orthostatic hypotension) and peripheral neuropathy (loss of deep tendon reflexes and loss of light touch sensation in her feet).

The 72-year-old retired electrician has symptoms (abnormal sensation, particularly at night) and signs (absent vibration and pinprick sensation in legs) of peripheral diabetic neuropathy.

The 23-year-old librarian has retinopathy. The findings on funduscopic examination are classic for background retinopathy.

The urinary albumin excretion rate of the 28-year-old medical student is elevated, indicating that she has signs of diabetic nephropathy. Her hypertension may also be due to the renal complications of diabetes.

The 58-year-old basketball coach has peripheral vascular disease as evidenced by exercise-induced leg pain (claudication) and decreased pulses in his left leg. His neurologic examination is normal, so he does not have clinical evidence of diabetic neuropathy.

■ REFERENCES

Atkinson MA, Maclaren NK: The pathogenesis of insulin-dependent diabetes mellitus. *N Engl J Med* 331(21):1428–1436, 1994.

Cryer PE: Hypoglycemia: the limiting factor in the management of IDDM. *Diabetes* 43(11):1378–1389, 1994.

Kahn CR: Insulin action, diabetogenes, and the cause of type II diabetes. *Diabetes* 43:1066–1084, 1994.

Nathan DM: Long-term complications of diabetes mellitus. *N Engl J Med* 328(23): 1676–1685, 1993.

Porte D Jr: Beta-cells in type II diabetes mellitus. *Diabetes* 40(2):166–180, 1991.

The Expert Committee on the Diagnosis and Classification of Diabetes Mellitus. Report of the expert committee on diagnosis and classification of diabetes mellitus. *Diabetes Care* 20(7):1183–1197, 1997.

Chapter 9

DISORDERS OF LIPID METABOLISM

Angeliki Georgopoulos, M.D.

▍CHAPTER OUTLINE

Case Study:
Introduction

A 47-year-old woman had a heart attack 6 months ago and is now returning to her physician's office for a follow-up visit. Her history revealed episodes of atypical chest pain approximately 2 months before her heart attack, but she has had no episodes since then. Her family history is positive for premature (before age 55 years) coronary artery disease. She was told recently that her father had elevated plasma cholesterol and that her paternal uncle had elevated triglycerides. She has no history of hypertension.

She has been feeling tired, and the cold weather has bothered her lately. She has no other health problems. She is still menstruating. She takes aspirin and nitroglycerin as needed. She has been exercising erratically for the past year. She works in a stressful job with frequent deadlines. She stopped smoking a year ago, and since the heart attack, she has been watching her fat and cholesterol intake. She drinks a glass of wine every night.

Physical examination revealed a 140-lb, 5' 7" woman, with a blood pressure of 130/82 mm Hg. Her heart rate and rhythm were normal. Her skin had bilateral xanthelasmas and no xanthomas. Examination of the neck showed normal carotid pulses and a smooth, enlarged thyroid gland. Her chest was clear, and she had no abnormal heart sounds or bruits. Her abdomen was normal. Her peripheral pulses were decreased on her right side. The results of her neurologic examination were normal except for slow reflexes.

▍LIPOPROTEINS

Classes of Lipoproteins
Chylomicrons
Very low-density lipoprotein (VLDL)
Intermediate-density lipoprotein (IDL)
Low-density lipoprotein (LDL)
High-density lipoprotein (HDL)

LIPOPROTEIN STRUCTURE

Cholesterol and triglycerides are useful lipids. Cholesterol is a component of cell membrane structure and a precursor of bile acid and steroid synthesis. Triglycerides are used for production and storage of energy. Since lipids are insoluble in water, they are carried in the plasma as lipid–protein structures called *lipoproteins*. Lipoproteins are classified and separated by their density or their electrophoretic mobility, which is determined by the ratio of lipid to protein (Figure 9-1).

FIGURE 9-1
COMPOSITION OF PLASMA LIPO-PROTEINS CLASSIFIED BY SIZE.
(*Source*: Adapted with permission from Bierman EL: Hyperlipoproteinemia. In *Current Concepts*. Kalamazoo, MI: Upjohn, 1984, p 6.)

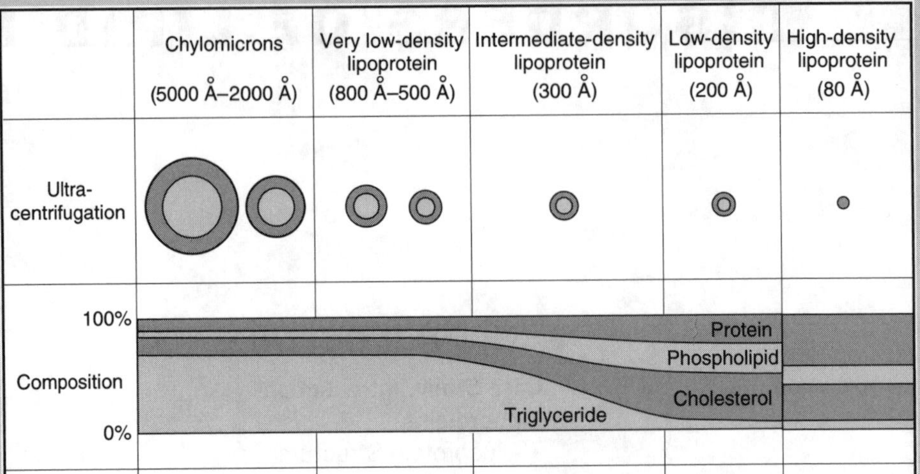

	Chylomicrons (5000 Å–2000 Å)	Very low-density lipoprotein (800 Å–500 Å)	Intermediate-density lipoprotein (300 Å)	Low-density lipoprotein (200 Å)	High-density lipoprotein (80 Å)
Ultra-centrifugation					
Composition	Triglyceride			Protein / Phospholipid / Cholesterol	
Apo-lipoprotein groups A	+				+
B	+	+	+	+	
C	+	+	±		+
E	+	+	+		±

Major Apolipoprotein Types and Subtypes
Apolipoprotein A (apo A-I, apo A-II, apo A-IV)
Apolipoprotein B (apo B-100, apo B-48)
Apolipoprotein C (apo C-I, apo C-II, apo C-III)
Apolipoprotein E (apo E-2, apo E-3, apo E-4)

Functions of Apolipoproteins
Solubilize lipids in plasma
Act as ligands for lipoprotein receptors (apo B and apo E)
Act as cofactors for enzymes (apo C-II and apo A-I)

The protein portion of a lipoprotein is called an apolipoprotein and is designated by a capital letter (apolipoprotein A = apo A). Each apolipoprotein category includes several protein molecules distinguished by roman numerals (e.g., apo A-I). Humans produce all of the apolipoprotein A, B, and C subtypes listed in the margin note. However, an individual's apo E isoform type is determined by two separate alleles (one from each parent). Homozygotes have only one isoform; heterozygotes have two. Apo E-3 and apo E-4 are the most common forms.

The composition of all lipoproteins is qualitatively similar but quantitatively different. All lipoproteins are spheres. They contain a core of nonpolar (totally insoluble) triglyceride and cholesterol esters. Their surface contains free cholesterol and the detergent-like phospholipids and apolipoproteins, which enable them to be soluble in plasma.

The various lipoproteins are distinguished by the proportions of their components (see Figure 9-1). Large, light lipoproteins like chylomicrons and very low-density lipoproteins (VLDLs) have cores that are rich in triglycerides. Small, denser lipoproteins such as low-density lipoproteins (LDLs) and high-density lipoproteins (HDLs), which contain more protein, have cores that contain mostly cholesterol esters. Chylomicron remnants and VLDL remnants, including intermediate-density lipoproteins (IDLs), are denser than chylomicrons and VLDLs but lighter than LDLs and HDLs. Remnants contain approximately equal proportions of cholesterol and triglycerides.

It is important to realize that the composition of circulating lipoprotein particles in the blood is not fixed; it changes through interactions with other lipoproteins, transfer proteins, and enzymes. There is heterogeneity in size and composition, even among lipoproteins classified in the same "family" of chylomicrons, VLDLs, remnants, IDLs, LDLs, and HDLs.

The major lipoprotein receptor that recognizes circulating lipoproteins and allows them to be removed from the circulation is the LDL receptor. This also is called the B/E receptor because it recognizes apo B and apo E. The hepatic LDL receptor is involved in lipoprotein clearance. A remnant receptor on liver cells also recognizes apo E.

Apolipoproteins E and B act as receptor ligands. Chylomicrons, VLDLs, remnants, and IDLs contain apo E and apo B. Apo E has a greater affinity for LDL receptors than apo B, so apo E mediates the cellular uptake of these lipoproteins. There is often more than one apo E per lipoprotein particle. LDL contains only apo B, so apo B is the LDL ligand for the LDL receptor. Ligand-binding by the liver receptors clears the lipoproteins from the circulation, but ligand-binding to cells in the blood vessel wall can result in foam cell formation, which initiates atherosclerosis.

Apo B–containing lipoproteins can be atherogenic (promote atherosclerosis). There is only one apo B per lipoprotein particle; therefore, the blood concentration of apo B reflects the number of potentially atherogenic particles in the circulation. Apo B is found in all lipoproteins except HDL. HDL, which contains large amounts of apo A-I, is considered antiatherogenic (prevents atherosclerosis).

Some apolipoproteins act as enzyme cofactors. Apolipoprotein C-II is a cofactor for the enzyme lipoprotein lipase (LpL), and apo A-I is a cofactor for the enzyme lecithin-cholesterol acyltransferase (LCAT).

LIPOPROTEIN METABOLIC PATHWAYS

Exogenous Pathway. The exogenous pathway involves metabolism of ingested fat (Figure 9-2). Dietary triglyceride is partially hydrolyzed in the intestine by pancreatic lipase before being absorbed. Triglycerides are reformed in intestinal cells and are incorporated into chylomicrons. Chylomicrons contain small amounts of dietary cholesterol, phospholipid, apo B-48 (one per particle), apo E, apo C-II, apo A-I, and apo A-IV.

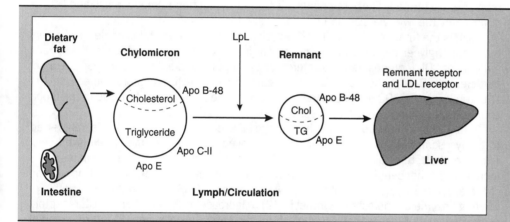

FIGURE 9-2
EXOGENOUS PATHWAY OF LIPOPROTEIN METABOLISM. LDL = low-density lipoprotein; Apo = apolipoprotein; LpL = lipoprotein lipase; Chol = cholesterol; TG = triglyceride.

Chylomicrons normally are present in the postprandial state but not in the fasting state. They are the biggest and lightest lipoprotein particles. Since they contain 80%–90% triglyceride, chylomicrons float to the top of a refrigerated tube of plasma.

Chylomicrons are transported to the circulation via the lymph. Circulating chylomicrons interact with plasma HDL and with LpL, an enzyme on the endothelial surface of blood vessel walls. In the presence of apo C-II, LpL hydrolyzes the triglyceride to release free fatty acids and produces remnant particles. The liberated free fatty acids are bound to albumin and used as fuel by peripheral tissues (muscle, adipose) and by the liver. In the liver, free fatty acids either are oxidized or used for synthesis of triglycerides. Free fatty acids provide energy (but not substrate) for gluconeogenesis.

Surface material liberated during chylomicron lipolysis (i.e., phospholipid, apolipoproteins other than apo B, free cholesterol) contributes to HDL formation. Chylomicron remnants are taken up by the liver via the apo E receptor and the apo B/E receptor. The ligand for both receptors is apo E.

Endogenous Pathway. In contrast to the exogenous pathway that operates only after fat ingestion, the endogenous pathway is always active (Figure 9-3). It involves VLDL synthesis in the endoplasmic reticulum (ER) of the liver. This synthesis is driven by fatty acids, which are used for triglyceride synthesis, and apo B-100. These VLDL particles are secreted by the liver and carry endogenous triglyceride and cholesterol to the circulation.

VLDL contains 50%–60% triglycerides and some cholesterol, apo B-100 (one per particle), apo C-II, and apo E (can be many per particle). The metabolic fate of VLDL in the circulation is similar to that of chylomicrons. VLDL interacts with HDL and is hydrolyzed by LpL. During hydrolysis, surface material is transferred to HDL, and free fatty acids are transferred to peripheral tissues and the liver. During hydrolysis, VLDL

Role of Lipases in Lipid Metabolism

Pancreatic lipase hydrolyzes dietary triglyceride in intestine.
Lipoprotein lipase hydrolyzes triglyceride in chylomicrons and VLDL in blood vessel walls.
Adipose tissue lipase hydrolyzes triglyceride in adipose tissue to release stored fat; it is inhibited by insulin and stimulated by epinephrine.

Chylomicrons deliver dietary fat to tissues for fuel. **Chylomicron remnants** deliver dietary cholesterol to the liver.

FIGURE 9-3
ENDOGENOUS PATHWAY OF LI-POPROTEIN METABOLISM. Chol = cholesterol; TG = triglyceride; VLDL = very low-density lipoprotein; LDL = low-density lipoprotein; IDL = intermediate-density lipoprotein; Apo = apolipoproteins; LpL = lipoprotein lipase.

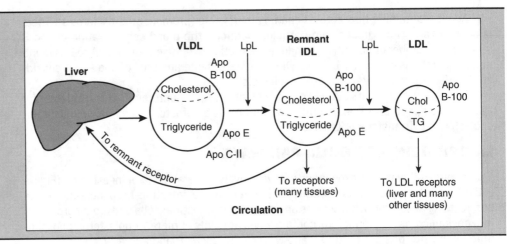

Circulating LDL delivers cholesterol to cells where it can be used for synthesis of plasma membranes, bile acid production (liver only), and steroid hormone synthesis (adrenals, ovaries, testes, skin).

remnants are formed. These remnants are further hydrolyzed to produce IDL and LDL or removed by the liver via LDL and remnant receptors.

LDL is the final product of VLDL lipolysis. The LDL core contains cholesterol esters but little triglyceride. LDL is the major carrier of cholesterol in the blood. Surface material of LDL includes free cholesterol, phospholipid, and only one apolipoprotein per particle: apo B-100. Apo B-100 is the ligand for liver LDL receptors. Defects in the structure of apo B-100 or the LDL receptor lead to the accumulation of LDL in the blood and increased blood cholesterol levels.

When LDL is taken up by cells through the LDL receptor (Figure 9-4), it is transferred to the lysosomes where free cholesterol is released and used for membrane synthesis. The free cholesterol also enters a regulatory pool. As the size of this regulatory pool increases, further cellular accumulation of free cholesterol is prevented by: (1) inhibition of the enzyme 3-hydroxy-3-methylglutaryl-coenzyme A (HMG-CoA) reductase, the rate-limiting enzyme of cholesterol synthesis, (2) a decrease in the number of LDL receptors on the cell membrane, so that less cholesterol can enter the cells, and (3) esterification of

FIGURE 9-4
LOW-DENSITY LIPOPROTEIN (LDL) RECEPTOR-MEDIATED PATHWAY OF REGULATION OF INTRACELLULAR CHOLESTEROL. LDL interacts with receptors, is taken up by the cell, and is degraded in lysosomes to amino acids and cholesterol. The accumulating cholesterol (1) suppresses additional cholesterol synthesis by feedback inhibition of 3-hydroxy-3 methylglutaryl coenzyme A (HMG-CoA) reductase, (2) is converted into cholesterol esters by acyl CoA:cholesterol acyltransferase (ACAT); and (3) down-regulates LDL receptors so less cholesterol is removed from plasma. (*Source:* Adapted with permission from Goldstein JL, Hobbs HH, Brown MS: Familial hypercholesterolemia. In *The Metabolic and Molecular Bases of Inherited Disease,* 7th ed. Edited by Scriver C, Beaudet A, Sly W, et al. New York, NY: McGraw-Hill, 1995, p 1981.)

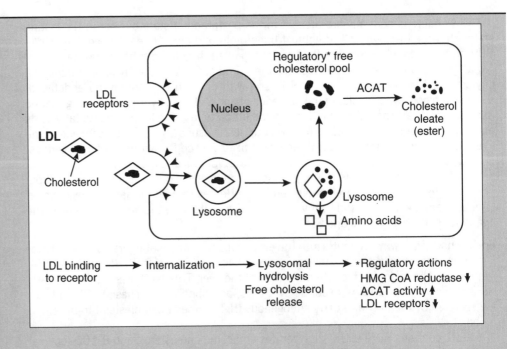

free cholesterol with fatty acids to cholesterol esters by the enzyme acyl-CoA:cholesterol acyltransferase (ACAT).

If the cellular uptake of LDL occurred only through this pathway, atherosclerosis would not develop. It is hypothesized that development of atherosclerosis involves lipoprotein uptake by unregulated pathways. Unregulated uptake of oxidized LDL by scavenger receptors is one example of this.

Remnant particles (both chylomicron and VLDL) also are potentially atherogenic. They can remain in the circulation for a long time if there are abnormalities in apo E or in the liver receptors. When this happens, the remnants become cholesterol enriched by ongoing transfer of cholesterol from HDL in exchange for triglycerides. This transfer is facilitated by cholesterol ester transfer protein (CETP). The cholesterol-rich remnants can be taken up by cells of the blood vessel wall and can cause atherosclerosis.

Reverse Cholesterol Pathway. In contrast to the exogenous and endogenous pathways that deliver cholesterol to the cells and can lead to the development of atherosclerosis, the reverse cholesterol pathway removes cholesterol from the cells and eventually from the body (Figure 9-5). This process involves nascent HDL, a discoidal form of HDL, which contains mostly apo A-I and phospholipids. Nascent HDL is secreted by the liver and intestine and is formed by the surface components released during lipolysis of triglyceride-rich lipoproteins. The apo A-I in nascent HDL binds to a cellular receptor and initiates the process of free cholesterol transfer from the cell.

LCAT is the enzyme in the circulation that esterifies lipoprotein free cholesterol to cholesterol esters by transferring fatty acid from phospholipid. **ACAT** is the enzyme that catalyzes the reaction of free cholesterol with fatty acid to form cholesterol esters in the cell.

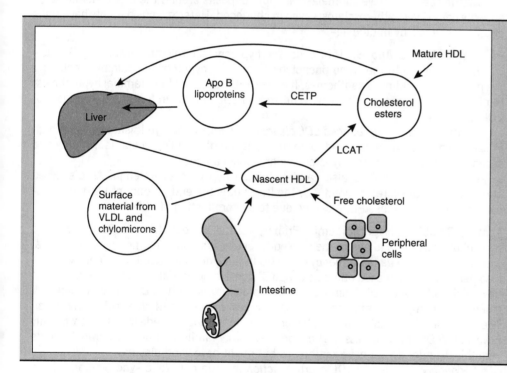

FIGURE 9-5
REVERSE CHOLESTEROL PATHWAY MEDIATED BY HDL. CETP = cholesterol ester transfer protein; LCAT = lecithin-cholesterol acyltransferase; HDL = high-density lipoprotein; VLDL = very low-density lipoprotein.

Free cholesterol, phospholipid, and apo A-I in nascent HDL form a good substrate for LCAT, the enzyme that esterifies the free cholesterol to cholesterol esters. Uptake and esterification of free cholesterol render the nascent HDL particle spherical.

The cholesterol esters in HDL are exchanged for triglyceride in apo B–containing lipoproteins (i.e., VLDL, IDL, LDL, chylomicron remnants), which are still in the circulation. As mentioned above, the transfer is facilitated by CETP. Both HDL and apo B–containing lipoproteins are taken up by specific liver receptors, so that the cholesterol can be delivered to the liver for disposal. Some of the cholesterol is used for synthesis of bile acids, which are excreted into the intestine and leave the body through the stool.

Cholesterol is removed from the body when it is delivered to the liver and excreted as bile acids.

■ HYPERLIPIDEMIA

Hyperlipidemia refers to elevated plasma levels of cholesterol, triglyceride, or both. Hyperlipidemias are due to increased lipoprotein production, decreased clearance of lipoproteins, or a combination of both. The defect can be primary (genetic), secondary (due to diseases or drugs), or a combination of the two. The major risks of untreated hyperlipidemia are atherosclerosis and pancreatitis.

TYPES OF HYPERLIPIDEMIA

Isolated Hypercholesterolemia. Since LDL cholesterol is the major carrier of cholesterol in the blood, isolated hypercholesterolemia usually is due to decreased clearance or overproduction of LDL.

Primary causes of decreased LDL clearance include genetic defects in LDL receptors and genetic defects in apo B, preventing interaction with LDL receptors.

Familial Hypercholesterolemia. Familial hypercholesterolemia is a monogenic, autosomal dominant disorder caused by a defect in the LDL receptor. The frequency in the United States is 1:500 individuals. Hypercholesterolemia is present in infancy and worsens with age. Homozygotes have extremely high cholesterol levels (500–1000 mg/dL); heterozygotes have cholesterol levels of 350–500 mg/dL. Patients have xanthomas (lipid deposits) over tendons, especially over the Achilles tendon and tendons of the hands. They can also have xanthelasmas (lipid deposits around the eyes). Homozygous patients have severe atherosclerosis even in childhood. Heterozygous patients have signs of atherosclerosis by middle age.

Familial Defective Apo B. This cause of hypercholesterolemia (frequency 1:500–1:700) presents with the same phenotype as familial hypercholesterolemia, including the presence of tendinous xanthomas. It can be differentiated from familial hypercholesterolemia by in vitro studies that show decreased LDL binding in fibroblasts with normal LDL receptors.

Secondary causes of reduced LDL clearance include hypothyroidism and a diet high in saturated fats, which can lead to down-regulation of the LDL receptors. Primary and secondary causes of isolated hypercholesterolemia can coexist.

Overproduction of LDL also causes isolated hypercholesterolemia. As discussed above, LDL is not secreted directly by the liver but is the end product of VLDL metabolism. Therefore, increased LDL can be due to overproduction of VLDL.

Familial Combined Hyperlipidemia. Primary VLDL overproduction resulting in isolated hypercholesterolemia is one of the consequences of familial combined hyperlipidemia, which occurs with a gene frequency of 1:100 in the United States. Individuals with this disorder produce increased numbers of apo B–containing particles. Family members can have high VLDL and LDL (combined hyperlipidemia) or high VLDL alone or high LDL alone, depending on the efficiency of VLDL removal versus the efficiency of LDL removal. The diagnosis of familial combined hyperlipidemia cannot be made in patients who only have high VLDL or LDL unless the lipid profile of other family members is known. Patients with this disorder do not have xanthomas but might have xanthelasmas.

Secondary causes of VLDL overproduction include nephrotic syndrome and drugs such as glucocorticoids and anabolic steroids.

Isolated hypercholesterolemia from any cause is associated with an increased risk of atherosclerosis but not pancreatitis (see Table 9-1).

The **major risks of hyperlipidemia** are **pancreatitis** as a result of high levels of triglyceride from chylomicrons and **atherosclerosis** as a result of high levels of cholesterol (and sometimes triglyceride) from apo B–containing lipoproteins.

Major Causes of Isolated Hypercholesterolemia

Decreased LDL Clearance
Primary (genetic) causes
  Defective LDL receptors (familial hypercholesterolemia)
  Defective apo B (cannot interact with LDL receptors)
Secondary causes
  Hypothyroidism
  High-fat diet (down-regulates LDL receptors)

Increased VLDL Leading to LDL Overproduction
Primary (genetic) causes
  Familial combined hyperlipidemia with increased cholesterol only
Secondary causes
  Nephrotic syndrome
  Glucocorticoids
  Anabolic steroids

Case Study:
Continued

Since this woman had atherosclerosis at an early age (less than 55 years) and the physical examination revealed xanthelasmas, she was screened for hyperlipidemia. Her lipid levels were high with total cholesterol, 287 mg/dL (desirable < 200 mg/dL) and triglycerides, 295 mg/dL (desirable < 150 mg/dL). She does not have isolated hypercholesterolemia.

Her history of cold intolerance and physical findings of an enlarged thyroid gland and slow reflexes were consistent with the presence of hypothyroidism. Her low thyroxine (T_4) level of 3.8 μg/dL (normal: 5.0–11.5 μg/dL) and her high thyroid-stimulating hormone

(TSH) level of 27 mU/L (normal: 0.3–5.0 mU/L) confirmed the diagnosis of primary hypothyroidism.

A primary (genetic) basis for her hyperlipidemia is indicated by her family history of hyperlipidemia and the early onset of her atherosclerosis. She also has a secondary cause for decreased cholesterol clearance (hypothyroidism). Additional laboratory testing revealed no other secondary causes. Plasma glucose, liver function tests, creatinine, urinalysis, and complete blood count (CBC) were normal.

Case Study:
Continued

Isolated Hypertriglyceridemia. Since VLDL is the major carrier of triglyceride in the fasting state, modest, isolated fasting hypertriglyceridemia (a triglyceride level in the 200–400 mg/dL range) is due to VLDL elevation. Either increased VLDL production, decreased VLDL clearance (decreased lipolysis), or both are responsible. Two genetic disorders result in the isolated hypertriglyceridemia phenotype: familial hypertriglyceridemia (gene frequency 1:500) and familial hypercholesterolemia (gene frequency 1:100) [Figure 9-6].

Familial Hypertriglyceridemia. The hypertriglyceridemia is due to production of a *normal number* of very large VLDL particles with extra triglyceride at the core. Since there is only one apo B per particle, apo B levels are not increased. These particles are poorly lipolyzed by LpL. They are too large to be taken up easily into blood vessels; thus, this disorder is not atherogenic.

Familial Combined Hyperlipidemia. This disorder is described in the preceding section, the triglyceride elevation is due to production of an *increased number* of small, dense apo B–containing VLDL particles and remnants that are easily taken up by blood vessels. This disorder is atherogenic.

Secondary causes of hypertriglyceridemia include diabetes, renal disease, and drugs. These are common and must always be ruled out.

Diabetes. Insulin deficiency or insulin resistance results in the activation of hormone-sensitive lipase, which increases lipolysis within adipose tissue. The excess free fatty acids are released into the circulation and are delivered to the liver, which incorporates them into triglycerides. The triglycerides are then packaged into VLDL. Insulin deficiency

---

Major Causes of Isolated Mild-to-Moderate Hypertriglyceridemia

Increased VLDL Production, Decreased Catabolism, or Both

Primary (genetic) causes
   Familial hypertriglyceridemia
   Familial combined hyperlipidemia
Secondary causes
   Diabetes
   Renal failure
   Drugs such as alcohol, glucocorticoids, estrogen, β-blockers, and diuretics

---

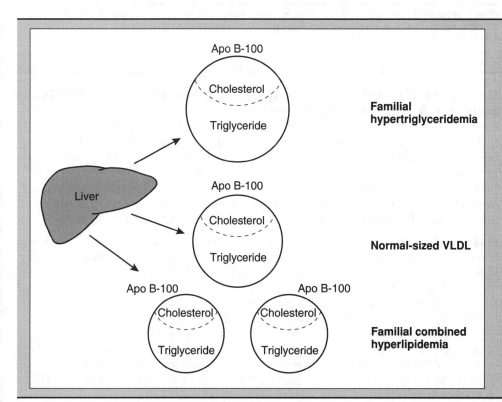

FIGURE 9-6
TYPES OF HYPERTRIGLYCERIDEMIA. Note the large size but normal number of particles in familial hypertriglyceridemia. Note the small size and increased number of particles in familial combined hyperlipidemia. Apo = apolipoprotein; VLDL = very-low-density lipoprotein. (*Source:* Reprinted with permission from Chait A, Brunzell JD: Endocrine system syllabus. Seattle, WA: Washington University School of Medicine, 1994, p 17.)

or insulin resistance also impairs action of LpL, resulting in decreased clearance of VLDL from the circulation. Additional metabolic abnormalities, including decreased remnant clearance, also exist. Hypertriglyceridemia improves with diabetes control.

Renal Disease. Nephrotic syndrome is associated with increased VLDL production. Impaired VLDL lipolysis by LpL and decreased clearance of VLDL can also contribute to the hypertriglyceridemia associated with renal failure. The clearance defect involves remnant lipoproteins as well.

Drugs. Alcohol increases VLDL production. Alcohol is converted to acetate, which serves as a metabolic fuel, and oxidation of free fatty acids is decreased. The free fatty acids are converted to triglycerides and incorporated into VLDL instead. Increased glucocorticoids cause insulin resistance, which increases VLDL production. Estrogen increases VLDL production and VLDL clearance. If VLDL clearance is impaired, VLDL and triglyceride levels increase. Diuretics and β-blockers also are associated with increased triglyceride levels. The mechanisms are not clearly understood.

There are no xanthomas. Modest triglyceride elevation is not associated with an increased risk of pancreatitis. However, the combination of a primary disorder and a superimposed secondary disorder can result in severe triglyceride elevation, which changes the clinical picture (see below). The risk for atherosclerosis depends on the cause of the hypertriglyceridemia (Table 9-1).

Table 9-1
Classification and Clinical Manifestations of Hyperlipidemia

LIPID ELEVATION	LIPOPROTEINS	PANCREATITIS	ATHEROSCLEROSIS	TYPE OF XANTHOMAS[a]
Cholesterol only	LDL	No	Yes	Tendinous and tuberous
Triglyceride only	VLDL	No	Variable	Rare tuberous
Cholesterol and triglyceride	LDL and VLDL	No	Yes	
Cholesterol and triglyceride	Remnants[b]	No	Yes	Palmar and tuberoeruptive
Mainly triglyceride; some cholesterol	Chylomicrons[c]	Yes	Unlikely	Eruptive
Triglyceride level greater than cholesterol	VLDL and chylomicrons	Yes	Yes	Eruptive

Note. Xanthelasmas can be found with isolated cholesterol elevation or combined cholesterol and triglyceride elevation. LDL = low-density lipoprotein; VLDL = very low-density lipoprotein.
[a] Xanthomas are not always present.
[b] VLDL and chylomicron remnants.
[c] Presents in childhood.

Combined Cholesterol and Triglyceride Elevation with Cholesterol Predominance. This is a common hyperlipidemia due to VLDL and LDL elevation. Cholesterol elevation usually predominates (e.g., cholesterol, 290 mg/dL; triglyceride, 220 mg/dL). It is the result of increased VLDL production leading to increased LDL production. Clearance may also be decreased. The primary (genetic) cause is usually familial combined hyperlipidemia. Secondary causes include drugs (e.g., β-blockers, diuretics, steroids), renal failure, and nephrotic syndrome. It is not associated with xanthomas or an increased risk of pancreatitis, but it is associated with an increased risk of atherosclerosis (see Table 9-1). Xanthelasmas could be present.

Remnant Disease. Remnant disease, in which cholesterol and triglyceride elevations are of similar magnitude, is also called *familial dysbetalipoproteinemia*. This is a rare disorder due to an increased number of remnants of triglyceride-rich lipoproteins (i.e., VLDLs, chylomicrons). The remnants are enriched in cholesterol, resulting in similar proportions of cholesterol and triglycerides. The remnants accumulate owing to combined defects of overproduction and decreased clearance. Overproduction is due either to a genetic defect, such as familial combined hyperlipidemia, or a secondary cause, such as diabetes. The decreased clearance is due to a genetic defect in apo E, the ligand mediating the binding of the remnants to liver receptors for clearance. Patients with this disorder are usually homozygous for the apo E-2 isoform that has a defect in the receptor-binding region.

Usually, a secondary cause of remnant overproduction or decreased clearance is required to unmask this type of hyperlipidemia even in someone who is homozygous for the defective apo E-2. Patients with the disorder can have palmar or tuberoeruptive xanthomas. They are at an increased risk for atherosclerosis but usually not for pancreatitis (see Table 9-1).

Chylomicronemia Syndrome in Children. This is a rare disorder (< 1: 100,000) due to chylomicron elevation. Since chylomicrons contain mostly triglycerides, the triglyceride elevation is much greater than the cholesterol elevation. The disorder is due to a genetic defect resulting in decreased lipolysis of chylomicrons and VLDL. *LpL or its cofactor apo C-II is missing or defective.* On a typical Western diet that is high in fat, the triglyceride level is over 2000 mg/dL. These patients have hypertriglyceridemia from birth, and they are at risk for pancreatitis. Eruptive xanthomas occur on the trunk and the extremities. The risk of atherosclerosis could be increased later in life (see Table 9-1).

Chylomicronemia Syndrome in Adults. This is a common disorder characterized by increased cholesterol and triglyceride levels as a result of VLDL and chylomicron elevations. Since clearance of VLDL and chylomicrons share a common pathway, any defect in clearance can cause both to accumulate. The problem is compounded if it coexists with increased VLDL production. The increase in chylomicrons after a high-fat meal exacerbates the hyperlipidemia even further.

Occasionally this disorder occurs in patients who are homozygous for a genetic disorder causing hypertriglyceridemia. Most often, especially if the triglyceride level is greater than 1000 mg/dL, chylomicronemia syndrome is due to a combination of genetic and secondary causes. Diabetes is present in 50% of patients with adult chylomicronemia. Alcohol intake and steroid therapy are common contributing factors.

Patients can present with pancreatitis, eruptive orange xanthomas on the trunk and extremities, and lipemia retinalis on funduscopic examination (funduscopic examination reveals a cream-colored cast to retinal blood vessels due to the refraction of light by the high plasma chylomicron concentration). The underlying cause or causes determine whether or not the disorder is atherogenic (see Table 9-1).

CLASSIFICATION OF HYPERLIPIDEMIA: PHENOTYPE VERSUS GENOTYPE

Hyperlipidemias sometimes have been characterized according to the Fredrickson classification, which depends on lipoproteins present at a given moment: type I = increased chylomicrons; type IIA = increased cholesterol; type IIB = increased cholesterol and triglyceride; type III = increased remnants; type IV = increased VLDL; type V = increased VLDL and chylomicrons. These are phenotypes only, not genotypes.

The lipoprotein phenotype is like a picture: it represents the status of lipoprotein metabolism at a specific point in time and gives no information on the dynamics involved. Phenotypes can shift. For example, a patient with familial hypertriglyceridemia (type IV) who develops diabetes could develop chylomicronemia syndrome (type V) and shift back to modest hypertriglyceridemia only (type IV) if the diabetes is controlled.

A lipoprotein genotype can present as different phenotypes. For example, familial combined hyperlipidemia can present as increased cholesterol only (type IIA), increased cholesterol and triglyceride (type IIB), or triglyceride only (type IV).

SCREENING FOR HYPERLIPIDEMIA

Since hyperlipidemias increase the risk of pancreatitis and atherosclerosis, patients with coronary, peripheral vascular, or cerebrovascular disease and those with pancreatitis should be screened for hyperlipidemias. Patients with a family history of hyperlipidemias or premature atherosclerosis (before the age of 55 years in men and 65 years in women) should be screened also. Since hyperlipidemias are frequently associated with diabetes and renal failure, screening of patients with these diseases is recommended.

The following physical findings should also prompt hyperlipidemia screening: xanthomas, xanthelasmas, corneal arcus in a young person, lipemia retinalis, central obesity (associated with insulin resistance and VLDL excess), and turbid fasting plasma.

Candidates for Hyperlipidemia Screening

Medical history
Atherosclerosis (coronary, peripheral, cerebrovascular), pancreatitis, diabetes, and renal failure

Family medical history
Hyperlipidemia
Atherosclerosis in men (< age 55)
Atherosclerosis in women (< age 65)

Physical findings
Xanthomas, xanthelasmas, corneal arcus before 50 years of age, lipemia retinalis, central obesity, and turbid fasting plasma

Xanthelasma is also seen in individuals who do not have hyperlipidemia. This also is true of corneal arcus, which is common in the elderly.

Case Study: *Continued*	*As already noted, the patient had several indications for hyperlipidemia screening: atherosclerosis at a young age, a positive family history of premature atherosclerosis, and xanthelasmas on physical examination. A full fasting lipid profile was ordered.*

DIAGNOSIS OF HYPERLIPIDEMIA

The diagnosis of hyperlipidemia requires that a fasting lipid profile be done. The period of fasting should be 12–14 hours. Chylomicrons formed after the last meal should be cleared after this time if chylomicron disposal is normal. The lipid profile includes plasma triglyceride, total cholesterol, and HDL cholesterol levels. With this information, the LDL cholesterol level can be calculated using the Friedwald formula. The formula makes three assumptions: (1) the total cholesterol is the cholesterol present in VLDL, LDL, and HDL (no chylomicrons present); (2) most of the triglyceride is contained in the VLDL; and (3) the ratio of triglyceride to cholesterol in VLDL is approximately 5:1. The Friedwald formula for LDL cholesterol (CH) calculation is as follows:

$$LDL_{CH} = \text{total cholesterol} - (VLDL_{CH} + HDL_{CH})$$

$$VLDL_{CH} = \text{triglyceride}/5$$

Desirable Plasma Lipid Levels
Total cholesterol < 200 mg/dL (< 5.17 mmoL/L)
Triglycerides < 150 mg/dL (< 1.69 mmol/L)
LDL cholesterol < 130 mg/dL (< 3.36 mmol/L)
HDL cholesterol > 45 mg/dL (> 1.16 mmol/L)

If the triglyceride level is greater than 400 mg/dL, chylomicrons are present, and the formula cannot be used because chylomicron cholesterol would also have to be taken into account. A plasma refrigeration test should then be done to verify the presence of chylomicrons. If plasma containing chylomicrons is refrigerated overnight, the light chylomicrons will float to the top and form a creamy layer.

In patients with a triglyceride level greater than 400 mg/dL and in those with mixed cholesterol and triglyceride elevation, both cholesterol- and triglyceride-rich particles are atherogenic if the particles are remnants or if the triglyceride-containing VLDL particles are small, cholesterol enriched, and easily incorporated into blood vessel walls. In these cases, it is useful to consider the level of non–HDL cholesterol (total atherogenic cholesterol). This is calculated as:

$$\text{Total cholesterol} - HDL = LDL + VLDL + \text{remnants}$$

Case Study: *Continued*	*The patient's full fasting lipid profile revealed the following: total cholesterol, 287 mg/dL; triglycerides, 295 mg/dL; and HDL cholesterol, 41 mg/dL. From the Friedwald formula, her VLDL level was calculated as: 295/5 = 59 mg/dL (normal: < 30 mg/dL). Her LDL level was calculated as: 287 − (59 + 41) = 187 mg/dL. The LDL and VLDL cholesterol levels are both elevated, making it likely that the patient has an atherogenic disorder. Her non-HDL cholesterol was calculated as: 287 − 41 = 246 mg/dL (normal < 160 mg/dL). All of the patient's values are abnormal. The level of risk of atherosclerosis based on LDL and non–HDL cholesterol levels is shown in Table 9-2.*

Table 9-2
Atherosclerosis Risk Based on LDL and Non–HDL Cholesterol (mg/dL)

	LDL	**NON–HDL CHOLESTEROL**[a]
Category of risk		
Very high	≥ 190	≥ 220
High	≥ 160	≥ 190
Desirable (primary prevention)	< 130	< 160
Optimal (secondary prevention)	< 100	< 130

Note. LDL = low-density lipoprotein; non–HDL cholesterol = non–high-density lipoprotein cholesterol.
Source: Reprinted with permission from Havel RJ: Management of primary hyperlipidemia. *N Engl J Med* 332:1494, 1995.
[a] non–HDL cholesterol = LDL + VLDL + remnants = total cholesterol − HDL.

After the diagnosis of hyperlipidemia is made, it is important to assess whether there is a secondary cause. The following diseases are frequent causes of secondary hyperlipidemias and need to be ruled out: diabetes, hypothyroidism, renal failure, nephrotic syndrome, and liver disease. The following drugs can also cause secondary hyperlipidemia: alcohol, diuretics, β-blockers, estrogens, progesterone, androgens, corticosteroids, and retinoic acid.

If a secondary cause is found, it should be treated first. If correction of the secondary causes does not normalize the lipid profile, a coexisting primary disorder is presumed to exist. If no secondary cause is found, the hyperlipidemia is presumed to be primary (genetic). Family screening might be necessary to determine the genotype of the primary disorder.

TREATMENT OF HYPERLIPIDEMIA

Treatment of chylomicronemia decreases the risk of pancreatitis. Eruptive xanthomas resolve with treatment. Lowering plasma LDL has been shown in clinical trials to reduce the risk of fatal and nonfatal myocardial infarctions. Primary prevention refers to treatment of patients with no atherosclerosis, and secondary prevention refers to treatment of patients who already have atherosclerosis. Hyperlipidemia treatment can result in some regression of atherosclerotic lesions as well as regression of tuberous and tendinous xanthomas.

Treatment of Hypercholesterolemia. The National Cholesterol Education
Program (NCEP) guidelines for prevention of atherosclerosis by lowering LDL cholesterol levels are listed below.

NCEP Guidelines for Primary Prevention. For primary prevention, criteria for treatment are based upon the number of risk factors for atherosclerosis present: age, gender, family history of premature atherosclerosis, smoking, diabetes, hypertension, and low HDL (Table 9-3). Diabetes is counted as two risk factors because in patients with diabetes atherosclerotic events occur earlier, are more severe, and are more likely to be fatal. High HDL (> 60 mg/dL) is a negative risk factor, which can be subtracted from the total number of risk factors.

> **Evaluation of Hyperlipidemia**
> Is hyperlipidemia present?
> Which lipids and lipoproteins are elevated?
> Is there a family history of hyperlipidemia? (a primary disorder?)
> Is there a secondary cause for the hyperlipidemia?
> Is this a combined primary and secondary hyperlipidemia?

Male more than 45 years old
Postmenopausal female or female more than 55 years old
Family history of premature coronary heart disease
  In men less than 55 years old
  In women less than 65 years old
Cigarette smoking
Hypertension (blood pressure > 140/90 mm Hg) or treatment for hypertension
Diabetes mellitus (counts as two risk factors)
Low HDL (< 35 mg/dL)
HDL greater than 60 mg/dL is a negative risk factor

Note. HDL = high-density lipoprotein.

Table 9-3
Major Risk Factors for Development of Atherosclerosis

If two or more risk factors are present, the patient is at a high risk for atherosclerosis and a more rigorous plan for treating LDL cholesterol is followed. The desirable *goal* if two or more atherosclerosis risk factors are present is an LDL cholesterol level of less than 130 mg/dL. The treatment plan outlined below is recommended.

1. Treat secondary causes of hyperlipidemia.
2. Adjust calories to achieve ideal body weight, starting with phase 1 of the American Heart Association (AHA) diet. Decrease fat to less than 30% of calories, consisting of 10% each saturated, monounsaturated, and polyunsaturated fat. Decrease cholesterol intake to less than 300 mg a day. If the AHA step 1 diet fails to lower the LDL cholesterol level sufficiently, the stricter AHA step 2 diet can be used. This diet restricts monounsaturated and polyunsaturated fat to less than 20% of calories, saturated fat to no more than 7% of calories, and cholesterol to less than 200 mg a day.
3. Prescribe 20 minutes of exercise (at least) daily, when feasible.
4. Insist that the patient quit smoking.
5. Control hypertension.
6. Try diet and exercise for at least 1 year before adding drugs. Use drugs if the patient fails to reach the LDL cholesterol goal with diet and exercise.

If the patient has two or more atherosclerotic risk factors, add drugs if the LDL cholesterol level remains greater than or equal to 160 mg/dL. If the patient has fewer than two atherosclerotic risk factors, is a male more than 35 years old, or is a postmenopausal female, add drugs if the LDL cholesterol level remains greater than or equal to 190 mg/dL. If the patient has fewer than two atherosclerotic risk factors, is a male less than 35 years old, or is a premenopausal female, use drugs if the LDL cholesterol level is greater than or equal to 220 mg/dL.

NCEP Guidelines for Secondary Prevention. The desirable goal is an LDL cholesterol level less than 100 mg/dL. The treatment plan outlined below is recommended.

1. Follow the steps of diet, exercise, hypertension control, and smoking cessation outlined above for primary prevention.
2. Try diet and exercise alone for 3–6 months before starting drugs.

Drug Therapy for Hypercholesterolemia. The first choice for drug therapy for hypercholesterolemia is either an HMG-CoA reductase inhibitor or niacin, unless niacin is contraindicated (patients with diabetes, abnormal liver function tests, or bleeding ulcer). Niacin decreases production of VLDL, the precursor of LDL. HMG-CoA reductase inhibitors decrease cholesterol synthesis. A bile acid sequestrant such as colestipol or cholestyramine also can be used. Bile acids are synthesized from cholesterol in the liver. Bile acid sequestrants bind bile acids in the intestine so that they cannot return to the liver via the enterohepatic circulation. Both bile acid sequestrants and HMG-CoA reductase inhibitors decrease the liver cell pool of free cholesterol, which results in an increase in liver LDL receptors and increased removal of LDL cholesterol from the plasma. Gemfibrozil, which increases VLDL disposal, is not indicated for treatment of isolated hypercholesterolemia (Table 9-4).

Table 9-4
Drugs Used to Treat Hyperlipidemia

DRUG	ACTION	INDICATION	CONCERNS
Niacin	Decreases VLDL production	Increased VLDL and LDL (Increased triglyceride and cholesterol)	Increased blood glucose. Increased liver enzymes and uric acid, flushing, and gastrointestinal side effects
Gemfibrozil	Increases VLDL and chylomicron disposal	Increased VLDL and chylomicrons (increased triglycerides)	Increased liver enzymes, rare myositis
Fish oil	Decreases VLDL production	Increased chylomicrons (increased triglycerides)	Rare bleeding if combined with anticoagulants or aspirin
HMG-CoA reductase inhibitors ("statins")[a]	Decrease cholesterol synthesis	Increased LDL (increased cholesterol)	Increased liver enzymes, rare myopathy
Bile acid sequestrants	Increase cholesterol loss from intestine	Increased LDL (increased cholesterol)	Malabsorption of other drugs, gastrointestinal side effects

Note. VLDL = very low-density lipoprotein; LDL = low-density lipoprotein; HMG-CoA = 3-hydroxy-3-methylglutaryl-CoA.
[a] Fluvastatin, lovastatin; pravastatin, simvastatin, and atorvastatin.

Treatment of Isolated Hypertriglyceridemia. The desired plasma triglyceride level is less than 150–200 mg/dL. A treatment plan is outlined below.

1. Treat secondary causes.
2. Institute life-style changes as outlined above for treatment of hypercholesterolemia.
3. Institute caloric adjustment to achieve ideal body weight.
4. Restrict not only total and saturated fat but also simple sugars and alcohol, which increase VLDL production.
5. Drug treatment depends on the nature of the underlying hyperlipidemia. If it is an atherogenic disorder like familial combined hyperlipidemia, treat with gemfibrozil or niacin (see Table 9-4). An alternative to gemfibrozil is fish oil.

Treatment of Combined Cholesterol and Triglyceride Elevations Including Remnant Disease. Since in this disorder the lipid elevations are due to either LDL and VLDL cholesterol or remnant lipoproteins and all of them are potentially atherogenic, a non–HDL cholesterol treatment goal is more appropriate than a LDL cholesterol goal. The desirable level of non–HDL cholesterol is less than 160 mg/dL for primary prevention. The optimal level for secondary prevention is less than 130 mg/dL (see Table 9-2). A treatment plan is outlined below.

1. Treat secondary causes.
2. Institute life-style changes as indicated above for isolated hypercholesterolemia and hypertriglyceridemia.
3. The initiation of drug treatment depends on the level of non–HDL cholesterol and the presence or absence of atherosclerosis or the number of atherosclerotic risk factors present. Start with niacin unless niacin is contraindicated. Alternative drugs include an HMG-CoA reductase inhibitor or gemfibrozil alone or in combination with a bile acid sequestrant (see Table 9-4).

Treatment of Chylomicronemia. The risk of pancreatitis in patients with chylomicronemia syndrome is low if triglycerides are lowered to less than 1000 mg/dL in patients with no previous history of pancreatitis, and to less than 500 mg/dL in patients with a previous history of pancreatitis. In children who lack LpL or its cofactor apo C-II, the main treatment involves restriction of fat intake to 10%–20% of calories. Medium-chain fatty acids can be used for cooking since they do not form chylomicrons. In adults with chylomicronemia, a secondary cause such as diabetes is usually present and needs to be treated first. Restriction of fat and increased exercise also are recommended. The drug of choice for this disorder is gemfibrozil (see Table 9-3). An alternative therapy to gemfibrozil is fish oil.

Treatment of Low HDL Levels. A low HDL cholesterol level is a risk factor for atherosclerosis, but effective treatment for this condition is limited. Treatment involves addressing the factors that raise HDL, namely increasing exercise when possible, estrogen replacement in postmenopausal women if not contraindicated, and treating elevated triglyceride levels. Niacin can raise HDL in some patients.

Case Study:
Resolution

This patient's cholesterol and triglyceride levels were elevated to a similar degree. A combination of increased VLDL and LDL levels is possible. This phenotype is seen in patients with familial combined hyperlipidemia. Given the family history of cholesterol elevation in her father and triglyceride elevation in her uncle, the diagnosis of familial combined hyperlipidemia is very likely. Another possibility is VLDL overproduction due to her familial combined hyperlipidemia coupled with apo E-2 homozygosity, which hampers remnant clearance (remnant disease). Special tests of her apo E isoforms and tests to measure remnants would be required to be certain of the diagnosis.

This patient should be treated for her hypothyroidism first. If her lipid levels are still elevated as a result of primary hyperlipidemia and she has remnant disease, niacin, which decreases VLDL production, or gemfibrozil, which increases VLDL disposal, would be the first drugs of choice. If the patient has combined LDL and VLDL elevation, treatment choices would be niacin, an HMG-CoA reductase inhibitor, or a combination of gemfibrozil and a bile acid sequestrant. Combinations of gemfibrozil or niacin and an HMG-CoA reductase inhibitor result in an increased risk of myopathy.

■ REVIEW QUESTIONS

Directions: For each of the following questions, choose the **one best** answer.

Questions 1 and 2

A 22-year-old student who had an asthma attack was treated with prednisone, a glucocorticosteroid, which was to be tapered over the next month. She attended a health fair a few days later where her cholesterol was tested and found to be elevated. She was referred to her physician who ordered a lipid profile and found a total cholesterol of 255 mg/dL, triglyceride of 295 mg/dL, and high-density lipoprotein (HDL) of 58 mg/dL. The physician consulted a lipid expert to interpret the results.

1. The lipid expert knows that this patient has

    (A) isolated low-density lipoprotein (LDL) elevation (LDL > 130 mg/dL)
    (B) combined LDL and very low-density lipoprotein (VLDL) elevation (LDL > 130 mg/dL and VLDL > 30 mg/dL)
    (C) chylomicron elevation
    (D) isolated VLDL elevation (VLDL > 30 mg/dL)
    (E) combined VLDL and chylomicron elevation

2. If asked whether this is a primary disorder that needs to be treated with lipid-lowering drugs, the lipid expert would most likely reply that

    (A) it is a primary disorder that should be treated with drugs
    (B) it is a secondary hyperlipidemia, and no drugs are necessary
    (C) it is a combined primary and secondary hyperlipidemia, and no drugs are necessary
    (D) it is not known whether this is a primary or secondary disorder, and no drugs are necessary
    (E) it is not known whether this is a primary or secondary disorder, but drugs should be started

3. A 38-year-old obese man with severe coronary atherosclerosis goes to his physician for an evaluation of his hyperlipidemia. He has no tendinous xanthomas or xanthelasmas. His blood glucose, urinalysis, liver, thyroid, and kidney function tests are normal. He is taking no medications other than nitroglycerin as needed. His father, who had high cholesterol and high triglycerides, died at age 40 of a massive heart attack. His 45-year-old sister just had coronary bypass surgery. She has normal cholesterol but high triglycerides. The patient's physician orders a fasting lipid profile, which reveals: total cholesterol, 338 mg/dL; triglycerides, 125 mg/dL; and HDL, 31 mg/dL. The most likely diagnosis for this patient is

    (A) familial defective apo B
    (B) familial combined hyperlipidemia
    (C) familial hypertriglyceridemia
    (D) familial remnant disease
    (E) combined familial and secondary hyperlipidemia

4. A child is brought to the emergency room with severe abdominal pain after attending a birthday party where he ate a cheeseburger, French fries, and a milk shake. Physical examination reveals epigastric tenderness and a vesicular rash on his buttocks and trunk. The physician's diagnosis is pancreatitis. Which of the following lipid disorders is this child most likely to have?

    (A) Familial hypercholesterolemia
    (B) Familial combined hyperlipidemia
    (C) Familial lipoprotein lipase (LpL) deficiency
    (D) Familial defective apo B
    (E) Familial remnant disease

5. A 42-year-old computer analyst recently had a heart attack. His overnight refrigerated plasma had a creamy layer on top. His fasting lipid profile is as follows: total cholesterol, 289 mg/dL; triglycerides, 3325 mg/dL; HDL, 13 mg/dL; and blood glucose, 250 mg/dL (normal: 70–110 mg/dL). His lipid values can best be explained by

(A) LDL overproduction and decreased clearance by the liver
(B) normal clearance of chylomicrons but failure to lipolyze VLDL into LDL
(C) complete lipolysis and clearance of chylomicrons
(D) up-regulated LDL receptors and increased LDL clearance
(E) overproduction and decreased clearance of VLDL and chylomicrons

6. A 25-year-old healthy woman on no medications asks her physician for a prescription for oral contraceptives. Her mother has hyperlipidemia. Her physician orders a lipid profile. Total plasma cholesterol is 180 mg/dL, HDL cholesterol is 35 mg/dL, and triglycerides are 355 mg/dL. Her urinalysis, blood glucose, liver, thyroid, and kidney function tests are normal. The physician's diagnosis is most likely

(A) familial hypertriglyceridemia
(B) familial hypercholesterolemia
(C) familial dysbetalipoproteinemia
(D) secondary hypertriglyceridemia
(E) chylomicronemia syndrome

▌ANSWERS AND EXPLANATIONS

1. The answer is B. VLDL cholesterol is calculated by dividing the triglyceride level by 5 (295 mg/dL ÷ 5 mg/dL = 59 mg/dL). To calculate the LDL level, the Friedwald formula can be used because the triglycerides are below 400 mg/dL.

LDL = total cholesterol − (VLDL + HDL) = 255 mg/dL − (59 mg/dL + 58 mg/dL) = 138 mg/dL

2. The answer is D. Glucocorticosteroids cause insulin resistance, which can result in increased VLDL and LDL production. It is impossible to know if this is a secondary disorder only or a combined primary and secondary disorder because no family history concerning lipid levels is available and the secondary disorder has not resolved. After the steroids are discontinued, a lipid profile should be repeated to determine whether a primary hyperlipidemia is present. At this point, since the patient is young and has no known atherosclerosis, drug treatment should not be initiated.

3. The answer is B. Since the patient's sister has triglyceride elevation with normal cholesterol, his father had both cholesterol and triglyceride elevations, and the patient has isolated hypercholesterolemia, distractors A, C, and D are incorrect. Secondary causes are not likely given his normal laboratory tests and no intake of drugs affecting lipids. Different members of a family with familial combined hyperlipidemia can present with isolated cholesterol elevation, isolated triglyceride elevation, or a combination of the two.

4. The answer is C. Pancreatitis in a child who also has eruptive xanthomas is likely to be due to an inability to clear chylomicrons after eating a fatty meal. Deficiency of LpL or its cofactor apo C-II can cause chylomicronemia in a child. None of the other disorders listed result in chylomicronemia.

5. The answer is E. An adult patient with plasma triglycerides above 1000 mg/dL and a creamy layer on top of refrigerated plasma has elevated chylomicrons and VLDL due to combined overproduction and clearance defects. A secondary cause of hyperlipidemia, such as diabetes, and an underlying primary disorder, such as familial hypertriglyceridemia or familial combined hyperlipidemia, usually are present.

6. The answer is A. Since the patient's abnormality is isolated triglyceride elevation of less than 400 mg/dL, chylomicrons should not be present. The patient is taking no medications, and her laboratory profile reveals no secondary cause for triglyceride elevations. Distractors B and C are excluded since her cholesterol is normal. Estrogen causes increased VLDL production but also increases VLDL turnover. If the physician prescribes an estrogen-containing oral contraceptive, the patient should repeat a fasting lipid profile to be sure that she does not develop marked hypertriglyceridemia. Estrogen also raises HDL, which would be beneficial.

▌REFERENCES

Brown G, Albers JJ, Fisher LD, et al: Regression of coronary artery disease as a result of intensive lipid-lowering therapy in men with high levels of apolipoprotein B. *N Engl J Med* 323:1289–1298, 1990.

Dammerman M, Breslow JL: Genetic basis of lipoprotein disorders. *Circulation* 91:505, 1995.

Expert Panel on Detection, Evaluation, and Treatment of High Blood Cholesterol in Adults (Adult Treatment Panel II): Summary of the second report of the National Cholesterol Education Program (NCEP). *JAMA* 269:3015, 1993.

Goldstein JL, Hobbs HH, Brown MS: Familial hypercholesterolemia. In *The Metabolic and Molecular Bases of Inherited Disease*, 7th ed. Edited by Scriver C, Beaudet A, Sly W, et al. New York, NY: McGraw-Hill, 1995, p 1981.

Havel RJ, Rapaport E: Management of primary hyperlipidemia. *N Engl J Med* 332:1491, 1995.

Wong ND, Wilson PWF, Kannel WB: Serum cholesterol as a prognostic factor after myocardial infarction: the Framingham study. *Ann Intern Med* 115:687–693, 1991.

Wood PD, Stefanick ML, Williams PT, et al: The effects on plasma lipoproteins of a prudent weight-reducing diet, with or without exercise, in overweight men and women. *N Engl J Med* 325:461–466, 1991.

Chapter 10

OBESITY

Charles J. Billington, M.D.

■ CHAPTER OUTLINE

Case Study: Introduction

A 35-year-old man came to the clinic because high blood pressure was detected at a health fair screening program. He felt well and had no complaints. The patient said that he weighed approximately 250 lbs when he played football 15 years ago and has gained weight gradually since that time. He stated that he does not eat excessively. He is employed as a restaurant manager and has been working regularly. His job is sedentary, and his leisure pursuits include television, computers, and talking with friends. His mother, father, and brother are also obese. His maternal grandparents and his mother have type 2 diabetes mellitus. On examination, his blood pressure was 150/100 mm Hg, and his pulse was 82 beats/min. His height is 6', and his weight is 320 lbs. The remainder of his examination was unremarkable except for trace pedal edema bilaterally. Laboratory examination revealed a fasting plasma glucose of 115 mg/dL (normal: 70–105 mg/dL). An electrocardiogram (ECG) revealed mild left ventricular hypertrophy.

■ INTRODUCTION

The recognition that obesity poses a risk to health and life dates back to Hippocrates. Although much attention has been directed toward the medical consequences of obesity in recent years, the prevalence of obesity is increasing. The most recent National Health and Nutrition Examination Survey (NHANES III) in 1990–1991 indicates that one-third of Americans are obese and that this proportion has risen substantially in the last 15 years. The previous survey (NHANES II) conducted in 1976–1980 and studies from 1960–1962 showed that 25% of Americans were obese.

Recognition of genetic influences on body weight and the greater availability of drugs for the treatment of obesity have reinforced concerns about obesity as a public health issue. Former Surgeon General C. Everett Koop, who directed public attention to the problems of smoking and drugs, now heads an organization called "Shape Up America" whose mission is to focus attention on the problems of obesity and lack of fitness.

DEFINITIONS

Obesity is defined as excess accumulation of body fat. In normal adult men, 15%–22% of the body is composed of fat; in healthy adult women, 18%–33% of the body is composed of fat. Technically, men with more than 22% body fat and women with more than 33% body fat are obese. However, since total body fat is difficult to measure, obesity is usually defined either by reference to "ideal" body weight or by relating weight to height in the body mass index (BMI). Ideal body weight is determined from insurance company data correlating body weight (adjusted for sex, height, and to some extent, frame size) and survival.

Calculation of the Body Mass Index (BMI)
$$BMI = weight/height^2 = kg/m^2$$
$$BMI \simeq (pounds/inches^2) \times 702$$

The BMI is being used more frequently as the standard method of reference. Since normal body weight is more proportional to height squared than to height, the BMI is calculated by dividing weight in kilograms by the height in meters squared (kg/m^2). A close estimate of BMI can be made by dividing weight in pounds by height in inches squared, then multiplying the result by 702. The normal range for BMI is 19–25 kg/m^2. Obesity is defined as weight that is 20% above ideal body weight or a BMI of 27 (Table 10-1). The BMIs corresponding to a range of heights and weights are shown in Figure 10-1.

Table 10-1
Obesity Defined by Body Mass Index (BMI)

	BMI (kg/m²)
Normal weight	19–24.9
Slightly overweight	25–26.9
Mild obesity	27–29.9
Moderate-to-severe obesity	30–39.9
Morbid obesity	over 40

The distribution of body fat also is important. Upper body or abdominal obesity is associated with more medical problems than lower body obesity. Men are more likely to develop upper body (central) obesity, and women are more likely to develop lower body obesity. The distribution of body fat is influenced by genetic factors. However, the difference in fat distribution between the genders primarily is due to their gonadal hormones. Men produce mostly androgens, while women produce mostly estrogens. Thus, upper body obesity is called android or apple (shaped) obesity, while lower body obesity is called gynoid, gluteal, or pear (shaped) obesity. The most accurate measurements of upper body obesity are obtained with computed tomography (CT) or magnetic resonance imaging (MRI) of the abdomen, but these methods are too expensive for routine use.

Central Obesity (abdominal, apple, android obesity) is defined as a WHR > 0.85 in women and a WHR > 1.0 in men. Central obesity is responsible for most of the increased medical risk.

In clinical practice, upper body obesity is assessed by measuring the waist–hip ratio (WHR). The WHR is measured by comparing the girth at the narrowest point above the umbilicus to the greatest girth in the gluteal area. Women with a WHR greater than 0.85 and men with a WHR greater than 1.0 have central obesity.

BMI →	25	26	27	28	29	30	31	32	33	34	35	36	37	38	39	40
							Weight (in pounds)									
4' 10"	119	124	129	134	138	143	148	153	158	162	167	172	177	181	186	191
4' 11"	124	128	133	138	143	148	153	158	163	168	173	178	183	188	193	198
5' 0"	128	133	138	143	148	153	158	164	169	174	179	184	189	194	199	204
5' 1"	132	137	143	148	153	158	164	169	174	180	185	190	195	201	206	211
5' 2"	136	142	147	153	158	164	169	175	180	186	191	196	202	207	213	218
5' 3"	141	146	152	158	163	169	175	180	186	192	197	203	208	214	220	225
5' 4"	145	151	157	163	169	174	180	186	192	198	203	209	215	221	227	233
5' 5"	150	156	162	168	174	180	186	192	198	204	210	216	222	228	234	240
5' 6"	155	161	167	173	179	185	192	198	204	210	216	223	229	235	241	247
5' 7"	159	166	172	178	185	191	198	204	210	217	223	230	236	242	248	255
5' 8"	164	171	177	184	190	198	204	210	216	223	230	236	243	249	256	263
5' 9"	169	176	182	189	196	203	209	216	223	230	236	243	250	257	264	270
5' 10"	174	181	188	195	202	209	216	223	230	236	243	250	257	264	271	278
5' 11"	179	186	193	200	207	215	222	229	236	243	250	258	265	272	279	286
6' 0"	184	191	199	206	213	221	228	235	243	250	258	265	272	280	287	294
6' 1"	189	197	204	212	219	227	234	242	250	257	265	272	280	287	295	303
6' 2"	194	202	210	218	225	233	241	249	256	264	272	280	288	295	303	311
6' 3"	200	208	216	224	232	240	247	255	263	271	279	287	295	303	311	319
6' 4"	205	213	221	230	238	246	254	262	271	279	287	295	303	312	320	328

Height

Figure 10-1

BODY MASS INDEX (BMI) CALCULATED FOR A RANGE OF HEIGHTS (MEASURED IN FEET AND INCHES) AND WEIGHTS (MEASURED IN POUNDS). To determine the BMI for an individual, find that person's height in the left column. Find the weight closest to that person's weight along the row to the right. Go to the top of the column to find the closest BMI. For example, someone who is 5'6" and weighs 198 lbs has a BMI of 32. Someone who is 6'0" and weighs 210 lbs has a BMI of 28.5.

■ MEDICAL RISKS OF OBESITY

Obesity is a chronic disorder. Like hypertension and hypercholesterolemia, obesity primarily contributes to medical risk by enhancing the development of other serious conditions over a long period of time. Because obesity-related risk has a long "incubation period," the amount of prospective data acquired about obesity is limited. Some of the most extensive data come from insurance company studies, especially the Metropolitan Life Insurance Company; these data have been used to develop the desirable weight charts referred to above. These data also demonstrate a clear negative effect of increasing weight on all-cause mortality.

Insurance company records note the presence of obesity at one time only, that is, at the beginning of coverage, usually when individuals are relatively young. The Framingham Study, which has been accumulating data prospectively and at regular intervals since 1948, strongly confirms the adverse impact of obesity on mortality. Smaller studies of morbid obesity indicate that severe obesity confers a much greater risk.

Obesity increases the likelihood of developing a broad range of conditions, which are listed in Table 10-2. The cluster of closely associated disorders that make up the "insulin-resistance syndrome"—hyperinsulinemia, hyperglycemia (impaired glucose tolerance or diabetes), hypertension, hypertriglyceridemia, and low high-density lipoprotein (HDL) levels—is closely associated with central obesity and with atherosclerotic vascular disease. Obesity also increases the risk associated with surgical procedures.

Table 10-2
Conditions for Which Obesity is a Major Risk Factor

All-cause mortality	Diabetes mellitus
Coronary heart disease	Hypercholesterolemia
Stroke	Low HDL cholesterol
Sudden death	Gallstones
Congestive heart failure	Sleep apnea
Hypertension	Restrictive lung disease
Thromboembolic disease	Colorectal cancer
Osteoarthritis and gout	Endometrial and breast cancer

Note. HDL = high-density lipoprotein

The critical issue is whether weight loss significantly ameliorates the risks associated with obesity. There are short-term human studies showing that insulin resistance, diabetes, and lipid abnormalities improve with weight loss, but there is little long-term data in humans because it has been difficult to achieve weight loss for a long period of time. Nonetheless, it is believed that prolonged weight reduction would improve health and decrease mortality.

Obesity is defined as a BMI greater than 27, but **medically significant obesity** probably begins at a BMI above 30.

Data indicate that the risk associated with obesity rises continuously with weights above "ideal," but there is still uncertainty about the point at which obesity becomes serious enough to warrant medical intervention. One classification of obesity according to the level of risk for complications is shown in Table 10-3.

Table 10-3
Obesity Risk Defined by Body Mass Index (BMI)

NO COMORBID CONDITION[a]	BMI (kg/m²)
Minimal risk	< 30
Mild risk	30–34.9
Significant risk	35–39.9
Critical risk	over 40

COMORBID CONDITION[a] PRESENT	BMI (kg/m²)
Minimal risk	< 27
Mild risk	27–29.9
Significant risk	30–34.9
Critical risk	over 35

[a] Comorbid conditions: hypertension, diabetes mellitus, hyperlipidemia, smoking, cardiovascular disease, low levels of high-density lipoproteins, and sleep apnea.

This patient is at serious medical risk because of his obesity. With his height of 6' 2" (1.83 m) and his weight of 320 lbs (145 kg), his BMI is 43. The risks of obesity increase with the duration of obesity, and a younger individual is exposed to the risks of obesity for more years than an older person. This patient also has hypertension. Although he does not have diabetes at this time, he is at high risk for developing diabetes. His fasting plasma glucose is slightly elevated, and he has a strong family history of diabetes.

Case Study:
Continued

CAUSES OF OBESITY

Obesity results from excess caloric intake relative to energy expenditure. The scientific basis for this is not fully developed, but it is clear that human obesity results from interactions among genes, behavior, and the environment.

GENETIC FACTORS

Animal studies showing that obesity can be produced by a mutation in a single gene confirm that there are biologic mechanisms regulating body weight and fat mass. The most compelling evidence comes from the recent identification of leptin, a protein hormone secreted by adipose tissue that signals the brain about the amount of body fat. Leptin is the product of the *ob* gene. In the *ob/ob* mouse, an animal with monogenic obesity, a mutation in the *ob* gene results in a defective form of leptin that fails to provide the feedback signal to the brain. In the absence of normal leptin, the animal becomes obese. If leptin is administered to the *ob/ob* mouse, food intake is suppressed, energy expenditure increases, and the animal loses weight.

Obesity in other animals and in humans is not due to low levels of leptin. Leptin levels are high and are correlated with the percentage of body fat. It is possible that leptin resistance is an explanation for obesity. Animals such as the *fa/fa* rat and the *db/db* mouse, which lack normal leptin receptors, are obese. It also is possible that leptin levels are high in obese people because central regulatory systems are responding to other factors, and the leptin hormone signal is overridden. Little is known about how leptin levels are linked to food intake, but studies involving leptin and the leptin receptor have helped to elucidate genetic and neural mechanisms involved in obesity.

The best evidence for a strong genetic influence on the development of human obesity comes from studies of twins, that is, monozygotic versus dizygotic twins and twins reared together versus twins reared apart. The studies of Stunkard and others indicate that between 33% and 60% of the variance in body weight is due to genetic influences. Recent work from Bouchard and colleagues has confirmed a familial predisposition to obesity and indicates that fat distribution (upper body versus lower body) is genetically influenced. Studies of Pima Indian families suggest that metabolic rate is also partially genetically determined.

ACTIVITY AND ENVIRONMENT

Genetic factors account for some variance in body weight, but environment and culture contribute also. The marked increase in the prevalence of obesity in America during the last century is not due to a change in genetic makeup. Possible environmental causes of obesity are listed in Table 10-4. These include food intake driven by hunger created by advertising, a decline in overall physical activity and fitness, and the increase in sedentary leisure activities, such as watching television and using computers. There is an inverse relationship between socioeconomic status and the prevalence of obesity in

Human obesity is a group of heterogeneous disorders resulting from an interaction between genes, behavior, and the environment.

Both animal and human studies indicate a genetic component of obesity.

EXCESS FOOD INTAKE	REDUCED ENERGY EXPENDITURE
Genetic	Genetic
Abnormal neural regulation	Abnormal neural regulation
Learned behavior	Physical impairments and injuries
Social pressure	Automobile-based society
Wide availability of attractive foods	Sedentary occupations
Marketing of foods	Sedentary leisure activity
Boredom	
Depression	

Table 10-4
Probable Causes of Obesity

America. This is in sharp contrast to the strong direct relationship between socio-economic status and obesity in the developing world.

DIET COMPOSITION

The capacity for storing excess dietary carbohydrate as glycogen is limited. Excess dietary carbohydrate can be converted to fat, but this is a high-energy–requiring process. Excess dietary fat can easily be incorporated into body fat, and storage capacity in adipose tissue is very large. However, it is not clear that the fat content of the diet is a major contributor to obesity. The proportion of fat in the American diet has been steady or decreasing during the last 20 years, while the prevalence of obesity is increasing.

BRAIN CENTERS

Recent studies in animals have confirmed the essential role of the hypothalamus and other brain centers in regulating appetite, energy expenditure, and storage of fat. Injury to the ventromedial nucleus of the hypothalamus is associated with hyperphagia and major obesity. Injury to the lateral hypothalamus is associated with reduced food intake and weight loss. Leptin, insulin, and other metabolic and neural signals (especially from the autonomic nervous system) feed back to receptors in these brain regulatory centers (Figure 10-2), which integrate the information. Responses from these centers modulate eating behavior and energy metabolism. Numerous peptides and neurotransmitters are involved in these feedback systems.

FIGURE 10-2
FEEDBACK LOOPS THOUGHT TO REGULATE FEEDING AND ENERGY METABOLISM

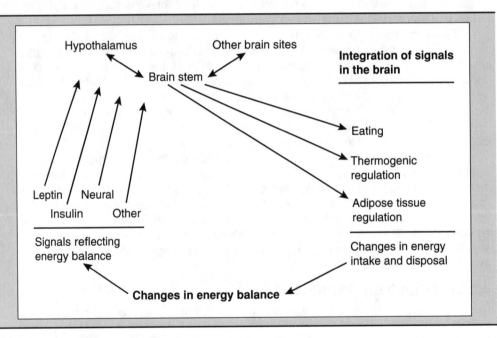

LIPOPROTEIN LIPASE

There is some evidence that the enzyme lipoprotein lipase, which functions as a "gatekeeper" for importing fatty acids into adipose tissue, also plays a key role in determining susceptibility to obesity. Lipoprotein lipase is required for hydrolysis of triglycerides in plasma chylomicrons and very low-density lipoproteins (VLDL) [see Chapter 9]. Hydrolysis releases free fatty acids, which can be stored in adipose tissue.

ENDOCRINE SYSTEM

Endocrine causes of obesity are very rare. Cushing's syndrome results in central obesity, which resolves when hypercortisolism is treated. The mechanism is not known. Androgens promote central fat deposition, but androgens alter the distribution of body fat more than the content. Weight gain associated with hypothyroidism primarily is due to the accumulation of tissue mucopolysaccharide rather than fat.

Increased carbohydrate intake results in increased insulin secretion. Insulin suppresses hormone-sensitive lipase and promotes uptake of free fatty acids into adipose

Endocrine causes of obesity are very rare. Cushing's syndrome and certain hypothalamic injuries cause obesity. Hypothyroidism does not cause obesity.

tissue for fat synthesis. Injected insulin also can result in increased food intake, which probably is due to hypoglycemia.

▌TREATMENT OF OBESITY

In many ways, the treatment of obesity is similar to the treatment of hypertension before the development of effective antihypertensive medication. Behavioral modifications, that is, permanent reduction of caloric intake and increased physical activity, remain the mainstays of therapy. The modifications in food choice and activity should be selected with the knowledge that they must be continued indefinitely. For most people there is no role for short-term "diets" that alter behavior radically for a short period.

Long-term behavioral changes are very difficult to maintain because established behavior patterns are difficult to alter and because homeostatic mechanisms operate to sustain usual weight. Calorie reduction leading to weight loss is accompanied by a reduction in basal metabolic rate, which makes it more difficult to sustain the weight loss. Fortunately, weight loss of 5%–10% improves glucose tolerance, hyperlipidemia, and hypertension even if weight remains far above the "ideal" level.

Intensity of treatment depends on the degree of obesity and the number of comorbid conditions (Table 10-5). In general, life-style changes are recommended for patients with modest increases in BMI and no comorbid conditions. Adoption of a low-fat diet may be helpful. Fat has a higher concentration of calories per weight (9 kcal/g) than carbohydrate and protein (4 kcal/g), so diets lower in fat are less efficient at providing energy to the body. Even simple changes such as increasing walking or fidgeting and restricting television viewing can help by increasing energy expenditure and decreasing exposure to food-related advertising. Drug therapy can be added for patients with severe obesity. Surgery may be appropriate for those with a BMI greater than 40 or those with a BMI greater than 35 and associated comorbidity. A combination of diet and exercise modification should continue even if additional therapy is required.

Diet and **exercise** remain the cornerstones of obesity therapy.

Recommendations for Treatment of Obesity
Make long-term changes in food and activity choices
Reduce calorie consumption by 400–500 cal/d
Reduce saturated fat intake
Increase vegetable and fiber intake
No eating between meals (no snacks)
No "junk" food (usually has high fat content)
Increase activity

BMI (kg/mg²)	COMORBIDITIES	TREATMENT
Greater than 27	Yes or no	Education about permanent life-style changes
Greater than 30	No	Education and behavior modification program
Greater than 30	Yes	Education, behavior modification program, and consider drugs
Greater than 35	Yes or no	Drugs appropriate; seek more aggressive intervention such as very low-calorie diet
Greater than 40	Yes	All of the above and consider surgery

Note. BMI = body mass index.

Table 10-5
Matching Obesity Therapy to Risk

Very low-calorie diets (VLCDs) can be effective and safe under the supervision of a physician for the short-term management of severe obesity. Treatment with these diets for more than a few weeks at a time rarely can be justified, except at specialized centers. Most authorities believe that an adequate protein source is needed to ensure safety. Monitoring of fluid intake, muscle cramping, muscle strength, electrolytes, uric acid, and the QT interval on the ECG is recommended.

Most of the drugs used for the treatment of obesity are associated with significant side effects, and the most effective drugs are associated with the most serious side effects. Therefore, drug treatment should be reserved for patients whose obesity is medically threatening. It can be difficult to identify when obesity represents a serious

Choosing pharmacologic intervention for obesity is a risk:benefit decision. Most of the drugs are associated with significant side effects.

Pharmacologic Treatments of Obesity
Anorectics suppress appetite. Thermogenics increase metabolic rate or energy expenditure. Malabsorptives interfere with food absorption.

threat for an individual patient. Drug treatment for patients with no comorbid conditions can be considered if the BMI is at least 30 but is more likely to be considered if the BMI is greater than 35. The existence of comorbid conditions such as diabetes or sleep apnea that respond to weight loss may lower the threshold for treatment.

PHARMACOLOGIC TREATMENT OF OBESITY

Pharmacologic management of obesity falls into three broad categories: (1) anorectic agents, which suppress appetite; (2) thermogenic agents, which increase metabolic rate, energy expenditure, or both; and (3) malabsorptive agents, which interfere with the absorption of food.

Anorectic Agents. Two classes of anorectic drugs have been used: serotonergic agents and noradrenergic agents; however, recently all serotonergic drugs were withdrawn from the market.

Serotonergic Anorectics. The serotonergic drugs were widely prescribed in the mid-nineties. The principal representatives of this class were fenfluramine, a racemic mixture of dextro and levo fenfluramine, and dexfenfluramine, the dextro isomer alone. Both of the drugs directly stimulate serotonin release and are also serotonin reuptake inhibitors, thus providing increased stimulation at serotonergic synapses by two mechanisms. The part of the brain in which these drugs worked is not clearly understood, but there is evidence in humans and in animals that serotonergic stimulation enhances the sensation of satiety.

These drugs did reduce food intake. There was also evidence of enhanced energy expenditure and thermogenesis, at least in animals. In clinical trials lasting up to 1 year, dexfenfluramine was associated with a sustained loss of 10% of body weight in responders. However, most patients regained whatever weight was lost if the drugs were discontinued.

The fenfluramines were withdrawn from the worldwide market in 1997 because of reports of valvular heart disease associated with and presumably induced by the drugs. The mechanism for the heart valve effects is unknown. An additional serious side effect was increased risk for primary pulmonary hypertension. This rare but potentially fatal complication occurred in approximately 20–30 patients per million patients taking the drugs. The mechanism for the increased risk for pulmonary hypertension was also unknown.

Other side effects include somnolence and fatigue, diarrhea, and the potential for rebound depression when the drugs are discontinued. Serotonergic anorectics may be associated with short-term memory problems in some patients, although this has not been evaluated in a disciplined way.

Other serotonergic agents, particularly those used for management of depression, occasionally have been associated with changes in appetite and weight loss. In general, these responses are feeble and not very useful clinically.

Noradrenergic Anorectics. This select group of agents appears to act at norepinephrine synapses within the brain. Examples of this type of medication include phentermine and mazindol. This class of agent is related to earlier amphetamine anorectics. Amphetamines clearly produce a reduction in appetite and possibly an increase in energy expenditure. However, the true amphetamines are associated with unacceptable side effects such as drug dependence, and their use in obesity management is now either discouraged or illegal. The attenuated amphetamines currently available for this type of treatment do have some stimulatory side effects, but there is little or no potential for abuse.

Other Approaches to Anorectic Therapy. Sibutramine, which is not yet approved by the Food and Drug Administration (FDA), appears to have both serotonergic and noradrenergic stimulatory properties. This drug has been very potent with respect to anorexia and weight loss in animal and human trials. Whether side effects, which may include hypertension, will be acceptable in long-term treatment is not known.

There is great interest in the therapeutic potential of leptin, the protein hormone from adipose tissue which appears to signal the brain that there is enough (or too much) fat. Leptin decreases food intake and increases energy expenditure in animals. However, obese humans have high leptin levels, and their sensitivity to pharmacologic doses of leptin is unknown.

A variety of brain neurotransmitters stimulate or suppress feeding, and vigorous attempts are being made to exploit these pharmacologically. For example, attempts are being made to produce antagonists to neuropeptide Y, a brain neurotransmitter that is a major stimulator of food intake. The success of this approach has yet to be determined.

Thermogenic Agents. These agents enhance energy expenditure and thus promote weight loss without affecting appetite. Thyroid hormone in pharmacologic doses was used for this purpose in the 1960s. Treatment with thyroid hormone did produce weight loss, indicating the potential for this style of therapy, but the side effects were unacceptable. These side effects were those expected with hyperthyroidism: cardiac arrhythmias, high-output heart failure, bone loss, muscle wasting, and mental disturbances.

The pharmaceutical industry is attempting to exploit a novel adrenergic receptor, the β_3-adrenergic receptor, to enhance thermogenesis. This β_3-receptor was found originally on brown adipose tissue in animals. Humans have β_3 responsiveness, but whether this occurs in brown adipose tissue is still uncertain. Agents that stimulate the β_3-receptor with minimal stimulation of classic adrenergic receptors do appear to be thermogenic in animal and human trials. It is not clear whether the enhanced thermogenesis will lead to long-term weight loss in humans, or whether these agents are specific for the β_3-receptor so that they will not stimulate β_1- and β_2-receptors and cause cardiac dysrhythmias.

The combination of caffeine or theobromine with ephedrine was noted to cause weight loss when it was used in Europe for management of asthma. Studies indicate that these drugs are thermogenic in humans. However, they are not used for weight management in the United States at the present time.

Malabsorptive Agents. These agents prevent ingested food from being absorbed into the body. In general, these agents interfere with carbohydrate absorption or with fat absorption. The fat substitute olestra works in this way, and other compounds are being tested. The major drawback for this approach is that carbohydrates and fat that are not absorbed in the small intestine usually are metabolized by bacteria in the large bowel, resulting in flatulence, diarrhea, and cramping. Furthermore, some of these metabolites and their associated calories are absorbed from the large bowel. The potential for malabsorptive agents in the management of human obesity is undetermined.

SURGICAL TREATMENT OF OBESITY

Concerns about the safety of gastric restriction surgery (gastric stapling) and the feeling that artificial willpower is not the business of the physician have limited the acceptance of obesity surgery in the medical community. However, current evidence indicates that surgery is the best long-term method of ameliorating, not curing, medically serious obesity until better medical therapies become available.

Surgery is appropriate for selected patients with medically severe obesity.

This patient qualified for pharmacologic treatment of his obesity on the basis of his risk profile. Drugs for treating obesity are more effective when they are combined with appropriate alterations in life style. His therapy should begin with negotiation of long-term changes in his choices of food and activity. Drug treatment can be added after that. Since most people regain lost weight when drug therapy is stopped, he should be made aware that he is likely to need long-term treatment. He also should be made aware of the long-term risks of these drugs.

Case Study:
Resolution

▌REVIEW QUESTIONS

Directions: For each of the following questions, choose the **one best** answer.

1. Aggressive treatment of obesity is not completely effective and may have risks. Which of the obese patients listed below is the most likely candidate for aggressive treatment?

    (A) An older, mildly obese woman whose diets have resulted only in short-term weight loss
    (B) A young man with type 2 diabetes whose twin has morbid obesity and sleep apnea
    (C) An older man with depression whose obesity is moderate but disfiguring to him
    (D) A young woman with heartburn, whose waist-to-hip ratio (WHR) is in the 0.7–0.8 range

2. A 30-year-old woman complains of fatigue. On physical examination the physician notes the following: height, 5'6"; weight, 210 lbs; and blood pressure, 140/95 mm Hg. In the course of the evaluation, the physician remarks on the patient's weight. She states that she does not want to do anything about her weight. Which of the following facts would strengthen the physician's case that she would benefit from weight reduction?

    (A) She has a high leptin level
    (B) She has not attempted to lose weight previously
    (C) Her waist-to-hip (WHR) ratio is 1.0
    (D) There is family history of obesity

3. The attorney general asks a physician's help in evaluating the advertising of a local weight loss business. Based on current data, which of the following claims is likely to be true?

    (A) The diet used by the weight loss program increases energy expenditure by stimulating β_3-receptors and suppressing thermogenesis
    (B) The weight loss program is 85% successful in decreasing body weight by 50% and maintaining this weight loss for several years
    (C) In this weight loss program, patients lose weight due to a combination of decreased caloric intake and exercise
    (D) The weight loss program converts android (upper body) obesity into less threatening gynoid (lower body) obesity

4. A potential side effect of catecholaminergic anorectic drugs is

    (A) behavioral stimulation
    (B) chronic obstructive pulmonary disease
    (C) hypertension
    (D) pulmonary hypertension

5. A young man asks his physician for a weight loss drug because he has a body mass index (BMI) of 29, asthma, and family history of obesity. In this case, the physician should

    (A) discuss long-term diet and activity changes only
    (B) discuss risks of the drugs and prescribe a drug if the patient agrees
    (C) enroll the patient in a behavior modification program and consider surgery
    (D) recommend exercise and a very low-calorie diet

■ ANSWERS AND EXPLANATIONS

1. The answer is B. The young man with type 2 diabetes is most likely to be severely obese since his identical twin is severely obese. Comorbidities such as diabetes increase the risk that his obesity will have major medical consequences. Since the man is young, the cumulative risk posed by his obesity is increased. The other individuals have mild-to-moderate obesity or have gynoid obesity (indicated by a low WHR), which is associated with less risk of major complications than central obesity.

2. The answer is C. The patient's high WHR indicates that she has central obesity, and women with central or android obesity experience significantly increased health risks. High leptin levels are seen in obesity but have no known effect on risk. Recent studies indicate that there is no increased medical risk from repeated attempts at weight loss resulting in cycles of weight loss and regain (so-called "yo-yo" dieting). Previous history regarding weight loss attempts does not affect the physician's case. A family history of obesity relates to cause, not risk.

3. The answer is C. Diet and exercise changes are the cause of all weight loss, even when they are supported by drugs or surgical therapy. No diet can increase metabolic rate in a way that produces weight loss, and if β_3-receptors could be stimulated sufficiently by diet, thermogenesis would be increased, not decreased. No medical treatment program can claim such a high percentage of weight loss in so many people over a sustained period. Mean weight reduction in responders to current pharmacologic therapy is 10% of body weight. There is no current method of changing fat distribution short of making major changes in the gonadal hormone milieu (i.e., substituting estrogen for androgens).

4. The answer is A. Behavioral stimulation is seen with catecholaminergic anorectics but usually not with the serotonergic agents. Chronic obstructive pulmonary disease is not related to obesity or its treatment. Hypertension is seen with obesity itself but is not a side effect of catecholaminergic agents. Pulmonary hypertension is associated with fenfluramine-type serotonergic anorectics.

5. The answer is A. The medical risk of obesity at the level of BMI of 29 does not warrant the risk of a very low-calorie diet, drugs, or surgery. Asthma is not one of the comorbid conditions that would justify an increase in the level of therapy. Even if the patient developed hypertension or one of the other comorbid conditions exacerbating the risk of obesity (see Table 10-3), his level of obesity would not add a large additional risk.

■ REFERENCES

Bouchard C, Tremblay A, Despres J-P, et al: The response to long-term overfeeding in identical twins. *N Engl J Med* 322:1477–1482, 1990.

Donahue RP, Abbott RD, Bloom E, et al: Central obesity and coronary heart disease in men. *Lancet* i:821–824, 1987.

Leibel RL, Rosenbaum M, Hirsch J: Changes in energy expenditure resulting from altered weight. *N Engl J Med* 332:621–628, 1995.

Lindpainter K: Finding an obesity gene—a tale of mice and men. *N Engl J Med* 332:679–680, 1995.

Manson JE, Willett WC, Stamper MJ, et al: Body weight and mortality among women. *N Engl J Med* 332:677–685, 1995.

National Institutes of Health Technology Assessment Conference: Methods for voluntary weight loss and control. *Ann Int Med* 119:641–770, 1993.

National Task Force on the Prevention and Treatment of Obesity: Long-term pharmacotherapy in the management of obesity. *JAMA* 276:1907–1915, 1996.

Pi-Sunyer, FX: Medical hazards of obesity. *Ann Int Med* 119:655–660, 1993.

Ravussin E, Lillioja S, Knowler WC, et al: Reduced rate of energy expenditure as a risk factor for body-weight gain. *N Engl J Med* 318:467–472, 1988.

Stunkard AJ: Current views on obesity. *Am J Med* 100:230–236, 1996.

Stunkard AJ, Harris JR, Pederson NL, et al: The body-mass index of twins raised apart. *N Engl J Med* 322:1483–1487, 1990.

Chapter 11
ENDOCRINOLOGY OF MALE REPRODUCTION

Charles J. Billington, M.D.

■ CHAPTER OUTLINE

Case Study:
Introduction

The patient is a 51-year-old man who presented with impotence. He reported approximately 10 years of nearly absent sexual function with a gradual decline in erection capability before that. He has been married for 25 years, and he and his wife have no children. Although working full-time, he complained of muscular weakness and general fatigue. His history included an assortment of minor surgeries and a bout with mumps at age 21 while in the military. His examination was remarkable for markedly reduced pubic and other body hair, eunuchoid fat distribution (fat around the hips rather than around the abdomen), and very small testicles. Laboratory examination revealed a very low testosterone level and high luteinizing hormone (LH) and follicle-stimulating hormone (FSH) levels.

■ ANDROGEN FUNCTIONS

The principal effects produced by the male reproductive axis result from gonadal androgen production and action. The androgens are classic steroid hormones. They are

Androgens Produce the Male Phenotype
Male body hair pattern
Male fat pattern (central fat deposition)
More muscle
Deeper voice
Bigger bones
Acne
Male sexual behavior

Time Course of Androgen Effects
Fetus: development of internal and external genitalia
Puberty: maturation of genitalia, secondary sex characteristics, growth spurt, and epiphyseal closure
Adult: maintenance of libido, fertility, strength, and bone mass

Androgens are critical for the maintenance of fertility.

Levels of Testicular Failure (Hypogonadism)
Problem at the level of the testes—primary hypogonadism
Problem at the level of the pituitary—secondary hypogonadism
Problem at the level of the hypothalamus—tertiary hypogonadism

synthesized primarily in the testes (adrenals contribute only a small fraction in men) and travel in the circulation mostly bound to carrier proteins. The major androgen produced by the testes is testosterone, which can be converted to the more active dihydrotestosterone (DHT) in target tissues and to estradiol in adipose tissue. Approximately 60% of the testosterone in the circulation is bound to sex hormone–binding globulin (SHBG), and approximately 38% is bound to albumin. The remaining 2% is unbound. The free testosterone, plus some testosterone that dissociates from its binding proteins, can enter target cells and bind to a cytoplasmic receptor. The complex is translocated to the nucleus where interaction with DNA results in messenger RNA (mRNA) synthesis and, eventually, protein synthesis.

At various points in development, androgens produce the male phenotype: male internal genitalia, penis, scrotum and descended testicles, male pattern body hair, male fat pattern (central or intra-abdominal fat deposition), increased muscle mass, vocal cord elongation and thickening, and increases in bone mass. Androgens appear to be largely responsible for the skin changes resulting in acne. In addition, there are androgen effects on sexual behavior and on behavior in general.

The critical function of the male gonadal system, from a species perspective, is the androgen contribution to fertility and conception. Testosterone from the testes is essential for maintaining the germinal structures in which the sperm develop and mature. Hypogonadal men typically experience fertility disorders.

Once androgenization has occurred, the male phenotype tends to persist even if androgen levels decrease later. However, prolonged hypoandrogenization decreases male pattern body hair and muscle mass and may reduce the efficiency of erection, libido, and other sexual behaviors. With prolonged hypoandrogenization, the male fat pattern changes to a more female fat pattern (deposition of fat in the hips and thighs).

Impotence is another possible manifestation of androgen deficiency. Impotence is defined as the inability to achieve an erection adequate for successful intercourse. Male penile erection is a complex biologic event that is dependent on adequate arterial dilatation for blood flow into the corpora cavernosa. These events require normal neurologic and hormonal inputs to the penis and are affected by a long list of neurologic, vascular, and hormonal disorders, as well as systemic illnesses and drugs. Most impotence is multifactorial.

Hypogonadism is a prominent cause of impotence, although most impotent men are not hypogonadal and not all hypogonadal men are impotent. Impotent men should be tested for testosterone deficiency. If the cause of impotence is not obvious, they should be tested for thyroid disorders, hyperprolactinemia, and diabetes mellitus as well.

■ HYPOTHALAMIC-PITUITARY-GONADAL AXIS

The principal components of the male endocrine system—the *hypothalamic-pituitary-gonadal* (HPG) axis—are indicated in Figure 11-1. Hormone released from the hypothalamus stimulates hormone output from the anterior pituitary gland. Pituitary hormones stimulate the testes to produce testosterone, smaller amounts of other androgens, and inhibin, which elicit responses in their target tissues. Testosterone and inhibin exert negative feedback on both the pituitary gland and the hypothalamus. Pituitary hormones and input from higher centers in the central nervous system (CNS) also exert feedback on the hypothalamus. Defects at each point in the pathway illustrate the operation of that component and its contribution to the overall HPG axis.

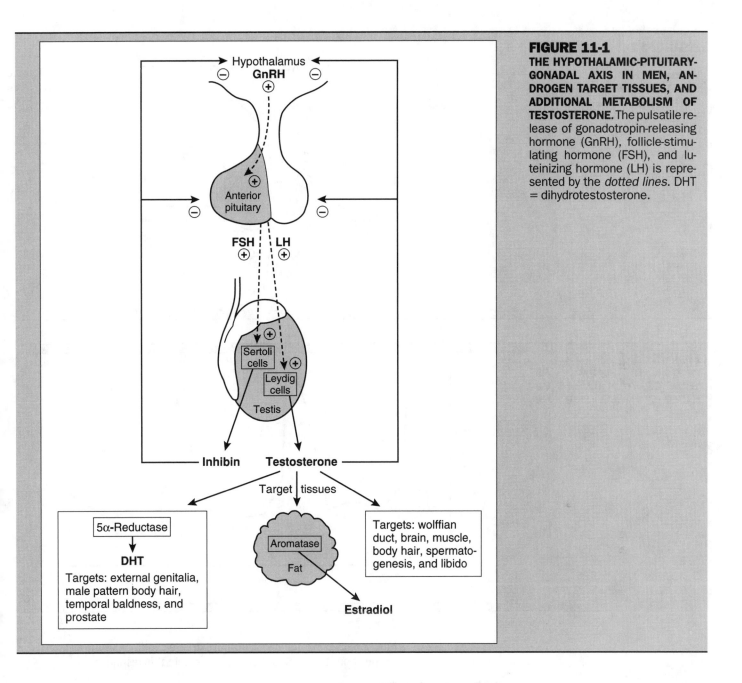

FIGURE 11-1

THE HYPOTHALAMIC-PITUITARY-GONADAL AXIS IN MEN, ANDROGEN TARGET TISSUES, AND ADDITIONAL METABOLISM OF TESTOSTERONE. The pulsatile release of gonadotropin-releasing hormone (GnRH), follicle-stimulating hormone (FSH), and luteinizing hormone (LH) is represented by the *dotted lines*. DHT = dihydrotestosterone.

■ HYPOTHALAMUS

PHYSIOLOGY

Gonadotropin-releasing hormone (GnRH), also known as luteinizing hormone–releasing hormone (LHRH), is synthesized in the hypothalamus and is secreted into the hypothalamic-pituitary portal system. Within the hypothalamus, GnRH-producing cells are located primarily in the paraventricular nucleus. These neurons are thought to receive modulatory input from other sites within the CNS, although the complete regulatory pathways have not yet been determined. Negative feedback on the hypothalamus is provided by testosterone and inhibin from the testes (Figure 11-2).

One feature of the HPG axis that deserves special mention is the hypothalamic pulse generator, which causes GnRH to be released into the hypothalamic-pituitary portal system in bursts. Pulsatile GnRH elicits pulsatile release of the gonadotropins LH and FSH from the anterior pituitary. Frequent sampling of GnRH from the pituitary portal system would reveal a pattern of serum concentrations like that shown in Figure 11-3. Men lacking normal pulse frequency or amplitude may be hypogonadal or infertile.

Hypothalamic gonadotropin–releasing hormone must be secreted in pulses to be effective. Pulses are secreted every 90–120 minutes.

FIGURE 11-2
THE HYPOTHALAMIC-PITUITARY LEVEL OF THE HYPOTHALAMIC-PITUITARY-GONADAL AXIS IN MEN. The pulsatile release of gonadotropin-releasing hormone (GnRH), follicle-stimulating hormone (FSH), and luteinizing hormone (LH) is represented by the *dotted lines*.

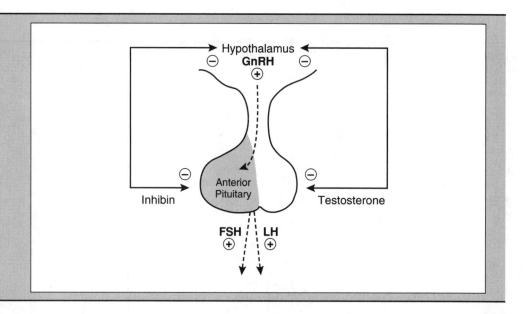

FIGURE 11-3
PATTERN OF PULSATILE RELEASE OF HYPOTHALAMIC GONADOTROPIN–RELEASING HORMONE.

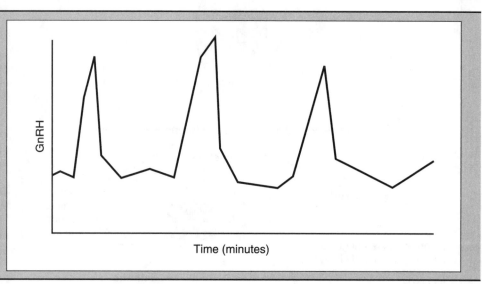

The HPG axis is functionally down-regulated during extreme conditions such as starvation or severe illness. Input from the CNS is thought to mediate this response.

HYPOTHALAMIC DEFECTS

Congenital abnormalities of the hypothalamus result in absent or defective GnRH or in abnormal GnRH pulses. Kallman's syndrome is the combination of congenital hypogonadotropic hypogonadism resulting from deficient GnRH production and an absent or defective sense of smell.

Acquired hypothalamic defects can be caused by tumors such as craniopharyngioma or metastatic tumors, injury from head trauma or radiation therapy, inflammation resulting from sarcoidosis, or infection such as tuberculosis. Severe illness and weight loss below the critical level needed to maintain the hypothalamic pulse generator also result in GnRH deficiency.

Manifestations of Hypothalamic Disorders. GnRH levels outside of the hypothalamic-pituitary portal system are too low to measure reliably. Defects at the hypothalamic level result in low or low-normal gonadotropin (LH and FSH) levels and low testosterone production. These "low-normal" gonadotropin values are inappropriately low, considering that testosterone feedback is missing. If the response to feedback mechanisms truly were normal, FSH and LH would be high in the presence of low testosterone.

Major Causes of Hypothalamic Defects

Congenital abnormalities
Starvation or severe illness
Tumors (craniopharyngioma, metastatic tumors)
Head trauma
Inflammation (sarcoidosis)
Infection
Radiation therapy

Defects at the hypothalamic level lower all hormones of the HPG axis.

The clinical consequences depend upon whether the hypogonadism is complete or partial and whether the onset occurs prenatally, before puberty, or after puberty.

Treatment Directed at the Hypothalamic Level. Full treatment, which includes restoring fertility, involves administration of pulsatile GnRH by a pump. GnRH cannot be given orally because peptide hormones are digested in the gastrointestinal tract. If it is not necessary to restore fertility, patients usually are treated with testosterone. Patients with inadequate GnRH pulses due to severe illness or weight loss respond to treatment of the underlying disease and to weight gain.

Administration of GnRH continuously results in down-regulation of pituitary LH and FSH secretion. This property has been exploited clinically. Long-acting *GnRH agonists* are used to produce chemical castration in men with prostate cancer because prostate cancer is androgen dependent. GnRH agonists also are used to treat central precocious puberty (see Chapter 14).

GnRH antagonists have been developed for use in many of the same situations. The antagonists may lower gonadotropin levels more effectively than the long-acting agonists. A combination of a GnRH antagonist and testosterone has the potential for functioning as a male contraceptive. The GnRH antagonist turns off spermatogenesis, which requires FSH, while the testosterone component preserves libido and potency.

The patient has obvious symptoms (muscle weakness, fatigue) and signs (impotence, reduced pubic and other body hair, female-type distribution of body fat, small testicles) of androgen deficiency. This was confirmed by his low level of testosterone. His history is compatible with infertility as well. He has no features suggesting that his androgen deficiency is due to an abnormality at the level of the hypothalamus. He has no history of trauma or irradiation. There is no history of headache or fever to suggest an enlarging central tumor or a central inflammatory process. He had normal sexual function until sometime in his 30s, which makes a congenital syndrome like Kallman's syndrome unlikely. The patient's elevated gonadotropin levels confirm his testicular failure and also indicate that his hypothalamus is functioning.

Case Study:
Continued

▍PITUITARY

PHYSIOLOGY

The gonadotropins LH and FSH are released from anterior pituitary gonadotroph cells in response to pulsatile stimulation by GnRH (Figure 11-2). LH and FSH are named for their actions on the ovary during the menstrual cycle. The structure of these hormones is the same in both sexes, and they function as trophic hormones for the gonads in both sexes. In men, these hormones stimulate the testes to produce testosterone and inhibin. Negative feedback provided by the testicular hormones regulates LH and FSH secretion.

PITUITARY DEFECTS

Pituitary cells secreting gonadotropins are very sensitive to damage, so FSH and LH secretion often is lost before thyroid-stimulating hormone (TSH) and adrenocorticotropic hormone (ACTH) secretion. HPG axis function frequently is lost when normal pituitary tissue is compressed by a pituitary adenoma, a craniopharyngioma, or a metastatic tumor. Prolactin-producing pituitary tumors are particularly likely to interfere with the HPG axis because prolactin inhibits LH and FSH release by suppressing the hypothalamic GnRH pulse generator.

The pituitary is very susceptible to damage by chronic meningitis, because it is located at the base of the brain. Tuberculosis and fungal infections also cause pituitary failure. Chronic inflammation due to arteritis or sarcoidosis, infiltrative disorders such as hemochromatosis, trauma from a basilar skull fracture, and radiation exposure when radiation treatment is given for other disorders are other causes of gonadotropin production.

It is very rare for a pituitary adenoma to oversecrete functional gonadotropins. Some adenomas secrete the α-subunit, which is common to both FSH and LH, but this is not active without the β-subunit.

Major Causes of Pituitary Defects
Tumors (pituitary adenoma, craniopharyngioma, metastatic tumors)
Inflammation (sarcoidosis, arteritis)
Infection
Infiltration (hemochromatosis)
Infarction
Trauma
Radiation therapy

Defects at the pituitary level lower plasma concentrations of FSH, LH, and testosterone.

Manifestations of Pituitary Disorders. Defects at the pituitary level result in secondary hypogonadism, with either low or inappropriately "normal" gonadotropin levels and low testosterone. As with hypothalamic lesions, clinical consequences depend upon whether the hypogonadism is complete or partial and the time of onset (prenatally, before puberty, or after puberty). A prolactin level should be measured if a pituitary disorder is suspected. If pituitary damage is extensive, patients also may have symptoms and signs of hypothyroidism (see Chapter 3), adrenal insufficiency (see Chapter 5), or both as a result of a lack of TSH and ACTH.

Treatment Directed at the Pituitary Level. If fertility is not a concern, men with secondary hypogonadism can be treated with testosterone. Men who are seeking fertility can be treated with episodic injections of gonadotropins. The usual preparation used is human chorionic gonadotropin (HCG), a placental hormone with a structure and actions similar to those of LH. HCG may be augmented with human menopausal gonadotropin (HMG), a mixture of LH and FSH.

Case Study:
Continued

This patient's laboratory values were not consistent with an abnormality at the pituitary level. The pituitary gland should respond to lack of negative feedback from testosterone by increasing output of LH and FSH, and the patient's high gonadotropin levels indicate that his pituitary gland was responding normally.

▌TESTICLES

PHYSIOLOGY

In the testes, LH acts on Leydig cells to stimulate testosterone production. FSH stimulates Sertoli cells to produce androgen-binding protein, which binds some of the testosterone. FSH also stimulates inhibin secretion from Sertoli cells. Inhibin, in turn, regulates FSH secretion by negative feedback (Figure 11-4). FSH and high local concentrations of testosterone are necessary for spermatogenesis and fertility, but libido and sexual performance respond only to testosterone. The mass of Leydig cells is small. Most of the testicular volume is made up of seminiferous tubules, which contain the maturing sperm, the germinal epithelium, and the Sertoli cells. Small testes generally indicate a deficiency in these elements.

FIGURE 11-4
ACTION OF PITUITARY GONADOTROPINS ON THEIR TARGET CELLS WITHIN THE TESTES. The pulsatile release of follicle-stimulating hormone (FSH) and luteinizing hormone (LH) is represented by the *dotted lines*.

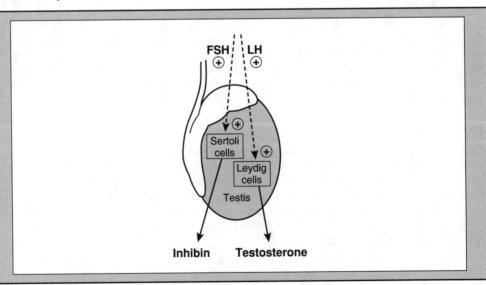

TESTICULAR DEFECTS

Developmental disorders such as Klinefelter's syndrome (47,XXY male) [see Chapters 13 and 14], other types of gonadal dysgenesis, cryptorchidism (testes fail to descend into the scrotum), gonadotropin resistance due to abnormal LH receptors or Leydig cell failure, enzymatic defects of testosterone synthesis, and myotonic dystrophy all result in primary hypogonadism.

Acquired testicular disorders cause primary hypogonadism by several mechanisms. Testicular tumors can damage testicles directly. Hypogonadism also can occur as a result of chemotherapy or radiation treatment. Testicles are more susceptible to trauma than many organs because of their exposed location. Testicular torsion results in twisting of the artery supplying the testicle. Some viral infections, especially mumps in a postpubescent man, and bacterial infections can produce orchitis (inflammation of the testes) severe enough to produce hypogonadism. Orchitis also can be caused by autoimmune disease. Hypogonadism associated with an episode of orchitis may not become manifest until years later.

Men do not have an abrupt decline in Leydig cell function with age equivalent to menopause in women in the absence of illness or testicular trauma. In healthy men, testosterone levels decline gradually with age, and free testosterone levels may fall by 40%; however, levels still remain within the normal range. Men whose aging changes are more severe can develop hypogonadism.

Manifestations of Testicular Disease. Testicular defects result in low testosterone levels. LH and FSH levels are high because the pituitary is no longer suppressed by negative feedback. As with hypothalamic and pituitary disorders, symptoms and signs depend on the degree of androgen deficiency.

If congenital disorders are partial or worsen slowly, early development can be normal. Men with Klinefelter's syndrome develop normally until puberty, when the testes fail. The increase in LH and FSH cannot elicit adequate Leydig cell testosterone synthesis or seminiferous tubule and germ cell development (see Chapters 13 and 14), and LH and FSH remain high. The testes remain small and become fibrotic. Body hair and external genitalia mature to varying degrees. Since the phenotype is so variable, a karyotype is required to confirm the diagnosis. Gynecomastia (breast tissue), impotence, and infertility are common complaints. Men who go untreated develop osteopenia because they produce too little testosterone to maintain bone mass.

In men whose aging changes are severe enough to produce hypogonadism, testosterone levels are low or low-normal. LH levels can be high but often remain within the normal range, possibly at somewhat higher levels than before.

Treatment of Gonadal Disorders. Most men with testicular failure are treated with testosterone. Testosterone replacement can restore libido and sexual function, increase muscle mass, reduce fatigue, and maintain bone mass. Testosterone contributes to the pubertal growth spurt in boys but also causes closure of the epiphyses. Therefore, boys who develop gonadal failure before puberty usually are not treated with testosterone until they are around 13 years old, to avoid premature epiphyseal closure resulting in short stature.

Androgen therapy is contraindicated in some men with prostate hyperplasia and in men with prostate cancer. Androgen replacement therapy does not cause prostate cancer but stimulates growth of hormone-sensitive cancers already present.

Major Causes of Testicular Defects
Developmental disorders
Tumors
Orchitis (infection, autoimmunity)
Chemotherapy
Radiation therapy

Testicular defects result in low testosterone with high gonadotropin levels.

The patient most likely has a testicular abnormality. His testosterone level was low, and his gonadotropin levels were high, indicating an unsuccessful attempt by the hypothalamic-pituitary system to correct his hypogonadism. This patient's hypogonadism was most likely due to orchitis caused by his mumps infection many years before. He also might have Klinefelter's syndrome or another form of gonadal dysgenesis. In some cases, adolescent males with Klinefelter's syndrome have normal pubertal development with testicular failure manifested later. A karyotype would be necessary to confirm this diagnosis.

Case Study:
Continued

ANDROGEN TARGET TISSUES

PHYSIOLOGY

Testosterone versus DHT
Both bind to the same androgen receptor.
Testosterone is required for the development of internal genitalia: epididymis and seminal vesicles.
DHT has greater receptor affinity and more androgen effect.
DHT is required for the development of external genitalia (penis, scrotum, prostate).

Two types of androgen target tissues exist—those that respond primarily to testosterone and those that require 5α-reductase action to convert testosterone to DHT for normal androgen action. Examples of these two types of tissue are shown in Figure 11-5. Testosterone and DHT bind to the same androgen receptor. DHT has much greater affinity for the androgen receptor than does testosterone, so tissues possessing an active reductase system show greater androgen effect.

Androgens such as testosterone can also be converted to estrogen. This requires the aromatase enzyme, which is found in adipose tissue. Much of the estrogen found in men is thought to be derived from this pathway. Estrogens can exert negative feedback on the hypothalamus and pituitary.

FIGURE 11-5
TESTOSTERONE ACTION. Note the enzymatic conversion of testosterone to dihydrotestosterone (DHT) and estrogen and the actions of DHT.

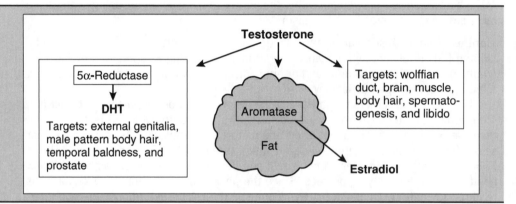

ANDROGEN TARGET TISSUE DEFECTS

The most dramatic target tissue disorders result from gene mutations that reduce androgen receptor function or reduce the efficiency of 5α-reductase so that conversion of testosterone to the more potent androgen, DHT, is decreased.

Excess conversion of testosterone to estrogen by the aromatase enzyme in men with excess adipose tissue is the most common target tissue abnormality. Although their testosterone levels remain much higher than their estrogen levels, these men show extra estrogen effects because the ratio of estrogen to androgen is increased above the normal range.

Fates of Testosterone in Target Tissues
Interacts directly with androgen receptors
Converted to DHT (requires 5α-reductase)
Converted to estradiol (requires aromatase)

Gene mutations resulting in loss of aromatase (loss of estrogen synthesis) or nonfunctional estrogen receptors (loss of estrogen action) were thought always to be lethal until recently. A man with a mutation in the estrogen receptor gene, who was totally resistant to estrogen, was described in 1994. His estrogen levels were high, but he was not able to respond to endogenous or exogenous estrogen. A man without functional aromatase was identified in 1995. His plasma estrogen levels were very low, but he responded to exogenous estrogen because his estrogen receptors were normal.

Manifestations of Target Tissue Defects. Clinical manifestations of abnormal androgen action can be dramatic. Men with a severe deficit or defect in androgen receptors are phenotypic females; this disorder is called "testicular feminization." They have high gonadotropin levels because the abnormal receptors in the pituitary cannot recognize testosterone feedback. Testosterone levels are high because the testes respond appropriately to high gonadotropin levels. Estrogen levels are high because the excess testosterone is converted to estrogen by aromatase in adipose tissue. This leads to breast development. These men have female external genitalia, a vagina ending in a blind pouch, and no internal genitalia except testes. They have sparse body hair because development of body hair depends on androgen action. Milder defects result in an androgynous phenotype (see Chapters 13 and 14).

A child with 5α-reductase deficiency appears female or has ambiguous external

Androgen Target Tissue Disorders
Androgen receptor deficiency
5α-Reductase deficiency
Gynecomastia
Aromatase deficiency
Estrogen receptor deficiency

genitalia at birth. A blind vaginal pouch is present. LH, FSH, and testosterone levels are near normal, and the internal genitalia develop normally. DHT levels are low, so masculinization of the external genitalia is incomplete. At puberty the level of testosterone rises dramatically. Secondary male sex characteristics develop, and the external genitalia become masculinized (see Chapters 13 and 14). The ratio of DHT to testosterone remains abnormally low. Affected individuals do not have acne or male pattern balding, and body hair is reduced. In areas where this genetic defect is common, a change from female to male gender identity at the time of puberty is accepted surprisingly well.

Gynecomastia is common in men of all ages, especially during puberty (see Chapter 14) and in men who are obese. True gynecomastia refers to the presence of firm ductal tissue under the areola; gynecomastia does not refer to fat in the breast area. Benign gynecomastia can be unilateral. LH, FSH, and testosterone levels in most men with gynecomastia are normal. Their estrogen levels are within the normal range but are thought to be increased relative to testosterone levels. The abnormality may be subtle.

Hypogonadal men who have low testosterone levels also have relatively increased estrogen levels, especially if they are obese. These men often have gynecomastia. Other causes of gynecomastia include drugs such as cimetidine, spironolactone, and flutamide, which are androgen-receptor blockers; hyperprolactinemia, which suppresses the hypothalamic pulse generator and decreases LH production; and some systemic diseases. Testicular tumors and feminizing adrenal tumors can cause gynecomastia, but these are rare.

The men described above with the aromatase and estrogen receptor mutations have normal adult male sexual development. They have normal or high testosterone levels, and yet their FSH and LH levels are high. This indicates that estrogen action is necessary for normal feedback inhibition of pituitary gonadotrophs in men. The young men with these conditions are very tall, with unfused epiphyses, low bone density, and high bone turnover characteristic of osteoporosis. Estrogen apparently is necessary for normal bone maturation in men as well as in women.

Treatment of Target Tissue Defects. Defects in reductase activity usually produce their most serious effects in utero. Full treatment would require prenatal diagnosis and a fetal DHT delivery system (or gene therapy), which is not available. If the disorder is recognized, and early gender assignment is male, infants are treated with surgery and testosterone to increase the size of the phallus. If the gender assignment is female, orchiectomy is performed, and estrogen treatment is given.

There is no therapy that restores androgen receptors. In individuals with testicular feminization, the phenotype and gender assignment are female. The testes must be removed because malignancy is likely to arise in intra-abdominal testes. Estrogen treatment is given so that secondary sexual characteristics develop.

Gynecomastia usually is asymptomatic and benign, needing no treatment except stopping the causative agent if possible. Weight loss may help, since estrogen is produced from androgens in adipose tissue. Testosterone-deficient men are treated with testosterone. If gynecomastia is painful, unilateral, and not centrally located under the nipple or develops rapidly, a mammogram should be obtained to rule out malignancy.

The patient has clear evidence of a major defect in androgen production, not a defect in androgen action. It is interesting to note that he did not have gynecomastia, even though he had a very low level of testosterone and his plasma estrogen level could be increased relative to his testosterone level. If he has a severe testicular defect, there might not be enough androgen to be aromatized to estrogen for breast development.

Case Study:
Continued

PHARMACOLOGIC TREATMENT WITH ANDROGENS AND ANTIANDROGENS

TESTOSTERONE REPLACEMENT THERAPY

Primary, secondary, and tertiary hypogonadism are usually treated with testosterone replacement.

Testosterone cannot be given orally because it is degraded quickly as it passes through the liver. 17α-Alkylated testosterone derivatives are active when given orally, but they cause liver toxicity. 17β-Testosterone esters, such as testosterone enanthate and testosterone cypionate, are less water soluble and have a much longer duration of action. These testosterone esters can be given intramuscularly at 2–3-week intervals. This often results in peak plasma levels above the normal range initially and trough levels below the normal range later.

Testosterone can be delivered more uniformly in transdermal patches, even though testosterone absorption across the skin is limited. Scrotal patches take advantage of thinner skin there. Scrotal patches produce normal testosterone and estradiol levels, but DHT levels are higher than normal because testosterone is converted to DHT in scrotal skin. The effects of high DHT levels on the prostate are not known. Larger testosterone patches applied to nonscrotal skin provide normal testosterone, DHT, and estradiol levels, but skin reactions to these patches can be a problem. Testosterone pellets, which are planted subcutaneously, provide normal testosterone, DHT, and estradiol levels for several months. They rarely are used in the United States because of the need for implantation and because pellets can be extruded spontaneously. More physiologic, sustained-release testosterone esters, implantable testosterone microspheres, and sublingual testosterone are being tested.

Testosterone causes increased growth of body hair and can cause acne and fluid retention resulting in leg edema. Whether testosterone replacement causes significant lowering of high-density lipoprotein (HDL) cholesterol in hypogonadal men is not known.

The prostate must be monitored in men given testosterone replacement therapy. A hemoglobin level should be monitored, especially in men likely to have hypoxemia (smokers and men with chronic obstructive lung disease or sleep apnea), because testosterone also stimulates synthesis of erythropoietin.

ANABOLIC USES OF ANDROGENS

Androgens cause nitrogen retention, increase protein synthesis, increase muscle mass, and stabilize bone mass in hypogonadal men. It is not clear whether androgens, alone or in combination with another anabolic hormone such as growth hormone, would benefit men with muscle wasting or bone loss due to underlying diseases or aging.

Androgens are used by athletes who are not hypogonadal. They hope to increase their muscle mass and strength to supranormal levels. These men usually use some form of testosterone or a testosterone derivative. In most cases, the doses used are several orders of magnitude higher than replacement doses of testosterone. The high doses suppress the hypothalamus and pituitary, which can lead to a low sperm count or testicular atrophy or both. Liver diseases, including tumors, have been reported in association with this abuse.

ANTIANDROGEN THERAPY

Antiandrogen Therapy at the Target Tissue Level
Androgen receptor blockers
5α-Reductase inhibitors

In some clinical situations the goal is to block androgen action at the target tissue level with antiandrogen therapy. Flutamide is an androgen receptor blocker that is used in the treatment of prostate cancer. Cyproterone acetate, another androgen receptor inhibitor, is not available in the United States. Finasteride, an inhibitor of 5α-reductase, is being evaluated for treatment of prostate cancer and benign prostatic hypertrophy. Finasteride inhibits DHT production, but plasma testosterone is maintained. It is hoped that 5α-reductase blockade can reduce prostate tissue without adverse effects on libido, sexual function, or bone mass.

TREATMENT OF IMPOTENCE

Impotence due to hypogonadism can be treated with testosterone replacement. Drugs causing or contributing to impotence (e.g., alcohol, opiates, spironolactone, estrogens, antihypertensive drugs, including diuretics and β-blockers, many antidepressants, antiandrogens) should be stopped if possible. Impotence caused by neurologic or vascular disorders, that impair blood flow to the penis can be treated with vasoactive drugs, such as intracavernous or intraurethral prostaglandin E_1 or a combination of intracavernous papaverine and phentolamine. Other treatments include vacuum devices that produce engorgement of the penis by reducing the surrounding pressure and surgically implanted penile prostheses.

The patient's testicular failure was treated with testosterone. This resulted in increased muscle mass and strength, a more typical male fat pattern, increased libido, and restoration of potency. He also developed mild acne and increased pubic and other body hair. He began to shave every day instead of once a week. He was happy with these results.

Fertility was not attainable in this patient. His testicles were very small, indicating that there was not enough testicular tissue to respond to gonadotropins.

Case Study:
Resolution

■ REVIEW QUESTIONS

Directions: For each of the following questions, choose the **one best** answer.

1. A 20-year-old man complains of lack of energy and impotence. He has little beard growth or body hair. Laboratory evaluation reveals a low testosterone level and high levels of luteinizing hormone (LH) and follicle-stimulating hormone (FSH). This patient is most likely to have

   (A) sarcoidosis of the hypothalamus
   (B) craniopharyngioma compressing the pituitary
   (C) history of head trauma
   (D) Klinefelter's syndrome (47,XXY)
   (E) congenital hypogonadotropic hypogonadism

2. A man presents to the clinic with impotence, decreased libido, listlessness, and muscular weakness. His laboratory examination shows low testosterone levels and low gonadotropin levels. This picture is consistent with a history of

   (A) finasteride use for prostate enlargement
   (B) mumps orchitis
   (C) prostate cancer treatment with androgen receptor blockade
   (D) pituitary tumor
   (E) Klinefelter's syndrome (47,XXY)

3. A medical researcher finds a new potent and long-lasting gonadotropin-releasing hormone (GnRH) agonist. Which of the following hormone patterns is consistent with the effects of this drug?

   (A) Low testosterone and low-to-normal gonadotropins
   (B) High testosterone and low-to-normal gonadotropins
   (C) Low testosterone and high gonadotropins
   (D) High testosterone and high gonadotropins

4. During a clinical trial of drug xx, many subjects have developed gynecomastia. The medical researcher's review indicates that many men treated with the drug have elevated testosterone associated with elevated levels of luteinizing hormone (LH) and follicle-stimulating hormone (FSH). Which of the following is consistent with this finding?

   (A) Drug xx activates the androgen receptor
   (B) Drug xx blocks the androgen receptor
   (C) Drug xx activates the estrogen receptor
   (D) Drug xx blocks the estrogen receptor

5. A physician who sees a patient with malnutrition would expect which of the following laboratory results?

   (A) Increased testosterone and decreased luteinizing hormone (LH)
   (B) Increased testosterone and increased LH
   (C) Decreased testosterone and decreased LH
   (D) Decreased testosterone and increased LH

■ ANSWERS AND EXPLANATIONS

1. The answer is D. Klinefelter's syndrome is a genetic disorder resulting in premature testicular failure. The hypothalamic and pituitary responses to low testosterone are normal so laboratory testing reveals high gonadotropin levels. In each of the other disorders, LH and FSH levels would be low because of a defect at the hypothalamic or pituitary level. Congenital hypogonadotropic hypogonadism coupled with anosmia (a defective sense of smell) is known as Kallman's syndrome.

2. The answer is D. With all axis hormones low, it is important to look for a hypothalamic or pituitary cause of the hypogonadism. Finasteride is a 5α-reductase inhibitor that blocks dihydrotestosterone synthesis in androgen target tissues. It would not interfere with hormones of the hypothalamic-pituitary-gonadal (HPG) axis. Mumps orchitis in adults causes premature testicular failure and low testosterone levels, but pituitary gonadotropin levels would be high. Androgen receptor blockade would result in high follicle-stimulating hormone (FSH), luteinizing hormone (LH), and testosterone. Klinefelter's syndrome also results in testicular failure with high gonadotropin levels.

3. The answer is A. Pulsatile release of GnRH is critical. A long-acting agonist of GnRH would down-regulate the system. LH and FSH levels would be suppressed, resulting in low testosterone levels.

4. The answer is B. When all axis hormone levels are high, target tissues, including the regulatory areas in hypothalamus and pituitary, are not getting an adequate androgen signal. Androgen receptor blockade is a way to acquire such a condition. The study subjects developed gynecomastia because they had high levels of testosterone that could be converted to estrogen by aromatase in peripheral tissues. Patients with testicular feminization who have deficient or defective androgen receptors due to a genetic defect have a similar hormone profile and have a female phenotype, including breast development.

5. The answer is C. In malnutrition or severe illness, the input from the central nervous system down-regulates the entire axis by suppressing normal pulses of GnRH from the hypothalamus.

■ REFERENCES

Bhasin S, Bremner W: Emerging issues in androgen replacement therapy. *J Clin Endocrinol Metab* 82:3–8, 1997.

Bhasin S, Storer TW, Berman N, et al: The effects of supraphysiologic doses of testosterone on muscle size and strength in normal men. *N Engl J Med* 335:1–7, 1996.

Braunstein GD: Gynecomastia. *N Engl J Med* 328:490–495, 1993.

Bulin SE: Aromatase deficiency in women and men: would you have predicted the phenotypes? *J Clin Endocrinol Metab* 81:867–871, 1996.

Ghusn HF, Cunningham GR: Evaluation and treatment of androgen deficiency in males. *Endocrinologist* 1:399–408, 1991.

Howard SS: Treatment of male infertility. *N Engl J Med* 332:312–316, 1995.

Quigley CA, de Bellis A, Marschke KB, et al: Androgen receptor defects: historical, clinical and molecular perspectives. *Endocr Rev* 16:271–321, 1995.

Rogol AD, Yesalis CE: Anabolic-androgenic steroids and athletes: what are the issues? *J Clin Endocrinol Metab* 74:465–469, 1992.

Smith EP, Boyd J, Frank GR, et al: Estrogen resistance caused by a mutation in the estrogen-receptor gene in a man. *N Engl J Med*. 331:1056–1060, 1994. (See also the accompanying editorial on pages 1088–1089.)

Spratt DI, Finkelstein JS, O'Dea L StL, et al: Long-term administration of gonadotropin-releasing hormone in men with idiopathic hypogonadotropic hypogonadism. A model for studies of the hormone's physiologic effects. *Ann Intern Med* 105:848–855, 1986.

Vermeulen A: Androgens in the aging male. *J Clin Endocrinol Metab* 73:221–224, 1991.

Chapter 12

ENDOCRINOLOGY OF FEMALE REPRODUCTION

Virginia R. Lupo, M.D., and Catherine B. Niewoehner, M.D.

■ CHAPTER OUTLINE

Case Study:
Introduction

J. Martin is a 22-year-old woman who came to the clinic because she had not had a menstrual period for 2 years. A long-distance runner on her college cross-country running team, this young woman was concerned because a recent x-ray of an injured left foot revealed several old stress fractures and loss of bone mineralization throughout her foot. She has always been healthy and active. She experienced menarche at the age of 13, and her periods were regular, occurring every 28 days, until she began training for a marathon 3 years ago. Her menses ceased for several months but resumed again after the marathon. Six months later she began her long-distance running again, and her menses ceased. She has a good appetite but maintains her weight with low-fat foods. She has not been sexually active during the past year. Her mother had autoimmune hypothyroidism and experienced menopause early. Her father and sister are well.

Physical examination revealed that her height was 5'6", and her weight was 98 lbs. Four years earlier her weight was 118 lbs. Breast development and body hair distribution were normal. Her pelvic examination was normal except for vaginal dryness and an atrophic vaginal mucosa. Cervical mucus was decreased and did not fern.

HYPOTHALAMIC-PITUITARY-OVARIAN HORMONE SYSTEM

The cyclic rise and fall of hormones resulting in ovulation and the potential for pregnancy each month is the result of intricately coordinated hormone secretion by the hypothalamus, pituitary, and ovaries, and the responses of the reproductive tract to these hormones (Figure 12-1).

FIGURE 12-1
HYPOTHALAMIC-PITUITARY-OVARIAN AXIS AND THE UTERUS. The uterus is the target organ for ovarian hormones. Most of the time, high levels of estrogen and progesterone inhibit follicle-stimulating hormone (FSH) and luteinizing hormone (LH) secretion by negative feedback. However, there is a period during the first half of the menstrual cycle when estrogen exerts positive feedback. GnRH = gonadotropin-releasing hormone.

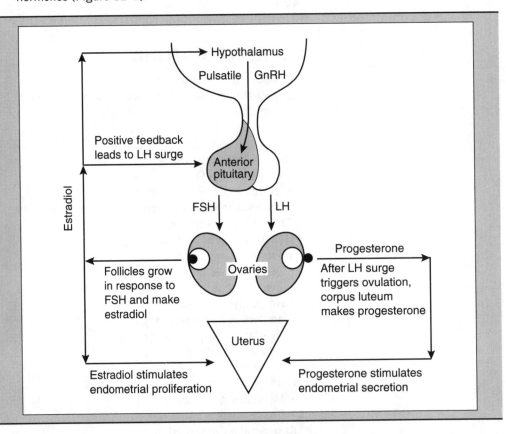

Variations in GnRH pulsatility determine whether the pituitary releases primarily FSH or LH into the general circulation.

HYPOTHALAMIC HORMONE SECRETION

The hypothalamic hormone regulating the pituitary-ovarian axis is gonadotropin-releasing hormone (GnRH), a 10–amino acid peptide synthesized in the arcuate nucleus of the medial-basal hypothalamus and in the preoptic area of the ventral hypothalamus. GnRH is transported by a network of portal veins to the anterior pituitary, where it binds to cell membrane receptors on the gonadotropin-producing cells (gonadotrophs) [see Chapter 2]. GnRH regulates the synthesis and release of the gonadotropins, follicle-stimulating hormone (FSH), and luteinizing hormone (LH). GnRH secretion is pulsatile, and GnRH action depends on the frequency and amplitude of these pulses.

Native GnRH has a half-life of several minutes, but substitutions of the amino acid at the sixth position markedly prolong the half-life of GnRH. Modification of other amino acids produces GnRH agonists or antagonists. Agonists increase gonadotropin secretion if they are administered in a pulsatile fashion, but sustained administration downregulates GnRH receptors, and release of FSH and LH is suppressed.

PITUITARY HORMONE SECRETION

FSH and LH are glycoprotein hormones produced in the gonadotrophs of the anterior pituitary. They have a common alpha chain, which is shared by another anterior pituitary hormone, thyroid-stimulating hormone (TSH), and by human chorionic gonadotropin (HCG), which is produced by the placenta during pregnancy. Each hormone has a unique beta chain, which binds to a specific receptor and accounts for the characteristic action of the hormone. The beta chains of LH and HCG are similar, but the beta chain of HCG is distinguished by a carboxy terminal tail of 24 extra amino acids. FSH and LH are secreted into the circulation in pulses in response to pulsatile secretion of GnRH. They stimulate production of ovarian hormones.

OVARIAN HORMONE SECRETION

Estrogen and progesterone are the major hormones secreted by the ovary in response to FSH and LH stimulation. Synthetic pathways for these steroid hormones are shown in Figure 12-2. The ovarian stromal cells also produce androgens in response to LH stimulation. Some ovarian androgens are secreted into the circulation, but most are converted to estrogens in the ovarian granulosa cells. The most active estrogen is estradiol, which is derived from testosterone by the enzymatic action of aromatase (see Figure 12-2). Since conversion of androgens to estrogens also occurs in adipose tissue, obese women often have higher estrogen levels than lean women.

Ovarian steroid hormones travel in the circulation mostly bound to carrier proteins. All of the hormones bind to albumin, but one-third of estrogen is bound to sex hormone–binding globulin (SHBG). The most active androgens, testosterone and dihydrotestosterone (DHT), are bound primarily to SHBG. Only the small fraction of free hormone is active.

Estrogen and progesterone have wide-ranging effects on tissues and metabolic processes. The major effects of these hormones are listed in Tables 12-1 and 12-2. Circulating estrogen and progesterone concentrations also regulate GnRH pulses and FSH and LH secretion by the pituitary, as described below. Ovarian androgens increase strength and libido and contribute to hair growth.

Table 12-1
Major Actions of Estrogens

Pubertal growth spurt	Maintain normal vasculature
Closing of epiphyses at puberty	Decrease bone resorption
Pubertal maturation of uterus and vagina	Reduce bowel motility
Proliferation of endometrial lining	Increase blood clotting factors
Breast development	Increase blood coagulation
Pigmentation of breasts and pubic area	Increase HDL cholesterol
Female distribution of body fat	Increase triglyceride turnover
Influence libido	Increase hepatic-binding protein synthesis
Maintain normal skin	Increase renin substrate

Note. HDL = high-density lipoprotein.

The ovaries also produce growth factors and polypeptide hormones such as inhibins, activins, and relaxin. They affect pituitary hormone secretion (inhibin decreases FSH secretion, and activin increases FSH secretion) and modulate hormone action. Their physiologic roles are not well understood.

Table 12-2
Major Actions of Progesterone

Breast development
Endometrial gland development
Maintains uterus during pregnancy
Inhibits lactation during pregnancy
Contributes to insulin resistance
Increases body temperature
Increases minute ventilation
Competes with aldosterone

■ NORMAL MENSTRUAL CYCLE

During childhood, the hypothalamus and the pituitary gland are very sensitive to negative feedback by circulating estrogen, and LH and FSH concentrations are low. As puberty approaches, this no longer is true (see Chapter 14). GnRH pulses increase in frequency and amplitude, and FSH and LH secretion rises. As puberty advances, the interplay between hypothalamic, pituitary, and ovarian hormones results in the series of events in the ovary and endometrium known as the menstrual cycle (Figure 12-3).

EVENTS IN THE OVARY

The ovary is composed primarily of three types of cells: germ cells (eggs or ova), squamous epithelial cells (granulosa cells), and stromal cells (theca cells). All of the ova that a

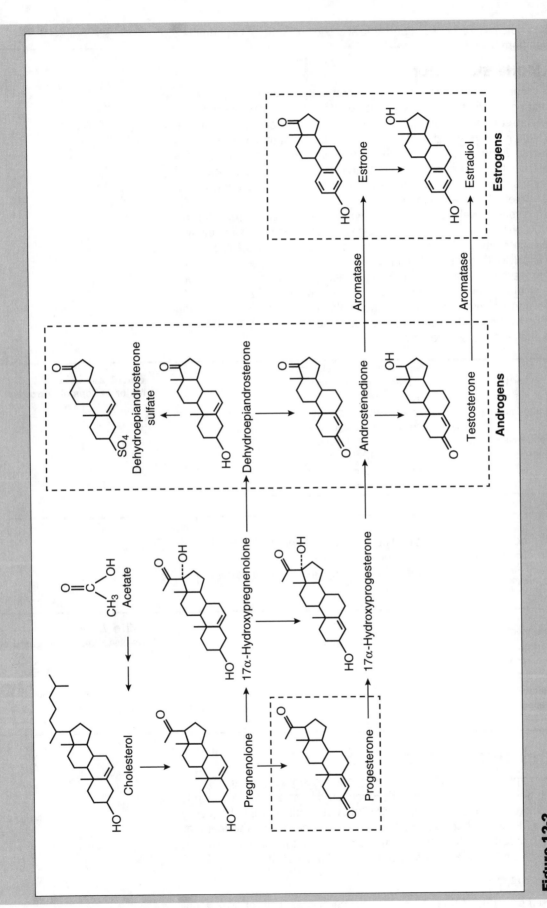

Figure 12-2

PATHWAYS OF OVARIAN STEROID HORMONE SYNTHESIS. Although pathways are shown as unidirectional for simplicity, steps from pregnenolone forward are reversible. The enzyme aromatase converts androgens into estrogens. Androgens also are converted to estrogens in peripheral tissues, especially adipose tissue. Testosterone is converted into the more active dihydrotestosterone by the enzyme 5α-reductase in peripheral tissues.

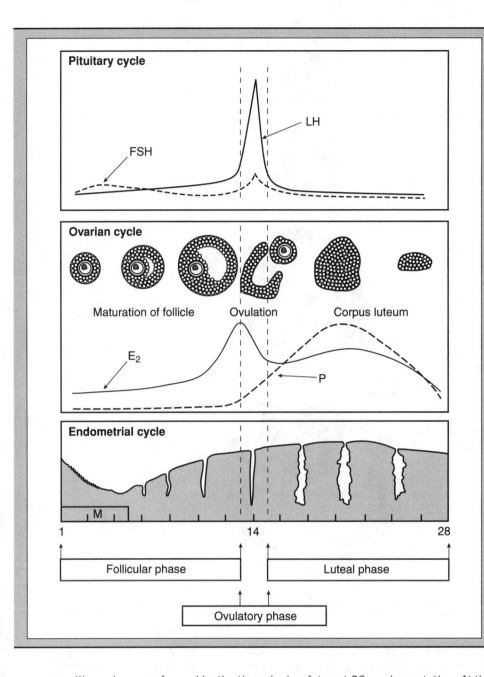

FIGURE 12-3
HORMONAL CHANGES DURING THE NORMAL MENSTRUAL CYCLE. The changes in pituitary hormone secretion, ovarian follicle development, hormone secretion, and the endometrial responses to ovarian hormones throughout the menstrual cycle are shown. FSH = follicle-stimulating hormone; LH = luteinizing hormone; E_2 = estradiol; P = progesterone; M = menses (the days of menstrual bleeding). (*Source:* Reprinted with permission from Rebar RW, Kenigsberg D, Hodgen GD: The normal menstrual cycle and the control of ovulation. In *Principles and Practice of Endocrinology and Metabolism.* Edited by Becker KL. Philadelphia, PA: J. B. Lippincott, 1990, p 789.)

woman will ever have are formed by the time she is a fetus at 20 weeks gestation. At that time, she has approximately 6 million primary oocytes with nuclei arrested in the diplotene phase of the first meiotic division. These oocytes do not proceed through meiosis until fertilization occurs, sometimes as long as 45 or more years later. The fact that these eggs have been exposed to environmental stresses for many years may explain the increase in poor reproductive function as women age and the exponential rise in chromosomal aneuploidy after the age of 35.

During gestation primary oocytes are incorporated into the basic unit of the ovary, the primordial follicle. A primordial follicle consists of a primary oocyte surrounded by a layer of granulosa cells held within a basement membrane (Figure 12-4). Stroma cells surround the follicle. From midgestation through childhood, a few primordial follicles develop into primary follicles with growing oocytes and then undergo atresia. Of the 6 million original primordial follicles, approximately 2 million are present at birth. By the time of the onset of menses during puberty (menarche), only 500,000 primordial follicles remain.

After menarche many primordial follicles emerge from the resting phase every month, probably due to changes in the local environment induced by FSH. Although the

Woman's Age	Approximate Number of Oocytes
20 weeks gestation	6,000,000
Birth	2,000,000
Menarche	500,000
55	0

Menarche is the onset of the first menses during puberty.

FIGURE 12-4
MATURATION OF THE SELECTED DOMINANT FOLLICLE PRIOR TO OVULATION. Schematic representation of (A) a primordial follicle, (B) an enlarging follicle surrounded by increasing numbers of granulosa cells, (C) an antral follicle, and (D) a fully developed follicle prior to ovulation. Note the development of a fluid-filled cavity in C and the thecal cells surrounding the follicle in B–D.

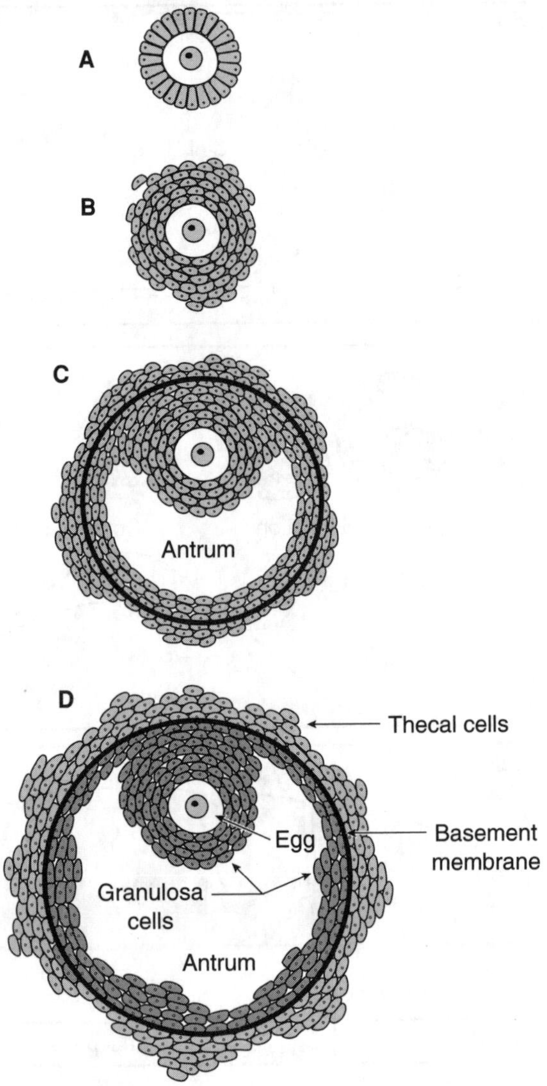

From menarche to menopause approximately one follicle per month develops to maturity and ovulation (a total of approximately 400 follicles).

beginning of a menstrual cycle is defined arbitrarily as the first day of menstrual blood flow, FSH levels actually begin to rise slightly before menses under the influence of tonic secretion of GnRH at a rate of one pulse per hour. As the level of FSH increases, a single dominant follicle is selected from the group of maturing, emerging primordial follicles. This follicle matures fully as it progresses toward ovulation (see Figure 12-4). The other emerging follicles undergo atresia. The factors responsible for selection of the dominant follicle are not understood.

Stimulation of the selected follicle by FSH causes granulosa cells to proliferate into a multilayered covering for the ovum. Fluid appears between the granulosa cells. This coalesces to form a fluid-filled cavity called the antrum. At the same time, the stromal cells around the follicle become more distinct, and a layer of stroma cells (known as theca cells) can be seen surrounding the follicle (see Figure 12-4). At the level of the ovary, the first half of the menstrual cycle is called the *follicular phase* because of the development of the dominant follicle (Table 12-3.)

FSH stimulates estrogen production by the granulosa cells. The rise in estrogen suppresses pituitary FSH secretion by negative feedback, and by the tenth day of the menstrual cycle, the FSH level begins to decline. However, since estrogen also induces the development of FSH receptors, FSH action is more efficient despite the lower FSH level, and estrogen production by the ovary continues to rise. The follicle continues to enlarge.

TIME OF MENSTRUAL CYCLE	OVARY	ENDOMETRIUM	MAJOR HORMONE	Table 12-3 Phases of the Menstrual Cycle
First half	Follicular phase	Proliferative phase	Estrogen	
Second half	Luteal phase	Secretory phase	Progesterone	

The rapid rise in estrogen secretion by the ripe ovarian follicle triggers a change in the pattern of GnRH secretion to rapid pulses. These rapid pulses stimulate the gonadotrophs to produce a surge of LH. There is a brief period of positive feedback, when the rising estrogen level also stimulates a midcycle rise in FSH. The LH surge is followed by ovulation, which occurs within the next 24 hours. At the time of ovulation, the follicle ruptures, and the egg and its surrounding granulosa cells (the cumulus) are extruded into the peritoneal cavity. Rupture of the follicle is not due to pressure, but to proteolytic digestion of the follicle wall.

The rise in estrogen, which peaks at ovulation, increases production and causes thinning of cervical mucus. This allows sperm to penetrate the cervix more easily. At this time, a drop of mucus on a slide dries in a ferning pattern (Figure 12-5), and a drop of mucus suspended between two glass slides can stretch as much as 10 cm without breaking. The ability of cervical mucus to stretch is referred to as *spinnbarkeit*. Ferning and spinnbarkeit are clinical signs of ovulation, which can be used to time intercourse for increased likelihood of conception or for contraception.

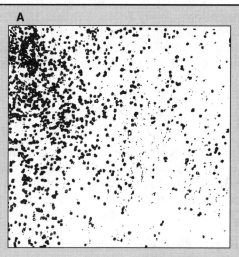
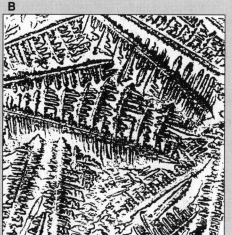

FIGURE 12-5
FERNING OF CERVICAL MUCUS.
(A) A smear of cervical mucus obtained from a normally menstruating woman on day 5 of the menstrual cycle. Lack of ferning is compatible with the low estrogen level at this time of the cycle. (B) A smear of cervical mucus obtained from the same woman just before ovulation when the estrogen level is high shows a ferning pattern. (*Source:* Reprinted with permission from Rebar RW: Practical evaluation of hormone status. In *Reproductive Endocrinology: Physiology, Pathology and Clinical Management,* 2nd ed. Edited by Yen SSC, Jaffe RB. Philadelphia, PA: W. B. Saunders, 1986, p 693.)

Some women note a sharp pain as a result of peritoneal irritation, which follows rupture of the ovarian follicle. This pain of ovulation occurring at midcycle is called *mittelschmerz*. Some women note an increase in libido due to increased ovarian androgen production induced by the LH surge before ovulation. A rise in basal body temperature immediately after rising in the morning can be observed in 95% of women who have just ovulated. This subtle sign of increased circulating progesterone confirms ovulation. Intercourse at the time of the temperature rise does not result in pregnancy as often as might be expected because maximal fertility occurs immediately *before* ovulation.

Maturation of two follicles that are fertilized after ovulation results in fraternal twins. There is a familial predisposition to multiple ovulation. Women prone to multiple gestations may have higher FSH levels or have FSH receptors that are more sensitive to FSH. Administration of high doses of exogenous gonadotropins in an attempt to induce fertility often results in maturation of several follicles. Identical twinning is not increased by exogenous gonadotropins.

Signs Indicating Ovulation
Mittelschmerz (pain due to follicle rupture)
Ferning of cervical mucus (estrogen effect)
Increased spinnbarkeit (estrogen effect)
Rise in basal body temperature (progesterone effect)
Increased libido (androgen effect)

After ovulation, the follicle antrum is filled with blood and lymph, and the wall of the follicle collapses. Blood vessels from the surrounding thecal layer invade the follicle. The granulosa cells remaining in the ruptured follicle enlarge and produce progesterone in response to the high level of circulating LH. These progesterone-rich cells appear yellow or luteinized. The luteinized granulosa cells together with the surrounding thecal cells form the corpus luteum, meaning "yellow body." At the level of the ovary, the period of the menstrual cycle after ovulation is called the *luteal* phase (see Table 12-3.)

Estrogen dominates the follicular phase of the menstrual cycle. The estrogen level remains high after ovulation, but progesterone dominates the luteal phase. Progesterone converts the lining of the uterus into an environment that can sustain a pregnancy (see below). Progesterone reduces production and causes thickening of cervical mucus even if estrogen is present.

During the luteal phase, pituitary secretion of LH and FSH is suppressed by the high levels of progesterone and estrogen (negative feedback). However, the corpus luteum cannot be sustained for long without LH and FSH support. The corpus luteum involutes, leaving a small white scar called the corpus albicans. When the corpus luteum fails, estrogen and progesterone levels fall, and the hypothalamus and pituitary gland are released from feedback inhibition. FSH starts to rise again. The endometrium cannot be sustained without progesterone; the endometrial lining is sloughed (see below), and another menstrual cycle begins.

If conception occurs, the placenta produces HCG, a hormone that acts like LH. HCG sustains the corpus luteum, which continues to produce progesterone to support the endometrium, and menstrual bleeding does not occur (see below and Chapter 15).

In many women, the menstrual cycle begins again every 28 days. Variation in the length of a menstrual cycle is almost always due to variation in the length of the follicular phase, not the luteal phase. The time from ovulation until the beginning of menses is usually 14 days. Variations resulting in a short luteal phase are a rare but treatable cause of infertility.

EVENTS IN THE ENDOMETRIUM

The cyclic rise and fall of estrogen and progesterone has predictable effects on the inner lining of the uterus (the endometrium), and it is the uterine response that determines the dating of the menstrual cycle (see Figure 12-3). Day 1 is the date of the onset of menses. At this time, the endometrial lining is being sloughed because estrogen and progesterone levels are too low to maintain it. However, FSH levels are rising, and estrogen levels soon increase in response.

At the end of menstrual blood flow, a thin basal layer of endometrium remains. Under the influence of rising estrogen levels during the ovarian follicular phase, endometrial glands proliferate from the stumps of glands remaining in the basal layer. Estrogen causes the glands to enlarge and become coiled, and the thickness of the lining of the uterus increases tenfold. Growth of the glands is accompanied by growth of the stroma and proliferation of spiral arteries from remaining basal arteries. A rich capillary network forms. All of this occurs in preparation for implantation of a fertilized egg. At the level of the uterus, the portion of the menstrual cycle preceding ovulation is called the *proliferative phase* (see Table 12-3).

After ovulation, the effects of progesterone on the endometrium predominate. Progesterone halts further growth in thickness and causes solidification and maturation of the endometrium. The endometrial glands cease to proliferate and begin secreting glycoproteins into the uterine cavity to create a favorable environment for implantation of the fertilized egg. At the level of the endometrium, the phase of the menstrual cycle from ovulation to menses is called the *secretory phase* (see Table 12-3).

If conception does not occur, and the corpus luteum involutes, progesterone levels fall precipitously, and there is no longer sufficient hormonal support for the spiral arterioles. The arterioles constrict, causing necrosis of the endometrial lining. Tissue sloughs off resulting in blood loss referred to as the menstrual period. In most women, bleeding lasts for 5 days. The average volume of blood lost during menses is 30 mL. Loss of more than 80 mL of menstrual blood each month usually results in anemia.

The changes in endometrial histology caused by estrogen and progesterone are sufficiently distinct to allow dating of the menstrual cycle that usually is accurate to within 48 hours.

■ DYSMENORRHEA AND PREMENSTRUAL SYNDROME

In some women, dysmenorrhea (painful menses) without any underlying pathology occurs during ovulatory menstrual cycles. The pain is cramping in nature and is thought to be due to uterine contractions caused by prostaglandins released as the endometrium is sloughed. Treatment includes inhibitors of prostaglandin release, suppression of ovulation with oral contraception, or both. Dilatation of the cervix during menses also is perceived by some women as cramping.

Premenstrual syndrome is a collection of recurrent symptoms (fatigue, irritability, mood swings, anxiety, depression, insomnia), which occur in some women mostly during the luteal phase of ovulatory menstrual cycles. Symptoms can persist into the follicular phase. The cause is uncertain. Although the luteal phase is associated with marked changes in the levels of FSH, LH, estrogen, and progesterone, no hormonal abnormalities have been identified in women with this syndrome.

Since Ms. Martin's height, breast development, body hair, age of first menses, and earlier menstrual cycles were normal, it was unlikely that her amenorrhea was due to a developmental abnormality. Her cervix and vagina were patent. She had obvious signs of estrogen deficiency, including vaginal dryness, an atrophic vaginal mucosa, and decreased cervical mucus, which did not fern. A pregnancy test was negative, as expected in view of the clinical evidence for estrogen deficiency. Additional tests were ordered to determine whether the problem was at the level of her hypothalamus, her pituitary gland, or her ovaries.	**Case Study:** *Continued*

■ MENSTRUAL CYCLE DYSFUNCTION

Normal menstrual cycles require normal function of the hypothalamus, pituitary, ovaries, and outflow tract. Failure of menses (amenorrhea) can be due to a problem at any of these levels. Causes of primary amenorrhea (failure of menses to occur at puberty) and secondary amenorrhea (cessation of menses after it has been established) are somewhat different. However, there is a great deal of overlap in the differential diagnosis (Table 12-4).

Table 12-4 **Major Causes of Amenorrhea**

Hypothalamic level
    Failure to attain or maintain critical level of
      body fat
    Severe stress
    Severe systemic illness
    Syndrome of anosmia and GnRH deficiency
Pituitary level
    Large pituitary tumors
    Hyperprolactinemia
    Postpartum necrosis
Ovarian level
    Ovarian dysgenesis (Turner's syndrome)
    Testicular feminization syndrome
    Chemotherapy
    Radiation damage
    Autoimmune disease

Outflow tract level
    Congenital obstruction
    Müllerian agenesis
    Recurrent endometrial infections
    Overvigorous curettage (Asherman's syndrome)

Note. GnRH = gonadotropin-releasing hormone.

PRIMARY AMENORRHEA

In the United States, the onset of first menses (menarche) occurs at an average age of 12 years and 8 months. Primary amenorrhea is defined as no menses by the age of 14 in the absence of the development of secondary sex characteristics (breast budding, pubic hair, axillary hair) *or* no menses by the age of 16 regardless of the presence or absence of secondary sex characteristics.

If a young woman appears healthy and has a family history of delayed sexual maturation, investigation may reveal that her pubertal development is just delayed (see Chapter 14). If secondary sex characteristics have developed, it is essential to be sure that the patient is not pregnant.

Primary Amenorrhea
No menses and no development of secondary sex characteristics by age 14
No menses by age 16

Hypothalamic Level. Hypothalamic primary amenorrhea most often is due to failure to accumulate enough body fat to reach the set point required for menarche. Body fat must reach this critical level so that GnRH pulses of sufficient frequency and amplitude can stimulate pituitary gonadotropin release. The mechanism by which the adipose tissue level regulates hypothalamic function is uncertain; the interaction of the adipose tissue hormone leptin with the central nervous system (CNS) is undergoing intense evaluation at this time (see Chapter 10). Hypothalamic primary amenorrhea is not unusual in teenage athletes, especially gymnasts, dancers, and young women running more than 20 miles per week. Hypothalamic amenorrhea is common in young women with anorexia nervosa who have very low levels of body fat due to a combination of starvation and exercise. Patients experiencing severe stress or severe systemic illness also are at increased risk of developing hypothalamic amenorrhea. Sexual maturation and menses usually respond promptly to decreased exercise, weight gain, or both or resolution of the underlying stress.

A rare CNS defect results in the combination of anosmia (absent sense of smell) and GnRH deficiency, which is analogous to Kallman's syndrome in men. FSH and LH levels and ovarian hormone levels are low in these women. These patients respond to GnRH agonists given in a pulsatile fashion that prevents down-regulation of receptors.

Pituitary Level. Craniopharyngiomas and other large pituitary tumors that destroy the pituitary gland by mass effects can cause primary amenorrhea. Patients with these tumors have low or low-normal FSH and LH levels and may have symptoms and signs of other pituitary hormone deficiencies as well (see Chapter 2). Treatment is directed toward removal of the underlying tumor whenever possible and estrogen and progesterone replacement.

Even small prolactin (PRL)-producing pituitary tumors can cause primary amenorrhea because high PRL levels interfere with GnRH pulses. There are many other causes of hyperprolactinemia, including renal failure, medications like the phenothiazines, and primary hypothyroidism. Phenothiazines suppress hypothalamic production of dopamine, which is a physiologic inhibitor of PRL secretion (see Chapter 2). Patients with primary hypothyroidism have high levels of thyrotropin-releasing hormone (TRH) and TSH. Normal TRH levels have little effect on PRL, but high levels of TRH stimulate PRL release. Hyperprolactinemia usually can be suppressed with dopamine agonists if treatment of the underlying disorder is not possible. This restores GnRH pulses and gonadotropin secretion.

Ovarian Level. If amenorrhea is due to absence or destruction of the ovaries, estrogen levels are low, and FSH and LH levels are high due to the absence of negative feedback by ovarian hormones.

Turner's syndrome or gonadal dysgenesis (karyotype 45,XO) is the most common congenital cause of primary amenorrhea. Loss of the second X chromosome results in ovaries that are fibrous streaks with few, if any, germ cells present at puberty. The pubertal growth spurt and secondary sexual characteristics do not develop in the absence of ovarian follicles, which are needed to synthesize estrogen. Although the outflow tract is intact, the uterus usually is quite small. Some of the other clinical features of this syndrome include a webbed neck, a shield chest, and an abnormal carrying angle (valgus deformity of the elbows) [see Chapters 13 and 14]. A karyotype is necessary to confirm the diagnosis, since the clinical features are quite variable, especially in women who are mosaics with karyotype 45,XX/45,XO.

Testicular feminization syndrome (karyotype 46,XY) is another congenital disorder that presents with primary amenorrhea. Patients with this disorder have a male genotype but a female phenotype due to the absence of functional androgen receptors. They have high FSH, LH, and testosterone levels because the pituitary lacks the receptors to recognize testosterone. Estrogen levels are high because testosterone is converted to estrogen in peripheral tissues. These patients have female external genitalia and female breast development but no ovaries or uterus and little body hair (see Chapters 13 and 14).

Environmental insults causing premature death of ovarian follicles and primary amenorrhea include radiation therapy and chemotherapy given for childhood malignancies. Amenorrhea due to ovarian failure is treated with estrogen and progesterone replacement.

Outflow Tract Level. If the problem is at the level of the outflow tract, secondary sex characteristics develop normally, because hypothalamic-pituitary-ovarian feedback loops are normal. Obstruction of menstrual flow can occur at several levels. An imperforate hymen results in monthly discomfort, which becomes progressively worse due to buildup of menstrual blood behind the intact hymen. Eventually a bulge can be noted on the perineum. This is an infrequent but easily corrected problem.

Disorders of müllerian duct development are of more concern. There may be no vaginal orifice. In these cases, surgical correction can be immensely rewarding, even if reproduction is not possible. Complete müllerian agenesis results in congenital absence of the uterus and proximal vagina.

SECONDARY AMENORRHEA

Secondary amenorrhea refers to amenorrhea occurring in a nonpregnant woman who has previously had menses and who is not expected to be experiencing menopause. Many of the conditions that cause primary amenorrhea also can cause secondary amenorrhea. As with primary amenorrhea, the problem can be at the level of the hypothalamus, the pituitary, the ovaries, or the outflow tract.

Hypothalamic Level. Lack of body fat, anorexia nervosa, severe weight loss, stress, or systemic illness cause secondary amenorrhea as well as primary amenorrhea (see above).

Pituitary Level. The same tumors that cause primary amenorrhea can cause secondary amenorrhea. Since mass lesions often affect the gonadotrophs before the cells producing TSH and adrenocorticotropic hormone (ACTH), women with these tumors may not have symptoms and signs of other pituitary hormone deficiencies. Hyperprolactinemia, which disrupts GnRH pulses, is a common cause of secondary amenorrhea. As indicated above, hyperprolactinemia can be due to a pituitary tumor, dopamine-suppressing drugs such as the phenothiazines, renal failure, and hypothyroidism, which results in an increase in TRH sufficient to stimulate PRL secretion.

Amenorrhea following childbirth can be due to postpartum necrosis of the pituitary gland. The pituitary gland normally hypertrophies during pregnancy because the rise in estrogen stimulates lactotrophs. If postpartum hemorrhage results in hypotension, the pituitary may undergo acute infarction due to lack of blood flow. Patients present with an inability to lactate, since milk production requires prolactin from the anterior pituitary (see Chapter 15). With modern obstetric care this catastrophe is very rare.

Women with secondary amenorrhea due to pituitary disorders have low or low-normal FSH and LH levels. Treatment is the same as the treatment for primary amenorrhea at the pituitary level, which is described above.

Ovarian Level. Women with Turner's syndrome can present with secondary amenorrhea rather than primary amenorrhea if follicle atresia is sufficiently delayed to allow the women to go through puberty. This is especially likely if women with this syndrome are mosaics of 45,XX and 45,XO. Premature ovarian failure (premature menopause) refers to ovarian failure in a woman under the age of 35. This can be due to autoimmune disease, chemotherapy, or radiation therapy, but the cause frequently is unknown.

If amenorrhea is due to ovarian failure, FSH and LH levels are high due to the absence of negative feedback by estrogen and progesterone. Ovarian failure is treated with estrogen and progesterone replacement.

Outflow Tract Level. Recurrent infections that cause destruction of the endometrial cavity and overvigorous curettage that denudes the endometrial lining result in scarring and amenorrhea if the endometrial glands are damaged too severely to respond to estrogen (Asherman's syndrome). The uterus is especially sensitive to vigorous curettage during the month after childbirth when the uterus is vascular and hypertrophied. Asherman's syndrome is treated by resecting some of the scar tissue and giving large doses of estrogen in an effort to stimulate regrowth of the endometrial lining.

EVALUATION AND TREATMENT OF AMENORRHEA

A flow diagram for the evaluation of amenorrhea is shown in Figure 12-6. After completing the history and physical examination to be sure that ovaries, a uterus, and a vagina are present and that the outflow tract is patent, a pregnancy test should be obtained regardless of the sexual history. A serum TSH level and a PRL level should be obtained even if other symptoms and signs of hyperprolactinemia and hypothyroidism are absent. These are common causes of amenorrhea, and other symptoms and signs may not appear until later in the course. Subtle elevations of TRH can stimulate enough PRL secretion to disrupt GnRH pulses in patients who are clinically euthyroid.

If the pregnancy test is negative and TSH and prolactin levels are within the normal range, a *progestin challenge* can be given to test for adequate estrogen activity. Progesterone or an oral progestin is given for several days and then withdrawn. Withdrawal bleeding occurring several days later indicates that enough estrogen is available to prepare the endometrium for the progesterone. The availability of estrogen indicates that the hypothalamus and pituitary are producing GnRH pulses and gonadotropins. Withdrawal bleeding also confirms that the endometrium is able to respond to estrogen and that the outflow tract is patent. If withdrawal bleeding occurs after a progestin challenge, amenorrhea is likely to be due to anovulation and progesterone deficiency.

FIGURE 12-6
EVALUATION OF AMENORRHEA.
If a patient presents with primary amenorrhea, it is necessary to make sure that the outflow tract is present. A karyotype may be necessary if the defect is at the level of the gonad. TSH = thyroid-stimulating hormone; FSH = follicle-stimulating hormone; LH = luteinizing hormone.

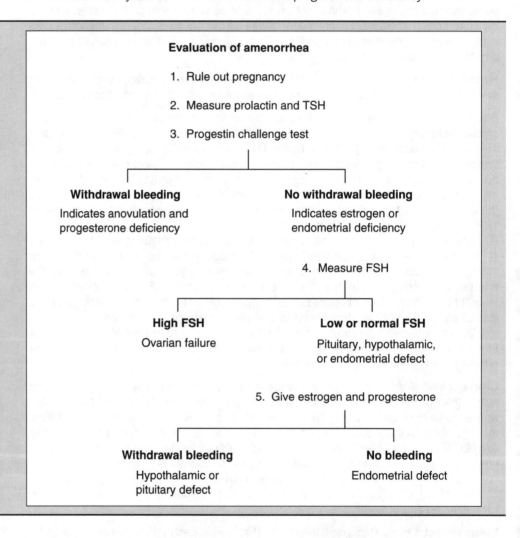

Evaluation of amenorrhea

1. Rule out pregnancy

2. Measure prolactin and TSH

3. Progestin challenge test

Withdrawal bleeding
Indicates anovulation and progesterone deficiency

No withdrawal bleeding
Indicates estrogen or endometrial deficiency

4. Measure FSH

High FSH
Ovarian failure

Low or normal FSH
Pituitary, hypothalamic, or endometrial defect

5. Give estrogen and progesterone

Withdrawal bleeding
Hypothalamic or pituitary defect

No bleeding
Endometrial defect

If amenorrhea is due to estrogen depletion, there will be no primed endometrium to respond to a progestin challenge. A serum FSH level helps to determine whether this is due to ovarian incompetence or to a problem at the pituitary or hypothalamic level. The FSH level is low or low-normal if the problem is at the pituitary or hypothalamic level. The FSH level is high if the problem is due to ovarian failure (Table 12-5). If the FSH level is high, it may be necessary to obtain a karyotype to diagnose Turner's syndrome or to rule out the presence of a Y chromosome remnant. If a karyotype reveals a Y chromosome remnant, the removal of the patient's gonads is required because remnants are likely to become neoplastic.

If the FSH level is normal, the problem may be the endometrium itself. If the endometrium is able to respond to hormonal stimulation, priming the endometrium with estrogen for 3 weeks and then giving and withdrawing progesterone should result in withdrawal bleeding.

LEVEL OF FAILURE	FSH	LH	ESTROGEN
Hypothalamus	Low[a]	Low[a]	Low
Pituitary	Low[a]	Low[a]	Low
Ovary	High	High	Low
Uterus	Normal	Normal	Normal

Note. FSH = follicle-stimulating hormone; LH = luteinizing hormone.
[a] Value may be low-normal.

Table 12-5
Amenorrhea: Hormone Relationships

Specific treatment of the underlying cause of amenorrhea is ideal but not always possible. Estrogen replacement stimulates the development of secondary sex characteristics and growth in girls with incomplete pubertal maturation. Progesterone is added to prevent the endometrial hyperplasia that results when estrogen replacement is given alone. Women without a uterus need not be given progesterone. Ovarian androgens usually are not replaced because they do not provide any additional increase in height, and virilizing side effects are common.

Even if sexual development is not an issue, hormone replacement is recommended for most women of premenopausal age with hypogonadism, regardless of whether the underlying problem is at the level of the hypothalamus, the pituitary gland, or the ovaries. Lack of estrogen results in osteopenia, and fractures may occur despite excellent physical conditioning. Women with hypogonadism also experience other consequences of estrogen deficiency that are common in postmenopausal women (see below).

If ovarian follicles are present, and the goal is ovulation and pregnancy, treatment with gonadotropins or pulsatile GnRH might be necessary. If the FSH level is greater than 40 mIU/mL and the LH level also is high, follicles probably are absent, and the woman is sterile.

The differential diagnosis for Ms. Martin's amenorrhea included hypothalamic amenorrhea, hypothyroidism, hyperprolactinemia, a pituitary tumor, or premature ovarian failure. Her thyroid function tests and TSH level were normal. Her PRL level also was within normal limits. A progestin challenge was not followed by withdrawal bleeding, indicating that her endometrium had not been prepared by estrogen.

Her FSH level should have been high in the absence of estrogen feedback, but the FSH level was low. This indicated that the hypothalamus or pituitary was the source of the problem, not the ovaries. Her clinical picture suggested hypothalamic amenorrhea due to loss of the critical fat mass required for normal GnRH pulses.

She was not willing to change her food intake or moderate her level of activity, so she was treated with an oral contraceptive containing estrogen and progesterone. After graduation from college, she obtained a job as a marketing executive with an athletic shoe company. She decreased her running to 18 miles per week and stopped using the oral contraceptive. Her weight increased to 115 lbs, and her menstrual periods resumed. Subsequently, she had two normal pregnancies.

Case Study:
Continued

DISORDERS OF ANDROGEN EXCESS

Women produce androgens in the ovaries and the adrenal glands. Testosterone and DHT are the most potent androgens, but since androgens can be interconverted in peripheral tissues, overproduction of any androgen can lead to symptoms and signs of androgen excess. Testosterone is converted to DHT in peripheral tissues by the enzyme 5α-reductase, and both hormones share the same receptor. Most dehydroepiandrosterone sulfate (DHEAS) is made in the adrenal glands rather than the ovaries.

Most testosterone and DHT in the circulation are bound to SHBG. Since androgens decrease hepatic synthesis of SHBG, androgen overproduction increases the proportion of the free hormone, which is the active form. Ingestion or application of anabolic steroids has the same effect as increasing endogenous androgen production. Estrogen increases SHBG production.

It is possible to have increased androgen action even if circulating androgen levels are normal, if a high level of 5α-reductase activity results in increased conversion of

Androgen	Relative Potency
Dihydrotestosterone	2.5
Testosterone	1.0
Androstenedione	0.15
DHEA	0.05
DHEAS	. . .

Factors Affecting SHBG

Decreased SHBG Synthesis	Increased SHBG Synthesis
Androgens	Estrogens
Obesity	Pregnancy
Hypothyroidism	Hyperthyroidism
Glucocorticoid excess	

Causes of Increased Androgen Effect

Increased endogenous androgen production (ovarian, adrenal, or both)

Exogenous androgen (anabolic steroids)

Decreased androgen binding (low SHBG)

Increased conversion of testosterone to dihydrotestosterone

Increased androgen receptor number or sensitivity

testosterone to the more active DHT. An increase in the number of androgen receptors can also result in increased androgen action.

Even mild androgen excess can cause hirsutism (excess hair growth) and acne. Some women develop oligomenorrhea or amenorrhea. High androgen levels result in temporal balding, deepening of the voice, clitoromegaly, and development of a male body habitus.

OVARIAN ANDROGEN OVERPRODUCTION

Ovarian androgen overproduction most often occurs in women with polycystic ovary syndrome (PCOS). Benign ovarian cysts also are sources of androgens. Ovarian androgen-secreting tumors, which can produce very high androgen levels, are rare.

Polycystic Ovary Syndrome. PCOS is a combination of androgen excess, anovulation, and insulin resistance that occurs in the absence of specific underlying ovarian or adrenal disease. The syndrome is associated with altered regulation of the pituitary-ovarian axis (Figure 12-7). The underlying cause is unknown; several factors probably perpetuate the syndrome.

LH levels are increased, although not necessarily above the normal range. In response, ovarian theca cells increase androgen production. The androgens are converted to estrogen in granulosa cells and in peripheral tissues. Estrogen production is chronic, not cyclic. The estrogen level remains in the early or middle follicular phase range, a level that continues to stimulate GnRH pulses. There is no late follicular phase burst of estrogen, no LH surge, no ovulation, and no corpus luteum to produce progesterone. With ongoing GnRH pulses and not enough progesterone feedback, LH secretion continues. The result is a vicious cycle resulting in menstrual irregularities and infertility. The continuous production of estrogen unopposed by progesterone results in endometrial hyperplasia. Bleeding occurs erratically as areas of the hyperplastic endometrial lining are sloughed. Low-level estrogen production and continuous androgen overproduction result in decreased SHBG, which increases the free androgen level. Some women have

FIGURE 12-7
METABOLIC ABNORMALITIES OF THE POLYCYSTIC OVARY SYNDROME. The underlying cause of the syndrome is uncertain. Note that once the syndrome is established, a vicious cycle perpetuates the anovulation and hirsutism. LH = luteinizing hormone; GnRH = gonadotropin-releasing hormone.

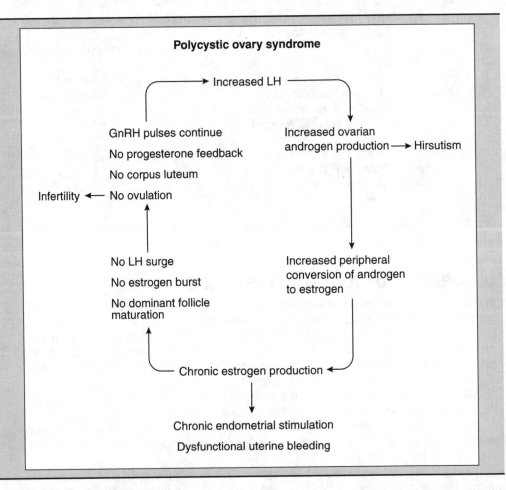

increased adrenal androgen production as well. Although women with PCOS have increased acne and hirsutism, they usually do not have more severe signs of androgen excess.

The insulin resistance associated with PCOS occurs mostly in muscle and adipose tissue, not the liver. The cause of the insulin resistance associated with the syndrome is uncertain. Insulin resistance is greater in obese women with PCOS but is present in lean women as well. Impaired glucose tolerance, type 2 diabetes, and hyperlipidemia are more common in patients with PCOS than in weight-matched controls.

Continuous LH stimulation results in hypertrophied thecal cells and enlarged ovaries. Since a dominant follicle is not selected each month, multiple follicles remain in the early developmental stages. Many small ovarian cysts are usually, but not always, visible by ultrasound or at surgery.

Women with PCOS are treated with low-dose oral contraceptives or periodic progestin therapy to interrupt continuous stimulation of the endometrium by unopposed estrogen. Women who wish to become pregnant are treated with an antiestrogen, such as clomiphene citrate, gonadotropin preparations, or pulsatile GnRH agonists in an attempt to break the cycle and allow the arrested menstrual cycle to proceed to ovulation. If present, obesity, hyperlipidemia, and impaired glucose tolerance also require treatment. Treatment of hirsutism is addressed below.

ADRENAL ANDROGEN OVERPRODUCTION

Congenital Adrenal Hyperplasia (CAH). This is the most common cause of adrenal androgen excess. CAH is caused by decreased activity of one of the enzymes required for production of cortisol (Figure 12-8 and Chapter 5). When plasma cortisol is low, the pituitary increases production of ACTH, which increases flux through the metabolic pathway leading to cortisol synthesis. Metabolites proximal to the dysfunctional or absent enzyme accumulate and are diverted into pathways leading to androgen synthesis. The most common enzymatic defect is 21-hydroxylase deficiency, followed by 11β-hydroxylase deficiency and 3β-hydroxysteroid dehydrogenase deficiency. If the enzymatic defect is severe, virilization of the genitalia occurs in utero and is apparent at birth. If the enzymatic defect is mild, patients present later with hirsutism alone or hirsutism coupled with abnormal menstrual cycles. Treatment with cortisol suppresses ACTH.

Signs of Androgen Excess
Hirsutism
Acne
Temporal balding
Deeper voice
Clitoromegaly
Male body habitus

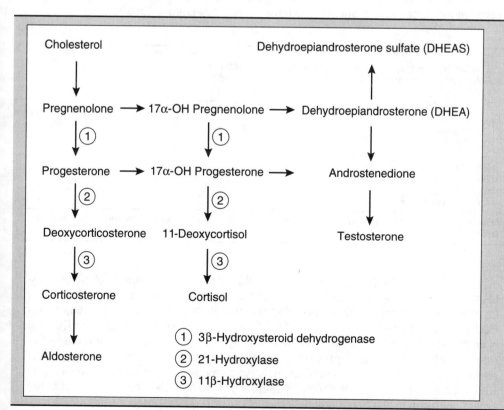

FIGURE 12-8
ADRENAL STEROID HORMONE SYNTHESIS. Pathways of adrenal steroid hormone synthesis are shown as unidirectional for simplicity, but steps from pregnenolone forward are reversible. Although a defect or deficiency of any of the enzymes shown can lead to congenital adrenal hyperplasia (CAH), the most common cause is 21-hydroxylase deficiency. This results in decreased cortisol synthesis and a compensatory increase in pituitary adrenocorticotropic hormone secretion, which leads to the accumulation of 17α-hydroxyprogesterone. Some of the excess 17α-hydroxyprogesterone is diverted to excess androgen synthesis.

Pituitary tumors producing ACTH (Cushing's disease) and tumors producing ectopic ACTH (Cushing's syndrome) also increase flux into adrenal androgen synthesis. Treatment of these disorders is discussed in Chapter 5. Adrenal androgen-secreting tumors, which can secrete very high levels of androgens, are rare.

HIRSUTISM

Hirsutism is the presence of excessive body hair in women.

Hirsutism, the presence of excessive body hair, is one of the earliest signs of increased androgen action. It is very difficult to differentiate between normal and excessive hair growth. Women develop more facial and body hair as estrogen levels decline with age and the ratio of circulating androgen to estrogen levels increases. Even a slight increase in body hair is very distressing for some women.

Androgen-responsive hair growth results from the interaction of DHT with its receptors in hair follicles. Before puberty most body hair is the fine, nonpigmented vellus hair, which is found all over the body. Terminal hair, which is coarse, pigmented, and responsive to androgens, is found only in the eyebrows and scalp. At the time of puberty, androgen levels increase dramatically, and vellus hair is converted to terminal hair. In women, this occurs mostly in the axillary and pubic regions, but if DHT production is excessive or the skin is unusually responsive to DHT, terminal hair appears on the lower face, periareolar areas of the breast, the chest, the back, the lower abdomen, and the inner thighs.

Most women with hirsutism have a combination of increased androgen production and increased hair follicle sensitivity to DHT. Women also can develop hirsutism if estrogen production is decreased by hyperprolactinemia or premature ovarian failure, which leaves the action of adrenal androgens relatively unopposed. Drugs such as minoxidil, phenytoin, diazoxide, cyclosporine, and danazol also stimulate hair growth.

Evaluation. A history and physical examination can be very helpful in the evaluation of hirsutism (Table 12-6). Benign forms of hirsutism often begin around the time of puberty, when gonadotropin production increases dramatically, and gradually become worse over time. Often there is a family history of hirsutism. Women who have mild, slowly developing hirsutism and regular menses are especially likely to have a benign underlying cause. Women with previously normal menstrual cycles who have rapidly developing hirsutism unrelated to puberty are more likely to have androgen-secreting tumors.

Table 12-6
Evaluation of Androgen Excess

History	Laboratory (serum values)
Duration and severity of symptoms and signs	Testosterone
Relationship to onset of puberty	FSH and LH
Family history	Prolactin
Frequency of menses	17α-Hydroxyprogesterone
Physical examination	Dexamethasone suppression test (if hypercortisolism is suspected)
Body habitus	DHEAS
Obesity	
Acne	
Breast development	
Body hair: amount and distribution	
Clitoromegaly	
Signs of hypercortisolism	

Note. FSH = follicle-stimulating hormone; LH = luteinizing hormone; DHEAS = dehydroepiandrosterone sulfate.

Laboratory evaluation of hirsutism should include measurement of serum testosterone; a very high level suggests an androgen-secreting tumor. LH and FSH are measured as indicators of pituitary-ovarian coordination and ovarian failure. Women with PCOS are likely to have a relatively fixed LH:FSH ratio of approximately 3:1. A PRL level is needed to rule out hyperprolactinemia. A 17α-hydroxyprogesterone level is obtained to rule out CAH caused by 21-hydroxylase deficiency (see Chapter 5). If signs of hypercortisolism are present, a workup for Cushing's syndrome with a dexamethasone suppression test should proceed as described in Chapter 5. A high DHEAS level suggests that the excess androgen is of adrenal origin.

Treatment. Treatment should be directed at the underlying cause of hirsutism if one can be found (Table 12-7). However, in many women it is difficult to determine whether the excess androgen is produced by the ovaries, the adrenals, or both.

Gonadotropin-stimulated ovarian androgen overproduction can be treated with oral contraceptives to suppress LH and FSH production. The estrogen component of oral contraceptives also stimulates SHBG synthesis so that less free androgen is available to interact with androgen receptors on hair follicles. Oral contraceptives with the least androgenic progestins should be used.

Treatment of hirsutism involves suppressing androgen secretion, blocking conversion of testosterone to dihydrotestosterone, or blocking androgen receptors.

Gonadotropin suppression	Antiandrogens
Oral contraceptives	Spironolactone
GnRH analogs	Flutamide
Adrenal androgen suppression	Cyproterone acetate[a]
Glucocorticoids	5α-Reductase inhibitors
	Finasteride
	Flutamide

Table 12-7
Treatment of Hirsutism

Note. GnRH = gonadotropin-releasing hormone.
[a] Not available in the United States.

Continuous administration of a GnRH analog decreases LH and FSH production by down-regulating pituitary GnRH receptors. Estrogen replacement must be added to prevent the consequences of estrogen deficiency, and a progestin must be added to prevent unopposed estrogen stimulation of the endometrium. A glucocorticoid, which inhibits ACTH production by negative feedback on the pituitary gland, is used to treat women with CAH.

Antiandrogens such as spironolactone, flutamide, and cyproterone acetate inhibit androgen binding to its receptors. Spironolactone is an aldosterone antagonist, which also interacts with the androgen receptor. Spironolactone does cause more frequent menses, but this can be controlled with an oral contraceptive. Flutamide is more expensive and more hepatotoxic. Cyproterone acetate is a potent progestin as well as an antiandrogen. It is available in Europe and Canada but not in the United States.

Finasteride prevents conversion of testosterone to DHT by inhibiting 5α-reductase. Finasteride should not be given to women who can become pregnant, because in animal studies it causes ambiguous genitalia in male offspring.

It is easier to suppress new hair growth than to eradicate established hirsutism. Most patients have some response to medical therapy, but this can take months to develop. All medications have dose-related side effects, so low-dose combined therapy may be better than high-dose monotherapy. Scoring systems to monitor treatment have been devised, but these are difficult to carry out accurately. It is just as helpful to ask whether a patient requires less shaving, plucking, waxing, or electrolysis to remove unwanted hair.

HORMONAL CONTRACEPTION

MECHANISMS OF ACTION

Hormonal contraception involves regular administration of estrogen, progestin, or both to prevent pregnancy, either by preventing ovulation or by creating an unfavorable climate for fertilization and implantation within the reproductive tract. A combination of estrogen and a progestin usually is given orally. The estrogen component suppresses pituitary FSH secretion by negative feedback. This prevents the development of a dominant follicle, thereby suppressing ovulation. Estrogen also increases the number of progesterone receptors, making the progesterone component more effective. Cyclic estrogen also stabilizes the endometrium to prevent irregular bleeding.

Naturally occurring estrogens are ineffective when given orally because they are metabolized rapidly by the liver. Synthetic ethinyl estradiol is used in almost all combined oral contraceptive preparations. The dose of ethinyl estradiol has fallen almost fivefold since oral contraceptives were introduced in the 1960s, and today women rarely take more than 35 μg/d.

The progesterone component of contraceptives acts at several levels. Progesterone suppresses pituitary LH secretion, which inhibits ovulation. Progesterone decreases fallopian tube motility, limiting the ability of a fertilized ovum to progress into the

Estrogen Component of Oral Contraceptives
Suppresses FSH secretion
Increases progesterone receptors

Progestin Component of Oral Contraceptives
Suppresses LH secretion
Decreases fallopian tube motility
Opposes estrogen action on the endometrium
Decreases and thickens cervical mucus

endometrial cavity and implant. Progesterone prevents estrogen-induced hyperplasia of the endometrium, making the uterine lining unfavorable for implantation of the fertilized ovum. Progesterone also causes cervical mucus to be tenacious and thick, which prevents sperm from penetrating the cervix.

Progesterone-only contraceptives offer hormonal contraception without exposure to estrogen. Progesterone alone suppresses LH but not FSH, so estrogen levels are not suppressed, and ovulation occurs in some women. Contraception depends on the effects of progesterone on cervical mucus and the endometrium.

Progesterone contraception can be given orally, intramuscularly, or in subcutaneous depot form. Naturally occurring progesterone is metabolized rapidly by the liver when given orally, but many synthetic forms of progesterone (progestins) are available. The newest progestins have very potent contraceptive action with less androgen activity and fewer masculinizing side effects than the progestins originally used.

Progesterone provides highly effective contraception for 3 months when given intramuscularly. When placed subcutaneously in pellets, progesterone is effective for up to 5 years. Progesterone also can be administered via a progesterone-impregnated intrauterine device or a vaginal ring. Resumption of regular ovulation may be delayed following use of depot forms of progesterone, so these should not be used in women who want only short-term contraception. Progesterone antagonists such as mifepristone, which produce a hostile environment for pregnancy by blocking the effects of progesterone on the uterus, are not available in the United States.

Long-acting GnRH agonists initially stimulate FSH and LH secretion but then downregulate GnRH receptors. Secretion of FSH and LH is suppressed, and ovulation is inhibited. GnRH agonists are effective but expensive, and prolonged use of this therapy alone results in a continuous low estrogen state with deleterious effects on bone and the cardiovascular system.

Most women take pills containing both estrogen and progesterone for 21 days each month. This interval is followed by 7 days with no medication to allow withdrawal bleeding. Fixed dose pills provide the same dose of estrogen and progesterone each day for 21 days. Variable dose pills alter the estrogen or progesterone doses every 10 days or every 7 days to minimize side effects while maintaining contraception. Emergency postcoital contraception requires a large dose of estrogen or combined estrogen and progestin, which probably prevents implantation.

SIDE EFFECTS

Many side effects of oral contraceptives are related to metabolic effects on the liver. Oral estrogen results in increased hepatic synthesis of clotting factors II and X and plasminogen and decreased synthesis of antithrombin. Estrogens also increase platelet aggregation (prostacyclin production is reduced). Since aging and cigarette smoking also result in a more hypercoagulable state, the risk of thromboembolic events caused by exogenous estrogen increases markedly in women over age 35 who smoke. The risk of cerebrovascular disease and myocardial infarction also is higher in this group. Women with a previous history of thrombophlebitis usually are not given oral estrogen.

Estrogen causes mild fluid retention, nausea, headache, and breast pain in some women. Estrogen increases plasma renin activity and salt and water retention, which exacerbates hypertension. Estrogen decreases low-density lipoprotein (LDL) cholesterol levels and increases high-density lipoprotein (HDL) cholesterol levels, which is beneficial, but estrogen also increases triglyceride and very-low-density lipoprotein (VLDL) synthesis, which can exacerbate underlying hypertriglyceridemia. Estrogen reduces bile flow and can cause cholestasis.

Progestins cause weight gain, and some women experience progestin-induced depression and fatigue. Older progestins decrease HDL cholesterol levels, but newer progestins with little androgen activity have less effect. Progesterone-only regimens are associated with irregular menstrual bleeding. Oral contraceptives can cause a mild, often transient, increase in insulin resistance similar to that seen in pregnancy (see Chapter 14).

Most studies show no effect of oral contraceptives on breast cancer and a protective effect on cancer of the ovary and the endometrium. The effect on cervical cancer is uncertain.

Contraindications to Estrogen-Containing Oral Contraceptives
Previous thromboembolic disease
Estrogen-sensitive malignancy
Known or suspected pregnancy
Unexplained vaginal bleeding
Smoking over age 35

The estrogen component of most pills is the same, but many progestins with different androgenic and metabolic side effects are available. Minor side effects of oral contraceptives are most pronounced during the first two cycles. Adjustments in the balance of estrogen and progestin and in the type of progestin should not be made until a period of acclimation has passed. Most women eventually find an oral contraceptive that works well for them.

At the age of 33, Ms. Martin's menstrual flow became lighter and more irregular. She returned to the clinic at the age of 34 having had no menses for 8 months. She was running approximately 14 miles per week. She felt well, although she complained of episodes of feeling too warm. Her libido had not changed, but intercourse had become painful because of vaginal dryness.

Her height was 5' 6", and her weight was 120 lbs. Her blood pressure was 110/60 mm Hg, and her heart rate was 60 beats/min. Significant findings during her physical examination included dry skin and a slightly enlarged thyroid gland. Her breast examination was normal. Her pelvic examination revealed atrophic vaginal mucosa, scant cervical mucus, which did not fern, and a normal uterus. Her ovaries were not palpable. A pregnancy test was negative. TSH and PRL levels were within normal limits. A progestin challenge was not followed by withdrawal bleeding.

Case Study:
Continued

■ MENOPAUSE

Menopause is the permanent cessation of menses, which occurs when the ovaries can no longer produce estrogen due to exhaustion of ovarian follicles. As indicated above, oocyte depletion is a lifelong process. Subtle ovulatory dysfunction is common after the age of 30, and fertility drops markedly as ovulation becomes less frequent after the age of 40. The follicular phase of the menstrual cycle becomes shorter, levels of FSH increase as estrogen production drops, and luteal phase defects become more and more frequent. Irregular uterine bleeding is common. Uterine bleeding may be decreased due to decreased estrogen production or increased if the remaining estrogen action is not opposed by adequate progesterone production during anovulatory cycles.

The *climacteric* is the entire period during which estrogen production is decreasing, starting with the first decrease in ovulation frequency and ending with generalized atrophy of all estrogen-sensitive tissues. Menopause is the specific point in time during the climacteric at which cessation of menses occurs.

If lack of menses is the diagnostic criterion, menopause can be ascertained only in retrospect. Usually the diagnosis is made after 6–12 months of amenorrhea in a woman who is over 45 years of age. A serum FSH level that is markedly elevated due to lack of estrogen feedback helps to confirm the diagnosis. The average age of menopause in the United States is 52 years. In general, menopause occurs later in obese women who have higher estrogen levels due to conversion of androgens to estrogen in body fat. Menopause occurs earlier in women who smoke cigarettes, perhaps because they tend to be thinner.

Ovarian failure is considered premature if menopause occurs prior to the age of 35. This can be caused by an autoimmune process directed at some component of the ovarian follicles or by radiation or chemotherapy. Often the cause is unknown.

EARLY CONSEQUENCES OF ESTROGEN DEPLETION

Episodes of vasomotor instability, called hot flashes or hot flushes, occur in 70%–80% of women during the perimenopausal period (Table 12-8). Women note sudden onset of flushing involving the head, neck, and chest. This is accompanied by a sensation of intense body heat, which is followed by perspiration. The core temperature increases by approximately 0.2°C, which elicits reflex vasodilatation followed by sweating. The heart rate increases slightly, and some women complain of palpitations. The duration of these episodes is highly variable. The flush lasts from a few minutes to an hour. Some women experience hot flashes for less than 1 year; others have hot flashes for 5–10 years. The severity of the associated symptoms ranges from barely noticeable to incapacitating.

Table 12-8
Consequences of Estrogen Depletion

EARLY CONSEQUENCES	LONG-TERM CONSEQUENCES
Vasomotor instability (hot flashes)	Loss of bone mass
Flushing	Osteoporotic fractures
Sweating	Increased central obesity
Increased heart rate	Increased cardiovascular disease
Sleep disturbance and fatigue	
Urogenital atrophy	
Atrophic vaginitis and cystitis	
Painful intercourse	
Thin skin that is less firm	
Decreased axillary and pubic hair	

Hot flashes are caused by the declining estrogen level at menopause, which somehow stimulates central thermoregulatory centers.

It is the declining estrogen level that stimulates central thermoregulatory centers and release of GnRH. Women who have always been estrogen deficient do not have hot flashes unless estrogen replacement therapy is withdrawn. Hot flashes are correlated with surges in serum LH levels, but LH secretion is not the cause of vasomotor instability. Women with a surgically absent hypothalamus do not produce LH, but they still experience hot flashes. GnRH agonists given continuously down-regulate GnRH receptors and suppress LH release but do not affect the incidence of hot flashes.

Hot flashes frequently are nocturnal. They cause sleep disturbances by rousing a woman completely or by altering her sleep state and limiting the adequacy of her sleep time. The sleep disruption is thought to be responsible for much of the fatigue, irritability, and depression experienced by some women at the time of the menopause. Hot flashes seem to be more severe in women who undergo surgical oophorectomy and have a rapid decline in estrogen levels as compared to women who undergo gradual ovarian decline with aging.

Estrogen depletion also causes urogenital atrophy. Many women develop atrophic urethritis and cystitis, with itching and burning and sometimes urinary frequency and incontinence. Vulvar and vaginal atrophy with decreased mucus production can result in burning, itching, painful intercourse, and vaginal bleeding related to a thin epithelium. Skin and hair also are affected by estrogen depletion. Skin becomes thinner and more wrinkled, and axillary and pubic hair become more sparse.

LONG-TERM CONSEQUENCES OF ESTROGEN DEPLETION

In premenopausal women, estrogen exerts a protective effect on bone mass. Estrogen suppresses parathyroid hormone–induced cytokine release by mononuclear cells, which decreases cytokine-mediated activation of osteoclasts. After the loss of estrogen at menopause, bone turnover increases, and osteoclasts dig more and deeper resorption cavities, which cannot be filled completely by osteoblasts. Estrogen deficiency is responsible for 75% of bone loss within the first 15 years of menopause. Thereafter, most bone loss occurs due to the aging process. Trabecular bone is more vulnerable to estrogen depletion than cortical bone, but both decrease markedly during the first decade after menopause. The loss of bone mass is associated with an increased risk of fractures of the wrist, spine, and hip (see Chapter 7).

Estrogen confers a protective effect on the cardiovascular system, which is lost after menopause. Estrogen increases HDL cholesterol and decreases LDL cholesterol. Estrogen also acts on endothelium and vascular smooth muscle to increase vasodilatation and blood flow.

After menopause women lose lean body mass. They develop more central obesity, which is associated with increased insulin resistance and increased atherosclerotic vascular disease.

HORMONAL TREATMENT OF MENOPAUSE

Estrogen replacement therapy after menopause decreases the vasomotor symptoms associated with hot flashes and reduces the symptoms and signs of urogenital atrophy. Estrogen replacement also helps to stabilize bone mass and prevents osteoporotic fractures (see Chapter 7). Case-control studies and ongoing epidemiologic studies indicate that postmenopausal estrogen use is associated with a 50% reduction in risk for cardiac disease and a reduction in risk for fatal strokes. The magnitude of this protection is not the same for all women. The protective effect is greatest for women with the greatest risk for cardiac disease and much less for women with no cardiac risk factors.

Unopposed estrogen replacement causes hyperplasia of the endometrium, which advances to adenocarcinoma in a small number of women. Progesterone is added to stabilize the endometrium and prevent hyperplasia. The impact of estrogen replacement therapy on breast cancer risk is the subject of extensive epidemiologic research at this time. Studies still are not conclusive.

Postmenopausal estrogen replacement therapy is available in many forms: oral, transdermal, and intravaginal. Vaginal estrogen preparations are used primarily by women who want relatively short-term relief from urogenital symptoms. Doses of estrogen used in hormone replacement therapy are lower than in the past. The dose of estrogen required for vasomotor symptom relief, osteoporosis prevention, and cardiac protection is almost sixfold lower than the estrogen content in the lowest dose oral contraceptives. Circulating estrogen levels during hormone replacement therapy are similar to the lowest estrogen levels during a typical menstrual cycle. Therefore, hormone replacement therapy is not contraindicated in smokers or in most women with a history of heart disease or thromboembolic disease. Whether or not estrogen should be given to women who have had breast cancer or who have a strong family history of breast cancer is uncertain. Optimal therapy requires balancing benefits versus risks on an individual basis.

Estrogen and progesterone can be given continuously or intermittently. Withdrawal bleeding occurs when the progestin is withdrawn. Continuous combined therapy results in endometrial atrophy and cessation of uterine bleeding after 1 year in most women, but breakthrough bleeding occurs during the initial months. The optimal duration of therapy is not certain. It appears that protection against osteoporosis stops shortly after estrogen ingestion stops.

Many women are reluctant to take hormone replacement therapy because of the side effects, the withdrawal bleeding, and fear of breast cancer. *Selective estrogen receptor modulators* (SERMs) have been developed in response to these concerns. These are synthetic compounds that take advantage of the different milieu around estrogen receptors in different tissues. They function as estrogen agonists in bone and heart but do not stimulate the uterus or the breast. Several of these compounds are in clinical trials. Tamoxifen, one of the early compounds in this class, antagonizes estrogen in the breast, but it has agonist activity in the endometrium as well as in bone.

Case Study:
Resolution

Ms. Martin's symptoms and signs indicated new estrogen deficiency, which was confirmed by the absence of withdrawal bleeding after a progestin challenge. Her FSH and LH levels were very high, in the postmenopausal range, indicating loss of almost all ovarian follicles. Her episodes of feeling too warm probably were hot flashes. The cause of her premature ovarian failure is not certain, but a familial autoimmune disorder is likely in view of her mother's autoimmune thyroid disease and early menopause.

Ms. Martin was started on estrogen replacement therapy and was given a progestin to counteract the effects of estrogen on the endometrium. Her vaginal dryness and discomfort during intercourse disappeared. She agreed to have a pelvic examination and a mammogram each year. She was particularly concerned about preventing osteoporotic fractures, because demineralization and stress fractures in her left foot had been noted years before despite her intense exercise. She planned to continue her current level of exercise and to increase her calcium intake.

■ REVIEW QUESTIONS

Directions: For each of the following questions, choose the **one best** answer.

Questions 1 and 2

A young woman, Anita G., comes to the clinic for a physical examination in order to obtain health insurance.

1. Based on this woman's history of regular menses, it is most likely that she is in the *late proliferative phase* of her menstrual cycle. If so, the physician would expect her to have

    (A) a high progesterone level, proliferative endometrium, and a suppressed luteinizing hormone (LH) level
    (B) a high progesterone level, secretory endometrium, and a developing corpus luteum
    (C) low estrogen and progesterone levels, many follicles developing, and a rising follicle-stimulating hormone (FSH) level
    (D) a high estrogen level, a well-developed dominant follicle, and a rising LH level
    (E) a low estrogen level, a well-developed corpus luteum, and a high FSH level

2. Several months later, Ms. G. returns to the clinic having had no menses for 6 weeks. Her pregnancy test is positive. If her pregnancy is to develop normally, which of the following must occur?

    (A) The pituitary must secrete high levels of human chorionic gonadotropin (HCG) to sustain the corpus luteum
    (B) The placenta must secrete high levels of LH and FSH to sustain the ovary
    (C) The corpus luteum must secrete high levels of progesterone to sustain the endometrium
    (D) The placenta must secrete high levels of estrogen to sustain the fetal pituitary
    (E) The pituitary must secrete high levels of prolactin (PRL) to sustain the placenta

3. An 18-year-old woman has never had a menstrual period. Her vagina and uterus are patent. A pregnancy test is negative. Thyroid function and the prolactin (PRL) level are normal. No bleeding follows a progestin challenge test. Based on this information, the physician is certain that

    (A) her LH level is high, but her FSH level is low
    (B) her müllerian duct inhibitory factor level is high
    (C) her human chorionic gonadotropin (HCG) level is high
    (D) her estrogen level is low
    (E) her gonadotropin-releasing hormone (GnRH) pulse generator is abnormal

4. Jennifer L. is a 32-year-old woman who had normal menstrual periods until she developed amenorrhea 6 months ago. She complains of fatigue, frequent flu-like illnesses, dry skin, and vaginal dryness during intercourse. Cervical mucus is scant and does not fern. Laboratory evaluation revealed the following: follicle-stimulating hormone (FSH), 3 IU/L (normal: 3–20 IU/L); luteinizing hormone (LH), 7 IU/L (normal: 8–28 IU/L); estradiol, 90 pmol/L (normal: 108–360 pmol/L); testosterone, 15 ng/dL (normal: 20–80 ng/dL); low free thyroxine index; thyroid-stimulating hormone (TSH), 1 µU/mL (normal: 0.5–6.0 µU/mL). The most likely cause for her amenorrhea is

    (A) congenital adrenal hyperplasia (CAH)
    (B) a large pituitary tumor
    (C) primary hypothyroidism
    (D) GnRH failure due to stress
    (E) chromosomal XO/XX mosaic

5. Sara T. is a 22-year-old woman who has always had irregular menstrual bleeding. Hirsutism has been increasing for several years. She has increased hair on her upper lip and chin, and a male escutcheon (hair extending from the pubis to the umbilicus). She has no temporal balding or clitoromegaly. Laboratory tests reveal the following: luteinizing hormone (LH), 22 IU/L (normal: 8–28 IU/L); follicle-stimulating hormone (FSH), 7 IU/L (normal: 3–20 IU/L); testosterone, 100 ng/dL (normal: 20–80 ng/dL); 17α-hydroxyprogesterone, normal; dehydroepiandrosterone sulfate (DHEAS), normal. She most likely has

   (A) polycystic ovary syndrome (PCOS)
   (B) an adrenal androgen-producing tumor
   (C) congenital adrenal hyperplasia (CAH)
   (D) an ovarian androgen-producing tumor
   (E) testicular feminization (testosterone receptor deficiency)

6. Julia R. consults her physician because an evaluation for infertility indicates that she has polycystic ovarian syndrome (PCOS). Which of the following factors is consistent with this diagnosis?

   (A) Decreased insulin resistance
   (B) Morbid obesity due to high progesterone production
   (C) Bone loss due to constant estrogen and androgen secretion
   (D) Increased luteinizing hormone pulses and ovulation frequency
   (E) Endometrial hyperplasia due to chronic estrogen secretion

Questions 7 and 8

Marion Z. is a previously healthy 52-year-old woman who has had no menses for 9 months. She is experiencing hot flashes and disturbed sleep and asks about hormone replacement therapy.

7. Further evaluation is most likely to reveal

   (A) high levels of follicle-stimulating hormone (FSH) and luteinizing hormone (LH)
   (B) 50% of her ovarian follicles remaining
   (C) absent gonadotropin-releasing hormone (GnRH) pulses
   (D) a low estrogen level but a high progesterone level

8. Risks and benefits of hormone replacement therapy for Ms Z. include which of the following?

   (A) High incidence of urethritis and vaginal atrophy
   (B) Lower risk of osteoporosis and lower risk of stroke
   (C) Higher level of low-density lipoprotein (LDL) cholesterol and increased atherosclerosis
   (D) Fewer hot flashes but increased sleep disturbances
   (E) Restoration of regular cycles and fertility

ANSWERS AND EXPLANATIONS

1. The answer is D. If a young woman is in the late proliferative phase of her menstrual cycle, ovulation will occur very soon. A well-developed dominant follicle that is producing estrogen is required for the LH surge, which precedes ovulation.

2. The answer is C. The endometrium cannot support ongoing development of the fetus unless progesterone production is sustained. During the first trimester, progesterone is produced by the corpus luteum, which is maintained by HCG produced in the placenta. After that, the placenta produces enough progesterone, and the corpus luteum is no longer necessary.

3. The answer is D. If the uterus is present, the outflow tract is patent, and no bleeding follows a progestin challenge, it is certain that there is not enough estrogen to prepare the endometrium for progesterone action. From the information given it is not possible to tell whether the problem is at the level of the hypothalamus, the pituitary gland, or the ovaries. The negative pregnancy test indicates that this woman's HCG level is not high.

4. The answer is B. Jennifer L. has clinical and laboratory evidence of pituitary failure. The vaginal dryness and nonferning cervical mucus indicate estrogen deficiency, which is confirmed by laboratory testing. The accompanying low or low-normal FSH and LH levels show that the problem is in the pituitary or hypothalamus, not the ovaries. Her fatigue and frequent flu-like illnesses suggest cortisol deficiency. Her fatigue, dry skin, and low-normal TSH level in the presence of a low thyroid hormone level indicate secondary hypothyroidism. GnRH failure due to stress is not accompanied by evidence of cortisol deficiency. CAH is unlikely. Her testosterone level is low, she has no signs of virilization, and even late-onset CAH is unlikely at 32 years of age. Amenorrhea due to Turner's syndrome or XO/XX mosaicism is the result of ovarian failure and is accompanied by high FSH and LH levels.

5. The answer is A. The long history of irregular menses, increasing hirsutism, and a LH:FSH ratio of approximately 3:1 are compatible with PCOS. The long duration of her irregular bleeding, lack of severe virilization, and a testosterone level that is not markedly elevated indicate that she does not have an adrenal or ovarian tumor. The normal DHEAS level also suggests that the androgen excess is not solely of adrenal origin. The normal 17α-hydroxyprogesterone level makes CAH unlikely. Testicular feminization results in primary amenorrhea because no ovaries and uterus are present.

6. The answer is E. Women with PCOS have increased insulin resistance, not decreased insulin resistance. Women with PCOS are not always obese, and progesterone does not cause morbid obesity. Chronic estrogen and androgen secretion protects women with PCOS from loss of bone mass. Women with PCOS usually are anovulatory; they do not have increased ovulation frequency. Chronic estrogen production that is unopposed by cyclic progesterone results in endometrial hyperplasia.

7. The answer is A. Ms Z.'s history is compatible with normal menopause, which is associated with marked depletion of ovarian follicles and low estrogen and progesterone production. The normal compensatory increase in FSH and LH requires GnRH stimulation.

8. The answer is B. Atrophic urethritis, vaginal atrophy, higher LDL cholesterol, increased risk of stroke and atherosclerotic vascular disease, increased risk of osteoporosis, hot flashes, and sleep disturbances are consequences of estrogen deficiency, not estrogen replacement. After menopause ovarian follicles are depleted, and it is not possible to restore fertility with hormone therapy.

■ REFERENCES

Baird DT, Glasier AF: Hormonal contraception. *N Engl J Med* 328:1543–1549, 1993.

Belchetz PE: Hormonal treatment of postmenopausal women. *N Engl J Med* 330:1062–1071, 1994.

Conn PM, Crowley WF: Gonadotropin-releasing hormone and its analogues. *N Engl J Med* 324:93–103, 1989.

Franks S: Polycystic ovary syndrome. *N Engl J Med* 333:853–861, 1995.

Godsland IF, Crook D, Simpson R, et al: The effects of different formulations of oral contraceptive agents on lipid and carbohydrate metabolism. *N Engl J Med* 323:1375–1381, 1990.

Haseltine FP, Wentz AC, Redmond GP, et al (eds): Proceedings of a symposium. An NICHD conference: androgens and women's health. *Am J Med* 98(Suppl 1A):1S–143S, 1995.

Rittmaster RS: Medical treatment of androgen-dependent hirsutism. *J Clin Endocrinol Metab* 80:2559–2563, 1995.

Writing Group of the PEPI Trial: Effects of hormone replacement therapy on endometrial histology in postmenopausal women. The postmenopausal estrogen/progestin interventions (PEPI) trial. *JAMA* 275:370–375, 1996.

Zhang Y, Kiel DP, Kreger BE, et al: Bone mass and the risk of breast cancer among postmenopausal women. *N Engl J Med* 336:611–617, 1997.

Chapter 13

GROWTH

Erica A. Eugster, M.D., and Joseph J. Sockalosky, M.D.

▮ CHAPTER OUTLINE

Case Study 1: *Introduction*	*A 6-year-old boy is referred to the growth clinic for evaluation of short stature. Six months ago his height was measured at 102 cm (less than the fifth percentile), and his weight was 16 kg. He has always been healthy. His birth history and growth and development have reportedly been normal. Family history revealed that his mother is 5' 1" tall and had menarche at 13.5 years. His father is 5' 5" tall and entered puberty at an "average" age. Physical examination revealed a normally proportioned boy with a height of 105 cm (thus his growth velocity is 3 cm in 6 mo = 6 cm/yr), weight of 17 kg, and no abnormal findings.*

▮ GROWTH PARAMETERS

Growth is a complex process resulting from the dynamic interaction of numerous factors, both endocrine and nonendocrine. An aberration in growth may be the first or only manifestation of a pathologic process. Body size and proportions have an important impact on an individual's psychological health and well-being.

Careful measurement and plotting of growth parameters on a standardized growth chart (Figure 13-1) at regular intervals are essential components of pediatric care. Height and weight are measured throughout childhood and adolescence. Head circumference usually is measured only during the first 3 years of life.

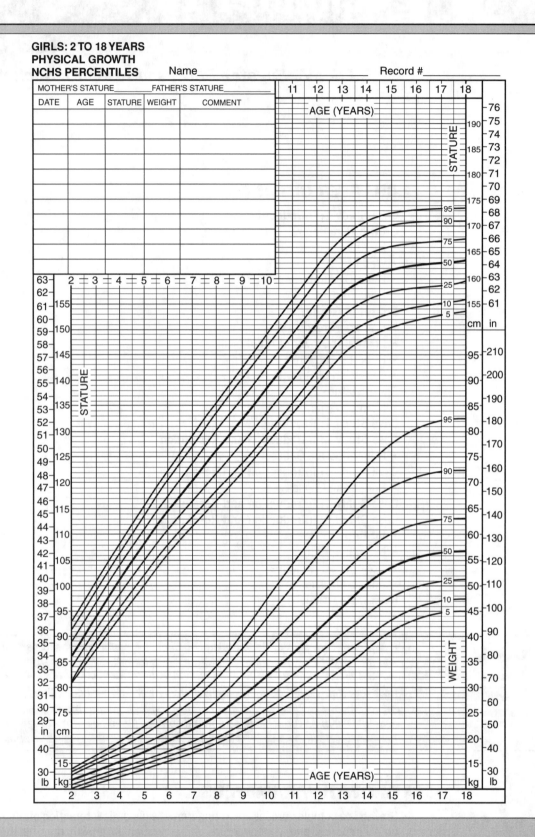

FIGURE 13-1
EXAMPLE OF A STANDARDIZED GROWTH CHART. NCHS = National Center for Health Statistics.

HEIGHT

Of all growth parameters, height is the one most affected by endocrine abnormalities. The most important factor in the evaluation of linear growth is the *growth velocity*, or rate of growth over time.

WEIGHT

Failure to thrive and obesity are the extremes of abnormal weight gain in children.

Failure to Thrive. Failure to thrive refers to poor weight gain in infancy and early childhood. The causes are many and are usually not endocrine; two exceptions are adrenal insufficiency and hyperthyroidism. Most cases of failure to thrive result from malnutrition, chronic disease, congenital anomalies, or psychosocial deprivation (Table 13-1).

FAILURE TO THRIVE	OBESITY
Malnutrition	Exogenous obesity
Inadequate intake	Syndromes
Malabsorption	Prader–Willi
Gastroesophageal reflux	Laurence-Moon-Biedl
Chronic disease	Hormonal abnormalities
Cystic fibrosis	Glucocorticoid excess
Congenital heart disease	Hypothalamic lesions
Inborn errors of metabolism	
Congenital anomalies	
Chromosomal abnormalities	
Syndromes	
CNS or neurologic disorders	
Psychosocial deprivation	
Hormonal abnormalities	
Hyperthyroidism	
Adrenal insufficiency	

Note. CNS = central nervous system.

Table 13-1
Major Causes of Abnormal Weight in Children

Obesity. Obesity results from an imbalance between energy intake and energy utilization. In most cases, obesity is due to a combination of genetic and environmental factors (so-called exogenous obesity) rather than to a hormonal imbalance or disease process (see Table 13-1). Children with exogenous obesity usually have a strong family history of obesity.

Obese children generally have tall stature, but the weight percentile is higher than the height percentile. These children may have lower energy needs or "slower metabolism" than the general population, but even if this is true, they consume more calories than their bodies require. In the case of very young children, caretakers are providing them with these calories.

Obesity also is seen in association with a number of syndromes. Affected individuals tend to have short stature, dysmorphic features, hypogonadism, or mental retardation. Examples of such syndromes include Prader-Willi and Laurence-Moon-Biedl syndromes.

Obesity in childhood rarely is due to a hormonal disorder other than glucocorticoid excess. Growth hormone (GH) deficiency and thyroid hormone deficiency usually do not result in significant obesity. Endocrine causes of obesity in children usually are associated with decreased linear growth.

Obesity can be due to a hypothalamic abnormality. In these cases, overeating is thought to be due to a lesion in the satiety center in the brain. Both congenital and acquired conditions cause this type of obesity.

First Law of Thermodynamics
$$\Delta U = Q - W$$
ΔU = stored energy (fat)
 Q = intake (calories consumed)
 W = work (calories burned)

Short or poorly growing obese children are more likely to have an endocrine disorder or a syndrome than tall or normally growing obese children.

HEAD CIRCUMFERENCE

Growth of the head is determined primarily by growth of the brain. Microcephaly and macrocephaly represent the two extremes of head size.

Microcephaly. Microcephaly is defined as a head size greater than 2 standard deviations (SD) below the mean head size for age. It often is associated with structural or functional abnormalities of the brain and reduced intellectual potential.

Microcephaly = head size 2 SD below the mean for age.
Macrocephaly = head size 2 SD above the mean for age.

A **bone age x-ray** can be used to predict height in children over age 7.

Macrocephaly. Macrocephaly is defined as a head size greater than 2 SD above the mean head size for age. The major causes of abnormal head size are listed in Table 13-2.

BONE AGE

A bone age x-ray is used to determine skeletal maturation, which is then compared to the chronologic age. An x-ray of the left hand and wrist is matched to standardized radiographs representing different ages for boys and girls (Figure 13-2). An x-ray of the hemiskeleton is used in the first 1–2 years of life. Normal bone age (bone age = chronologic age) implies the absence of a pathologic process affecting growth.

Table 13-2
Causes of Abnormal Head Circumference

MICROCEPHALY	MACROCEPHALY
Genetic factors	Hydrocephalus
Chromosomal abnormalities	Infection
Syndromes	Abscess
Intrauterine factors	Subdural effusion
Infection	Toxic or metabolic factors
Exposure to toxins	Lead
Perinatal or postnatal insult	Hypervitaminosis A
Ischemia	Mucopolysaccharidosis
Trauma	Traumatic causes
Infection	Subdural hematoma
Severe malnutrition	Hygroma
	Congenital anomalies
	Syndromes
	Familial

FIGURE 13-2
EXAMPLE OF A BONE AGE X-RAY. This is the standard for girls aged 5 years, 9 months. (*Source:* Reprinted with permission from Greulich WW, et al: *Radiographic Atlas of Skeletal Development of the Hand and Wrist,* 2nd ed. Stanford, CA: Stanford University Press, 1959, p 153.)

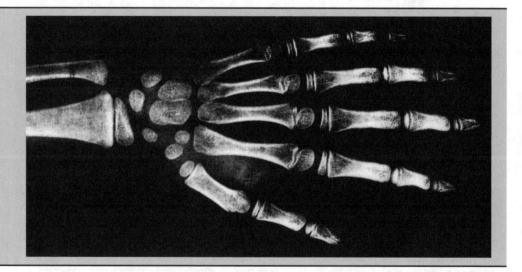

∎ PHASES OF GROWTH

Linear growth can be thought of as occurring in three distinct phases—prenatal, postnatal, and pubertal—each of which has unique characteristics.

PRENATAL GROWTH

Growth of the fetus is influenced by genetic and environmental factors and the hormonal milieu (Table 13-3).

Genetic Factors. Genetic factors include race, gender, parental size, and chromosomal abnormalities. Genetic forces tend to be more important after birth than during the prenatal period.

Environmental Factors. Environmental influences are the result of combined maternal and intrauterine forces. Maternal nutrition, alcohol use, smoking, infections, and other diseases have a strong impact on size at birth. The size of the mother is more important than the size of the father. This also is true in other species. For example, when

Shetland ponies are bred with Shire horses, the foal size is average for Shetlands if the mother is a Shetland pony. The foal size is average for Shires if the mother is a Shire horse (Figure 13-3).

GENETIC FACTORS		**Table 13-3**
Intrauterine environment	Hormones	**Major Influences on Linear Fetal Growth**
Placental function	Insulin	
Multiple gestation	Insulin-like growth factor I (IGF-I)	
Infection	IGF-II	
Exposure to toxins and teratogens	IGF-binding proteins	
Maternal factors	Chorionic somatomammotropin	
Body size	Other growth factors	
Parity		
Nutrition and general health		
Smoking		

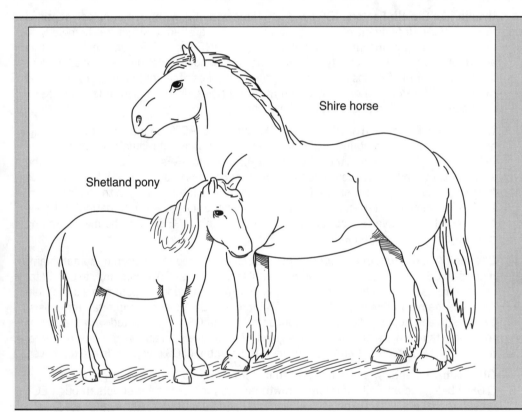

Shire horse

Shetland pony

FIGURE 13-3
The effect of maternal size on birth weight was demonstrated by breeding Shetland ponies and Shire horses. Foal size is average for Shetlands if the mother is a Shetland pony and average for Shires if the mother is a Shire horse. (*Source:* Adapted with permission from Walton A, et al: The maternal effects on growth and confirmation in Shire horse–Shetland pony crosses. *Proc R Soc Lond B Biol Sci* 124:311–335, 1938.)

Hormones and Growth Factors. Our understanding of growth factors is expanding rapidly. As the list of known growth factors increases, so does our appreciation for the complexity of their actions and interactions in the promotion of growth. Hormones that are known to have a major impact on somatic growth in the fetus include insulin and insulin-like growth factors I and II (IGF-I and IGF-II).

In general, the hormones that are essential for normal linear growth after birth (thyroid hormone, GH and others) do not have a significant role in the somatic growth of the fetus. However, these hormones have other important functions in fetal development. Thyroid hormone plays an important role in central nervous system (CNS) development and skeletal maturation. Glucocorticoids are necessary for pulmonary maturation, and androgens are necessary for normal male sexual differentiation. Metabolic effects of GH are listed in Table 13-4.

Insulin. Insulin exerts its influence through a number of anabolic actions primarily in the last trimester of pregnancy (Table 13-4). The importance of insulin is demonstrated by situations of insulin deficiency and excess. Infants with pancreatic agenesis have intrauterine growth retardation. Infants with leprechaunism (Donahue's syndrome) have an abnormal insulin receptor, resulting in lack of insulin action and severe growth retardation. These infants are short, with a skinny, wizened appearance as a result of a lack of subcutaneous fat. In contrast, infants born to diabetic mothers have macrosomia due to excess fetal insulin, which is secreted in response to the increase in maternal glucose crossing the placenta.

Table 13-4
Metabolic Effects of Insulin and Growth Hormone (GH)

	INSULIN	GH
Protein synthesis	Increases	Increases
IGF-I synthesis		Increases
Fat synthesis	Increases	Decreases
Lipolysis	Decreases	Increases
Glycogen synthesis	Increases	
Glycogenolysis	Decreases	Increases
Gluconeogenesis	Decreases	Increases

Note. IGF-I = insulin-like growth factor I.

Insulin-like Growth Factors. IGF-I and IGF-II are potent growth-promoting polypeptides in the fetus independent of GH. These proteins have striking structural homology to proinsulin and have insulin-like metabolic actions. IGF-I and IGF-II and their receptors are widely expressed in a variety of fetal tissues throughout gestation. Decreased placental expression of IGF-II has been found in animal studies of restricted fetal growth. IGF-I promotes differentiation of many different tissue types. At birth, serum levels of IGF-I have been found to correlate with birth weight.

IGF-Binding Proteins (IGFBPs). The IGFs circulate 99% bound to a family of six extracellular binding proteins (IGFBPs), which have important regulatory effects on the IGF system. They prolong the plasma half-life of the IGFs, and by controlling the availability of the IGFs to their receptors, they act as a reservoir of growth factors. These binding proteins have been shown to augment or diminish the activity of the IGFs in vitro. IGFBP-1 levels are increased in infants with intrauterine growth retardation and have been found to be inversely correlated with birth weight. IGFBP-3 is the major binding protein for IGF-I in postnatal life.

Chorionic Somatomammotropin. The placental hormone chorionic somatomammotropin (CS), also known as human placental lactogen, has 96% homology to GH. Fetal size at birth is normal when this hormone is missing, but evidence points to a direct role for CS in the promotion of fetal growth. CS increases DNA synthesis in fetal fibroblasts, myoblasts, and hepatocytes. Serum concentrations of CS are correlated with the size of the placenta and with fetal insulin-like growth factor levels. In animal studies, maternal malnutrition is associated with a decrease in the number of CS receptors in the fetal liver.

Other Growth Factors. Epidermal growth factor (EGF) and transforming growth factor α (TGFα) belong to a family of related growth factors that exert their effects through EGF receptors that are widely expressed in placental and fetal tissues. Although these growth factors are present in many tissues, their roles in human development are not well understood. Less well-characterized growth factors thought to be important in fetal growth include erythropoietin, fibroblast growth factor, nerve growth factor, and platelet-derived growth factor.

POSTNATAL GROWTH: PREPUBERTAL

After birth, infants often change percentiles on the growth chart by accelerating upward or by shifting downward to reach their genetically programmed growth channel. This process usually is complete by 2 years of age. Once children establish their position on the growth chart, they grow at predictable rates throughout childhood and adolescence. Since minor fluctuations in growth are normal, measurements should be obtained at no less than 6-month intervals. Growth rates also show seasonal variations, with the highest growth velocities occurring in the spring and summer.

Nonendocrine Factors. Important nonendocrine influences during the growing years include genetics, nutrition, general health, and psychosocial factors.

Endocrine Factors. Endocrine factors influencing prepubertal growth include GH, IGF-I, thyroid hormone, and insulin.

Linear growth velocity in the fetus reaches a peak of 2.5 cm/wk during the second trimester. If this continued, the linear growth rate would be more than 4 ft/yr!

From the age of 4 until puberty, children should be growing at a rate of at least 4.5 cm/yr.

Growth Hormone. After the first 6–9 months of life, GH is the primary mediator of linear growth. GH is a 191–amino acid polypeptide hormone of 22 kD secreted by the somatotrophs of the anterior pituitary gland. The gene for GH is on chromosome 17. GH exists in both free and bound forms. In the bound form, it is coupled to growth hormone–binding protein (GHBP), which is identical in structure to the extracellular domain of the GH receptor.

GH secretion is controlled by inhibitory and stimulatory factors and is modulated by feedback interactions within the GH axis (Figure 13-4). The primary stimulus for GH secretion is the hypothalamic peptide growth hormone–releasing hormone (GHRH).

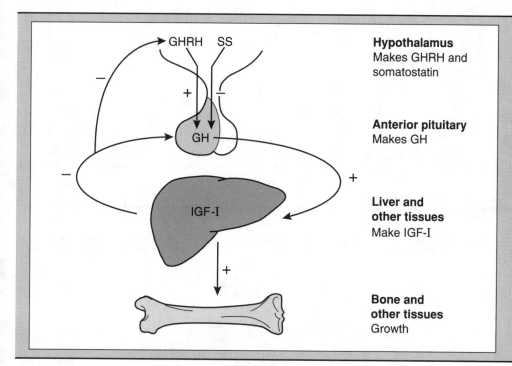

Hypothalamus
Makes GHRH and somatostatin

Anterior pituitary
Makes GH

Liver and other tissues
Make IGF-I

Bone and other tissues
Growth

FIGURE 13-4
GROWTH HORMONE FEEDBACK REGULATION. GHRH = growth hormone–releasing hormone; SS = somatostatin; GH = growth hormone; IGF-I = insulin-like growth factor I.

Numerous other substances stimulate GH secretion, including neurotransmitters, exercise, hypoglycemia, and sleep deprivation. GH is secreted in pulsatile fashion, with the highest pulses occurring during sleep. The amplitude of the pulses increases during puberty (Figure 13-5). The primary inhibitor of GH secretion is somatostatin (SS), also secreted by the hypothalamus.

GH has important physiologic effects on many different tissues. Primary sites of GH action are shown in Figure 13-6. Direct metabolic consequences of GH action include production of IGF-I in liver and nonhepatic tissues, increased protein synthesis, lipolysis, and glucose transport. GH helps to counteract hypoglycemia by stimulating gluconeogenesis and glycogenolysis (see Table 13-4). It also affects mineral metabolism, leading to increased sodium retention and increased intracellular potassium, magnesium, and phosphorus. Many of the effects of GH occur via the IGF system.

IGF-I and IGF-II. Postnatally, IGF-I and IGF-II are secreted in direct response to GH. These polypeptide growth factors have endocrine, paracrine, and autocrine actions. In addition, they exert negative feedback on the secretion of GH by acting at the pituitary and hypothalamus. Although plasma GH levels fluctuate widely, the IGFs are present at sustained concentrations.

Serum levels of IGF-I rise slowly throughout childhood. IGF-I stimulates the proliferation and differentiation of many different cell types. Together with GH, IGF-I stimulates skeletal growth directly by promoting differentiation and proliferation of chondrocytes within the growth plate. This process is thought to be initiated by the binding of GH to prechondrocytes, with subsequent production of IGF-I (Figure 13-7). Levels of IGF-I are decreased by malnutrition and are altered by a variety of disease states. Because of its insulin-like actions, IGF-I can cause hypoglycemia when given acutely.

Testing for **GH deficiency** involves administration of a substance known to stimulate GH release such as clonidine, arginine, or L-dopa, with subsequent measurement of GH response.

Neonates with GH deficiency may present with hypoglycemia because GH is important in glucose homeostasis. Their size is normal, indicating the absence of a GH effect on prenatal linear growth.

Serum levels of IGF-I are strongly correlated with GH secretion and can be useful in the diagnosis of GH deficiency.

FIGURE 13-5
PULSATILE SECRETION OF GROWTH HORMONE (GH) IN PREPUBERTAL AND PUBERTAL MALES. The figure shows the highest pulses occurring during sleep and increased pulse amplitude during puberty. (*Source:* Reprinted with permission from Kappy FI, et al: *The Diagnosis and Treatment of Endocrine Disorders in Childhood and Adolescence,* 4th ed. Springfield, IL: Charles C Thomas, 1994, p 50.)

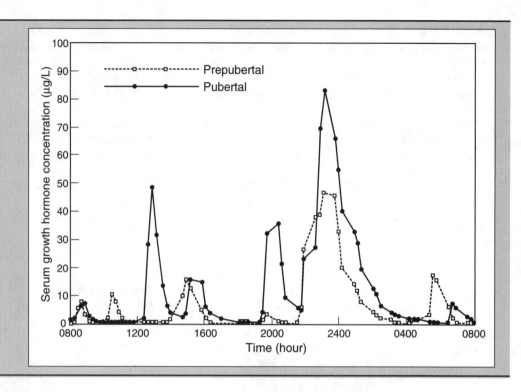

FIGURE 13-6
MAJOR SITES OF ACTION OF GROWTH HORMONE. IGF-I = insulin-like growth factor I. (*Source:* Reprinted with permission from Williams RH, et al: *Williams Textbook of Endocrinology,* 8th ed. Philadelphia, PA: W. B. Saunders, 1992, p 234.)

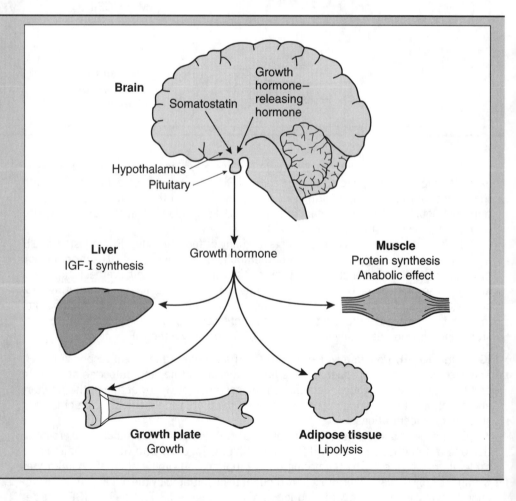

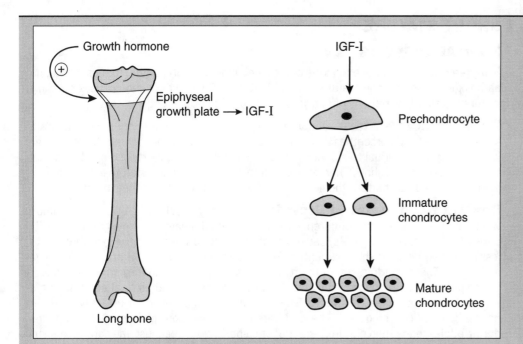

FIGURE 13-7
ROLE OF GROWTH HORMONE (GH) AND INSULIN-LIKE GROWTH FACTOR-I (IGF-I) IN THE DIFFERENTIATION AND PROLIFERATION OF CHONDROCYTES IN THE EPIPHYSEAL GROWTH PLATE. GH interaction with its receptors in the epiphyseal growth plate results in increased IGF-I messenger RNA and increased IGF-I. Increased IGF-I stimulates proliferation and maturation of chondrocytes.

IGF-II has 70% homology to IGF-I. IGF-II also causes differentiation and proliferation of cells. Serum levels decrease progressively after birth, and its postnatal importance is uncertain.

Thyroid Hormone. Normal levels of thyroid hormone are essential for normal linear growth and skeletal maturation. The growth-promoting actions of thyroid hormone occur via permissive effects on the GH/IGF axis. Thyroid hormone and GH have a synergistic effect on growth.

PUBERTAL GROWTH

The growth spurt of puberty is associated with an increase in the pulse amplitude of GH secretion and the production of androgens and estrogens. Sex steroids increase the production of GH. Sex steroids also increase muscle mass, adipose tissue, and bone density and stimulate the development of primary and secondary sex characteristics. By the end of puberty, boys have more lean tissue mass than girls, while girls have more adipose tissue mass than boys. Sex steroids also stimulate increased IGF-I production in cartilage and the maturation of osteoblasts, resulting in eventual fusion of the epiphyseal growth plates. Thyroid hormone also is necessary for normal growth during puberty. The pubertal growth spurt occurs earlier in girls than in boys (see Chapter 14.)

CESSATION OF GROWTH

Linear growth velocity gradually decreases after the pubertal growth spurt, and linear growth ceases when epiphyseal closure is complete. This occurs earlier in girls, who achieve approximately 95% of their adult height by the age of 13. Boys achieve approximately 95% of their adult height by the age of 14.5 years.

A child's final adult height can be estimated, if the heights of his or her parents are known, by calculating a midparental height range. Whether a child achieves or exceeds this range depends upon the timing and rate of progression of puberty and the presence of any conditions that might have an adverse effect on growth. The earlier puberty occurs and the more rapidly puberty progresses, the shorter the final adult height is likely to be.

Major Factors Affecting Growth from Birth to Puberty

Nonendocrine
Genetics
Nutrition
Physical health
Psychosocial factors

Endocrine
Insulin
GH
IGF-I
Thyroid hormone

Approximately 95% of total adult height has been reached when the bone age is 13 years in girls and 14.5 years in boys.

Midparental Height Range Calculation

For girls:

$$\frac{\text{Father's height} - 5'' + \text{mother's height}}{2}$$
$$= \text{mean height} \pm 2''$$

For boys:

$$\frac{\text{Mother's height} + 5'' + \text{father's height}}{2}$$
$$= \text{mean height} \pm 2''$$

▌SHORT STATURE

NORMAL VARIANTS

Many referrals to pediatric endocrine clinics are made for short stature. In most cases, no pathologic cause for short stature can be identified. The most common causes for short stature are simply variations of normal growth for the population.

Genetic Short Stature. Children with genetic short stature have heights that are at or below the third percentile for age. Their growth velocity is normal, and their bone age is also normal (i.e., equal to chronologic age). Their onset of puberty occurs at a normal age. Their parents are short. Therefore, children with genetic short stature achieve a final adult height that is short for the general population but normal for their families.

Constitutional Delay of Growth. Constitutional delay of growth is a common variation of normal growth. Children with constitutional delay have slow growth velocity during the first few years of life, causing them to shift downward on the growth chart to less than or equal to the third percentile. Subsequent growth velocity is normal. Bone age is delayed. These children enter puberty later than their peers, so they grow for a longer period of time. During puberty the growth spurt is normal, and their final adult height is within the normal range (Figure 13-8). There usually is a history of a family member having been a "late bloomer." These children may have more psychological problems during adolescence than children with genetic short stature because they are both short and sexually immature for their age.

Case Study 1: *Resolution*	*Previous growth data for the boy described in case 1 are plotted in the growth chart shown in Figure 13-9. His height has always been below the third percentile. His growth velocity is normal, indicating that no pathologic process is present. If a bone age had been done, it would have been equal to his chronologic age. This child has genetic short stature. A midparental height range calculation indicates that his expected adult height is:* $$\frac{(61 \text{ inches} + 5 \text{ inches}) + 65.8 \text{ inches}}{2} = 65.8 \text{ inches} \pm 2 \text{ inches}$$

Case Study 2: *Introduction and* *Resolution*	*Another 6-year-old boy is referred to the growth clinic for short stature. He has been healthy. According to his mother, his birth history and development were normal, and his height was at the 50th percentile at 12 months of age. Now he is noticeably shorter than his peers. This child's recent growth data are not shown but look identical to those of case 1. Family history revealed that his mother is 5' 3" tall and had late menarche at 17 years of age. His father is 5' 9" tall and had onset of puberty at an "average" age. The physical examination is completely normal. A bone age x-ray reveals that his bone age is more than 2 SD below the mean for his chronologic age.* *This child is shorter than his peers, but he appears healthy with no signs of systemic illness, hormone deficiency, or social deprivation. Although his height percentile shifted downward, his growth velocity is now normal for his delayed bone age. His family history indicates that his mother had constitutional delay of growth. It is likely that this child also has constitutional delay of growth. No treatment is needed. Counseling may be helpful later because of the expected delayed onset of sexual maturation compared with his peers.*

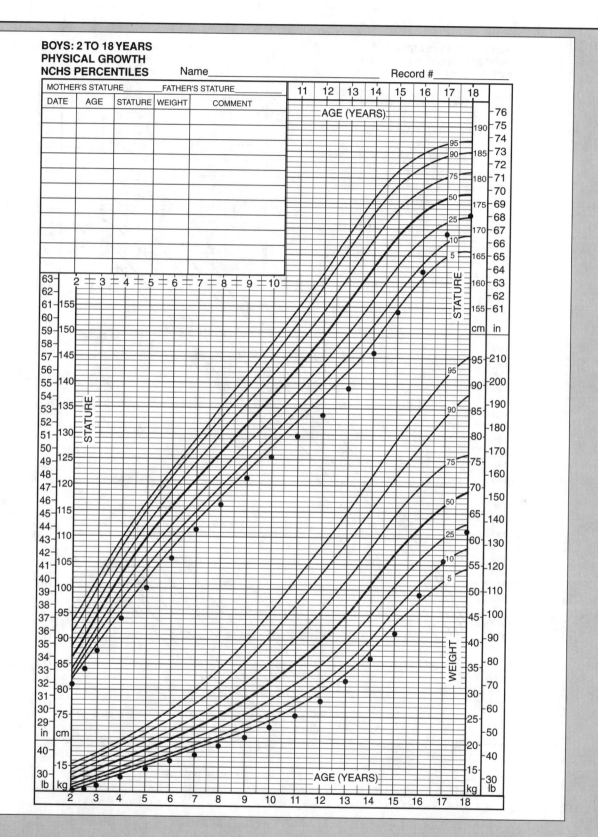

BOYS: 2 TO 18 YEARS
PHYSICAL GROWTH
NCHS PERCENTILES

FIGURE 13-8
GROWTH CHART FROM A PATIENT WITH CONSTITUTIONAL DELAY OF GROWTH. Children typically are short and have delayed puberty. Final height is within the normal range. NCHS = National Center for Health Statistics.

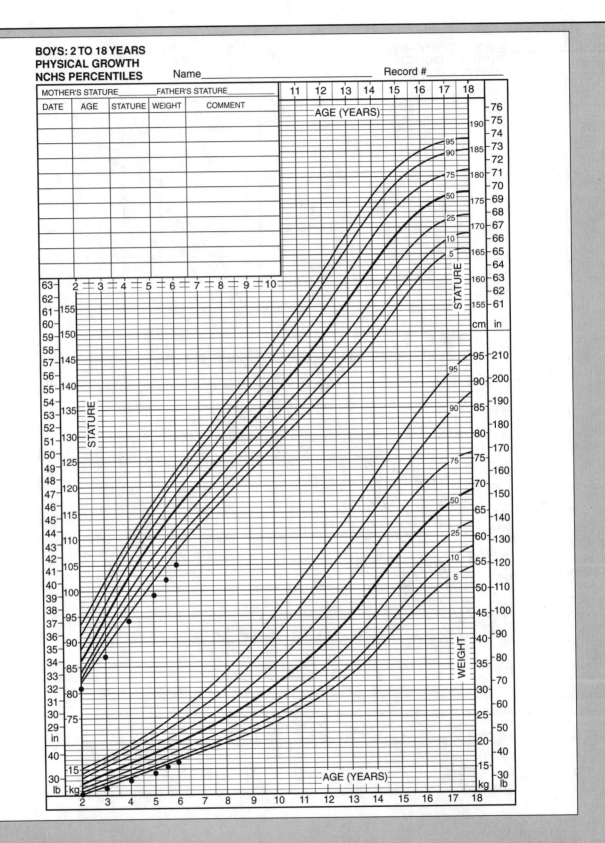

FIGURE 13-9
GROWTH CHART OF CASE 1. NCHS = National Center for Health Statistics.

NONENDOCRINE CAUSES

Chronic Disease. Any chronic disease can interfere with normal growth. In some cases linear growth failure is the initial or only manifestation of an underlying disorder. Examples of diseases that may be silent except for interfering with linear growth include inflammatory bowel disease, celiac sprue, renal insufficiency, and renal tubular acidosis.

Malnutrition. Nutritional deficiency is the most common cause for growth failure in the first 2 years of life. Poverty resulting in inadequate caloric intake is the most common cause of growth retardation worldwide.

Skeletal Dysplasia. Abnormal body proportions indicate that a skeletal dysplasia might be present. Over 100 types of skeletal dysplasia have been identified. The most common are forms of achondroplasia.

Chromosomal Abnormalities and Syndromes. Many syndromes and chromosomal abnormalities are associated with short stature. Examples include Down's syndrome, Prader-Willi syndrome, Williams', Bloom's, Russell-Silver, and Noonan's syndromes.

Turner's syndrome is an important cause of short stature in girls. Turner's syndrome is due to a missing or abnormal X chromosome, which results in gonadal dysgenesis (ovaries are fibrous streaks) and ovarian failure (see Chapter 14). Major physical findings associated with Turner's syndrome are illustrated by case 3. However, since the phenotypic expression of Turner's syndrome is extremely variable, a karyotype is required to make the diagnosis.

> If growth failure is due to malnutrition, the weight percentile decreases first. Linear growth is preserved initially but decreases as the chronicity and severity of malnutrition increase. Finally the head circumference becomes affected.

> Chromosome analysis is recommended for all girls with an abnormal growth velocity or height significantly below that expected for their families.

An 11-year-old girl is referred to the growth clinic for short stature. Her mother reports that her daughter always has been small for her age, but now the discrepancy between her daughter and her peers is increasing. Her mother remembers that her daughter's feet were puffy in the newborn period due to lymphedema. Otherwise, her health has been good except for chronic ear infections. She is doing well in school but has difficulty with math. Significant findings on physical examination include short stature, a low posterior hairline, a high-arched palate, prepubertal breasts, a shield-like chest, sparse pubic hair along the labia, an increased carrying angle of the arms (cubitus valgus), and hyperconvex fingernails. Further evaluation revealed no cardiac or renal abnormalities, although these are common in Turner's syndrome.

Her growth data are plotted in Figure 13-10. Figure 13-11 shows the same growth data plotted on a Turner's syndrome growth chart. This patient is growing at a rate that is typical for girls with Turner's syndrome. Treatment with synthetic GH was begun.

The average height for untreated women with Turner's syndrome is 56 inches. The short stature is not due to GH deficiency, but treatment with GH usually allows girls with Turner's syndrome to reach a height of 60 inches or more. Once an acceptable height has been reached, girls with Turner's syndrome are treated with estrogen and then a combination of estrogen and progesterone to induce sexual maturation and menses and prevent osteoporosis (see Chapter 14).

Case Study 3:
Introduction and Resolution

Intrauterine Growth Retardation. Intrauterine growth retardation is defined as a birth weight that is more than 2 SD below the mean adjusted weight for gestational age, race, and gender. Children with intrauterine growth retardation are a heterogeneous group with varied prognoses, depending on the cause and the time during gestation when the growth retardation occurred. Most "catch-up" growth, if any, takes place within the first 2 years after birth.

Psychosocial Dwarfism. Psychosocial dwarfism can be caused by emotional neglect (usually combined with poor nutrition) or by physical or psychologic abuse. Children with psychosocial dwarfism have been shown to be GH deficient, but they have little response to treatment with GH. Their endocrine abnormalities usually disappear within a few days after they are removed from a negative environment, and catch-up growth occurs.

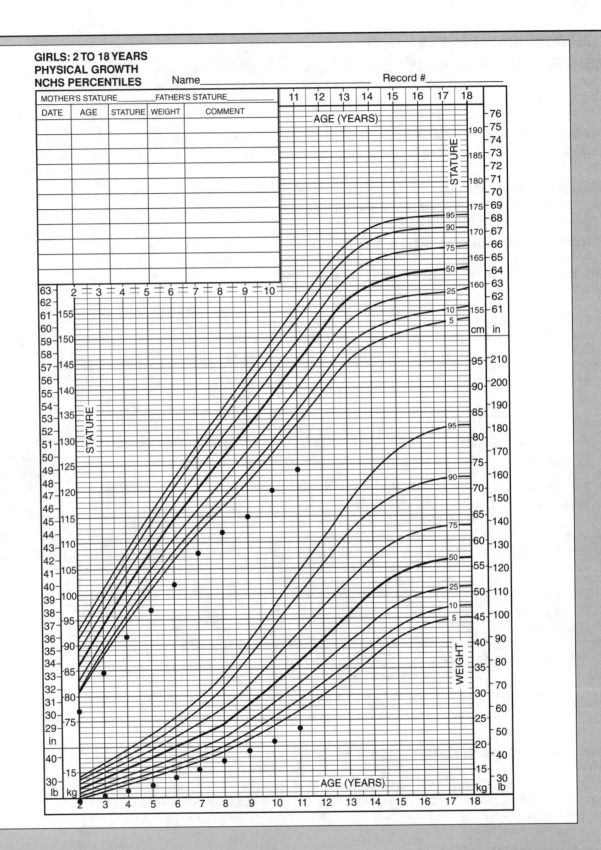

FIGURE 13-10
GROWTH CHART OF CASE 3. NCHS = National Center for Health Statistics.

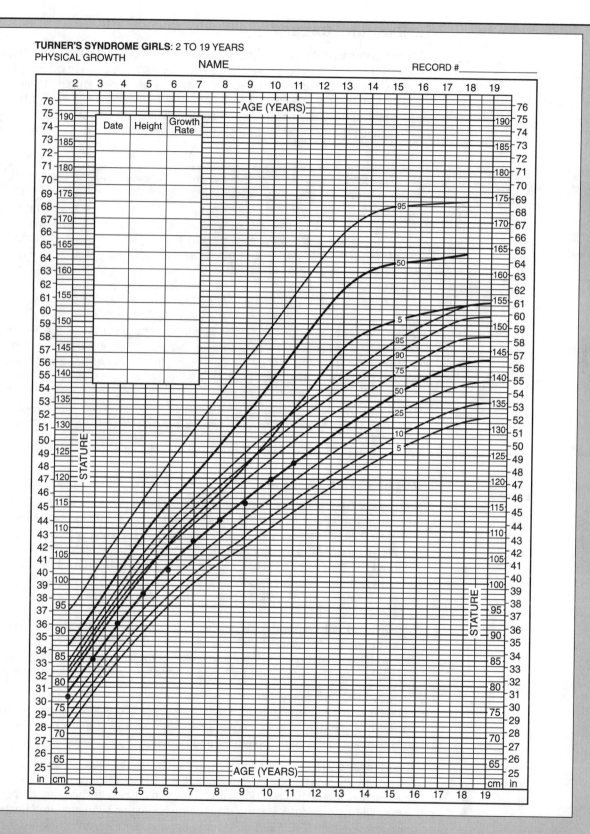

FIGURE 13-11
GROWTH DATA FROM CASE 3 PLOTTED ON A TURNER'S SYNDROME GROWTH CHART. The chart shows the normal percentiles superimposed on the percentiles for girls with Turner's syndrome. Although below the 5th percentile for the general population, this child is growing at the 50th percentile for girls with Turner's syndrome.

ENDOCRINE CAUSES

Hypothyroidism. A decrease in linear growth is one of the most sensitive indicators of thyroid hormone deficiency in children. This may occur while other symptoms and signs of hypothyroidism are so subtle that they go unrecognized. If hypothyroidism develops after age 3, intellectual development is within normal limits. The most common cause of hypothyroidism in children is autoimmune thyroiditis (Hashimoto's thyroiditis). Typical findings in children with hypothyroidism are illustrated in case 4.

Thyroid function testing should be done in all children being evaluated for abnormal growth.

Case Study 4:
Introduction and Resolution

A 9-year-old boy was referred to the growth clinic for evaluation of dry skin and poor growth. He also had some problems with constipation. His parents mentioned that he was tired all of the time, but they attributed his decreased energy to recent hot weather. Physical examination revealed an apathetic child with a slow pulse of 60 beats/min, blood pressure of 100/80 mm Hg, dry skin and hair, an enlarged thyroid gland, and deep tendon reflexes with a delayed relaxation phase. His intelligence was normal for his age. Growth data obtained from his medical record are shown in Figure 13-12.

This child's growth pattern could be the result of hypothyroidism or GH deficiency from a brain tumor. Laboratory studies revealed a thyroxine (T_4) level of 1.0 μg/dL (normal: 5.0–11.0 μg/dL) and a thyroid-stimulating hormone (TSH) level of 200 μU/L (normal: 0.4–5.0 μU/L), showing that he had primary hypothyroidism. Antimicrosomal and antithyroglobulin antibody titers were positive, indicating autoimmune thyroid disease. A bone age x-ray showed a delayed bone age.

He was treated with T_4 replacement, and normal growth resumed. If his initial thyroid tests had been normal, the next steps in his evaluation would have included GH stimulation testing and magnetic resonance imaging (MRI) of the brain to rule out a brain tumor.

GH or IGF-I Deficiency

Congenital GH Deficiency. Congenital GH deficiency can be hereditary or can be due to structural abnormalities of the pituitary gland or other midline structures. Therefore, congenital GH deficiency can occur alone or in association with deficiencies of other pituitary hormones. Families with autosomal recessive, autosomal dominant, and X-linked GH deficiency have been found. Examples of structural abnormalities include pituitary aplasia, pituitary hypoplasia, and septo-optic dysplasia. In some cases, the cause of congenital GH deficiency is unknown. Some of these cases might be due to deficiency of GHRH.

Children with congenital GH deficiency have normal length at birth. The growth rate slows during the first year of life, and decreased linear growth is quite apparent by the time a child is 2 years of age. Intellectual development is normal in children with isolated GH deficiency. They are at risk for hypoglycemia, especially during early infancy.

Acquired GH Deficiency. Acquired GH deficiency can cause growth failure at any age. Conditions that cause acquired GH deficiency include craniopharyngioma or other hypothalamic or pituitary tumors, cranial irradiation for brain tumors or leukemia, trauma, infection, autoimmune hypophysitis, and ischemia. Some cases are idiopathic.

Resistance to GH. Complete insensitivity to GH results in Laron dwarfism. This severe form of dwarfism is caused by mutations in the GH receptor gene and is inherited as an autosomal recessive disorder. Partial GH insensitivity may be the cause of short stature in some children previously classified as having idiopathic short stature. Affected children have low levels of GHBP and IGF-I and high levels of GH, reflecting resistance to GH. These children do not respond to exogenous GH treatment with an increase in IGF-I.

IGF-I Deficiency. Pygmies have normal plasma GH and IGF-II levels, but they have a congenital inability to produce IGF-I.

Diagnosis and Treatment of GH Deficiency. Basal GH levels vary throughout the day so the diagnosis of GH deficiency depends upon the lack of GH response to provocative

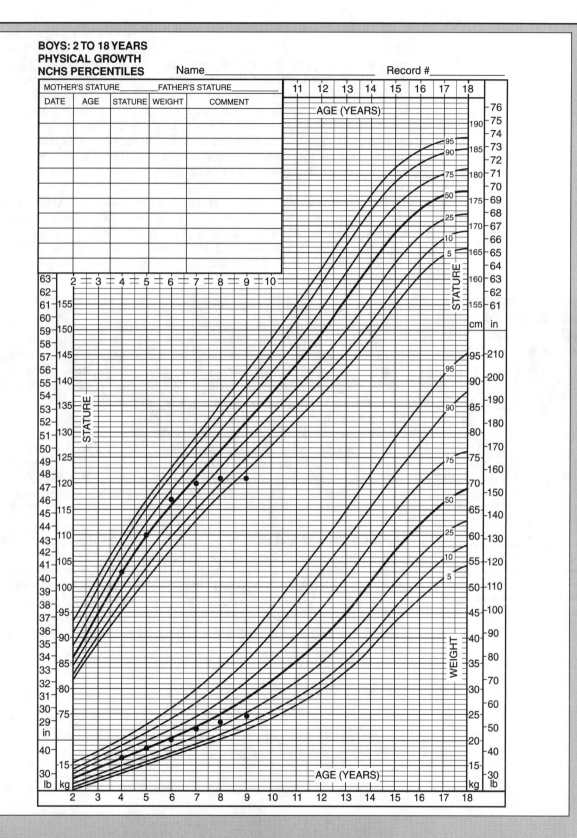

BOYS: 2 TO 18 YEARS
PHYSICAL GROWTH
NCHS PERCENTILES

FIGURE 13-12
GROWTH CHART FOR CASE 4. NCHS = National Center for Health Statistics.

testing. At least 10% of normal children fail to respond to a single stimulus, so two different methods must be used to confirm GH deficiency. Tests must be done when children are fasting because carbohydrate ingestion suppresses GH. Children with psychosocial dwarfism have low GH levels that may not respond to provocative testing.

GH should rise during sleep and after 10 minutes of vigorous exercise. Pharmacologic stimuli for GH release include arginine, clonidine, levodopa, glucagon, gonadotropin-releasing hormone (GnRH), and enough insulin to cause acute hypoglycemia. Clonidine can cause hypotension and drowsiness, L-dopa causes nausea, and insulin can cause hypoglycemia, seizures, or coma. IGF-I levels cannot be used to make the diagnosis of GH deficiency because IGF-I is very dependent upon nutrition and psychosocial status.

Children who are GH deficient require treatment with synthetic human GH. Treatment with synthetic GH currently is approved only for children with confirmed GH deficiency, growth failure due to renal insufficiency, or Turner's syndrome. However, synthetic GH and IGF-1 are available, and studies are being done to see whether children with other causes of short stature will benefit from treatment with GH.

| **Case Study 5:** *Introduction and Resolution* | At 15 months of age, a girl was referred to the growth clinic for abnormal growth. Although her initial height and growth rate were within the normal range, she had been "falling off" her growth chart since she was approximately 9 months of age (Figure 13-13). She was born at term, and development has been normal. She had problems with hypoglycemia in the newborn period but otherwise had been healthy. There was no family history of a growth disorder. The physical examination revealed a petite but otherwise normal child. A complete blood count, sedimentation rate, urinalysis, and serum chemistry screening were within normal limits. Her thyroid tests also were within normal limits. A karyotype was normal. Bone age was delayed.

There was no indication of systemic illness, malnutrition, or parental neglect. Her growth chart was compatible with a diagnosis of congenital GH deficiency. Because of continued abnormal growth velocity, this child underwent provocative testing. Test results confirmed classic GH deficiency, and she has been started on GH therapy. |

Marked increase in weight in association with severe slowing of linear growth is characteristic of **Cushing's syndrome** or **Cushing's disease**.

Glucocorticoid Excess. Glucocorticoid excess causes linear growth retardation in children. This may occur before other signs of hypercortisolism such as generalized obesity, muscle weakness, hypertension, and glucose intolerance become apparent (see Chapter 5). Cushing's disease and other causes of endogenous hypercortisolism do occur in children, but they are rare. Glucocorticoid excess in children usually is iatrogenic, since exogenous glucocorticoids are used to treat many conditions. The growth data plotted in Figure 13-14 are those of a 13-year-old girl who had an adrenocorticotropic hormone–producing pituitary adenoma (Cushing's disease).

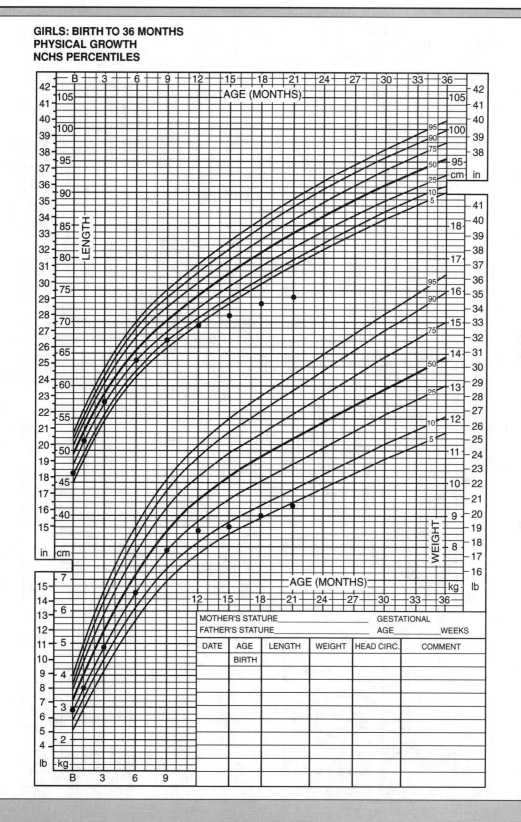

FIGURE 13-13
GROWTH CHART FOR CASE 5. NCHS = National Center for Health Statistics.

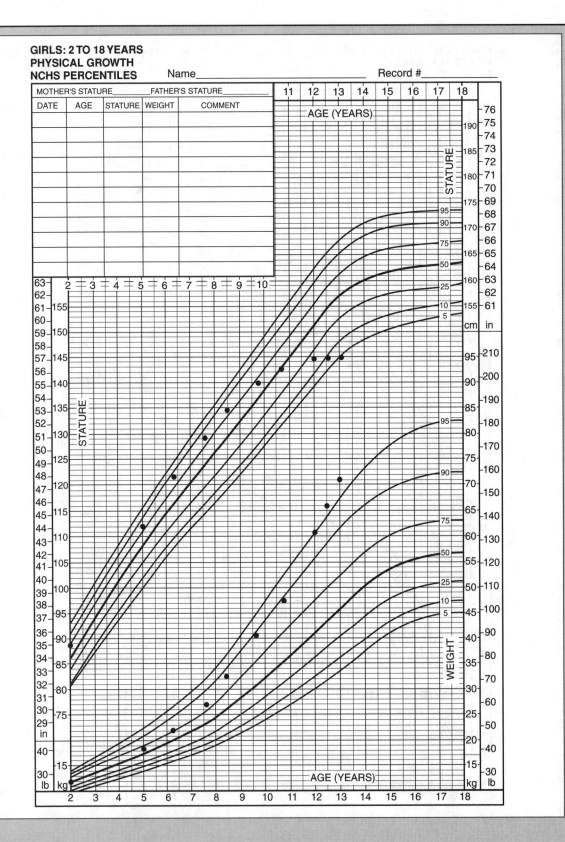

FIGURE 13-14
GROWTH CHART FROM A PATIENT WITH CUSHING'S DISEASE. Note the acceleration in weight coinciding with linear growth failure. NCHS = National Center for Health Statistics.

■ TALL STATURE

NORMAL VARIANT

Genetic Tall Stature. This represents a variation of normal growth in which height and weight are consistently above the 95th percentile. Growth velocity and bone age are normal, and there is a family history of tall stature. These individuals may achieve a final height at or above that of the general population, but their height is appropriate for their family.

NONENDOCRINE CAUSES

Syndromes or Chromosomal Abnormalities

Sotos' Syndrome. Children with Sotos' syndrome (also known as cerebral gigantism) have an acceleration of growth during the first few years of life along with characteristic facial features and developmental delay. The diagnosis is made by clinical criteria.

Klinefelter's Syndrome. This syndrome is seen in men with a 47,XXY karyotype (see Chapter 14). Most patients are diagnosed when they present with delayed puberty and hypogonadism. They often have gynecomastia.

Marfan's Syndrome. This autosomal dominant disorder is caused by mutations in the gene coding for fibrillin, a constituent of connective tissue. Typical findings include tall stature; arachnodactyly (long fingers and toes); and eye, cardiac, and skeletal abnormalities.

Homocystinuria. This is an autosomal recessive disorder, which is phenotypically similar to Marfan's syndrome. This condition is caused by deficiency of the enzyme cystathionine β-synthase, which is important in the metabolism of amino acids. Mental retardation, seizures, and vascular thrombosis are common.

ENDOCRINE CAUSES

Growth Hormone Excess. GH excess usually is due to a GH-secreting pituitary adenoma. This is an extremely rare cause of tall stature and growth acceleration in children. In adults, growth hormone excess causes acromegaly (see Chapter 2).

Precocious Puberty. Precocious puberty is present if signs of secondary sexual development appear before 8 years of age in girls and before 9 years of age in boys. Precocious puberty is an important cause of accelerated growth and tall stature in children. Bone age is advanced beyond chronologic age. Causes of precocious puberty are discussed in Chapter 14.

Paradoxically, untreated precocious puberty may ultimately result in short stature. Premature closure of the epiphyseal growth plates results from premature exposure to gonadal steroids. This is seen in the growth chart in Figure 13-15, which shows data from a patient with the onset of precocious puberty at the age of 5 years.

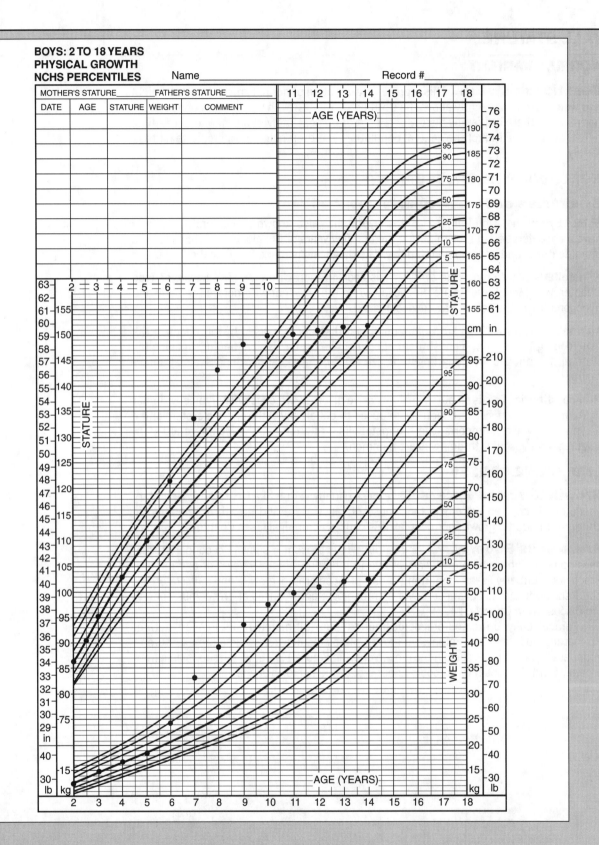

FIGURE 13-15

GROWTH CHART FROM A PATIENT WITH PRECOCIOUS PUBERTY. The chart shows the initial height acceleration followed by premature cessation of growth. NCHS = National Center for Health Statistics.

■ REVIEW QUESTIONS

Directions: For each of the following questions, choose the **one best** answer.

1. An 8-year-old boy is referred to the growth clinic for evaluation of obesity. Despite the fact that he "hardly eats anything," his weight has gone from the 75th percentile to well above the 95th percentile during the last 4–5 years. His height has gone from the 75th to the 90th percentile. Developmental history is normal. According to his mother, several relatives on the paternal side of the family are also "on the big side." What is the most likely diagnosis?

   (A) Hypothyroidism
   (B) Prader-Willi syndrome
   (C) Exogenous obesity
   (D) Growth hormone (GH) excess
   (E) Normal variant

2. A 14-year-old boy presents with complaints of short stature and pubertal delay. He has been healthy otherwise but states that he is the smallest boy in his class and that he is teased at school. His mother is 5′6″, and his father is 6′2″. His father reports that he grew 4″ in the military. On physical examination, the child is found to be well below the fifth percentile for height but is otherwise normal. Signs that puberty is just starting are noted. The most appropriate initial diagnostic test or tests would be

   (A) a bone age x-ray
   (B) luteinizing hormone and testosterone measurements
   (C) a karyotype
   (D) a head magnetic resonance imaging (MRI) scan
   (E) provocative growth hormone testing

3. An 18-month-old girl is referred to the growth clinic for growth failure. Her height has fallen from the 50th percentile at birth to the 10th percentile. Weight has decreased from the 50th percentile to below the 5th percentile. The child has otherwise been well. She lives at home with her mother, four siblings (ages 2 months to 7 years), her mother's boyfriend, and his two children. The most likely etiology for this child's failure to thrive is

   (A) growth hormone deficiency
   (B) insulin deficiency
   (C) thyroid hormone deficiency
   (D) nutritional inadequacy
   (E) congenital infection

4. A 10-year-old girl comes to an endocrinologist's office for evaluation of short stature. Her mother reports that she has always been small, but the difference from her peers has increased during the last several years. She has otherwise been well except for frequent ear infections. Her parents are of average height. A review of her growth chart reveals that her height has fallen from the 25th percentile to below the 5th percentile during the last few years. Weight has remained at the 25th percentile. Thyroid function tests, a complete blood count, sedimentation rate, urinalysis, serum electrolytes, and routine chemistries are normal. Her local physician has done a bone age x-ray, which is normal. Which of the following is the most essential next step in her evaluation?

   (A) Analysis of her caloric intake
   (B) Magnetic resonance imaging of the head
   (C) A karyotype
   (D) A stool sample for fecal fat
   (E) A skeletal survey

5. A 7-year-old boy is referred to the growth clinic because of concerns about his growth. He has been following the curve at approximately the fifth percentile. His mother's height is 5'1½", and his father's height is 5'6". His parents are interested in treatment with growth hormone (GH). Which would be the most appropriate management for this child?

   (A) Schedule the patient for GH stimulation testing now
   (B) Schedule GH testing if the child is still at the fifth percentile in a year
   (C) Prescribe GH at this time
   (D) Reassure the parents that the child is normal
   (E) Schedule other testing first before considering the use of GH

6. An 11-year-old girl presents with slow growth. Review of previous records shows that her height has fallen from the 75th percentile to the 25th percentile during the last 2 years and that she has not grown at all during the past 6 months. Weight has remained at the 50th percentile. She has otherwise been well, although her parents report that she has decreased energy and problems with constipation. They also report that she insists on wearing a sweatshirt even on a hot summer day. The most likely cause of this child's growth failure is

   (A) congenital growth hormone (GH) deficiency
   (B) Cushing's disease
   (C) constitutional delay
   (D) hypothyroidism
   (E) psychosocial deprivation

■ ANSWERS AND EXPLANATIONS

1. The answer is C. The fact that this child's linear growth has been normal indicates that his obesity is not due to organic pathology. The presence of a positive family history also is consistent with a diagnosis of exogenous obesity. No routine testing is indicated in such cases. A long-term, structured program of regular exercise combined with dietary intervention is the only effective therapy. Currently there is no approved pharmacologic treatment for obesity in children.

2. The answer is A. The finding of a delayed bone age would be consistent with a diagnosis of constitutional delay of growth and puberty. This should be suspected on the basis of the patient's presentation and family history. For most patients, reassurance and follow-up are all that are indicated. Some patients receive a short course of testosterone therapy to allow them to develop the physical changes of puberty if they are experiencing significant psychologic stress.

3. The answer is D. The weight percentile in this 18-month-old child has decreased more than the height percentile, which is consistent with a nutritional basis for failure to thrive. Initial management should consist of a 5-day diet history analyzed for caloric intake. In the first years of life, the average daily caloric requirement in children is 1000 kcal plus 100 kcal per year of life.

4. The answer is C. All girls with unexplained slow growth should have a karyotype to rule out Turner's syndrome. There is no evidence for malnutrition or malabsorption, and there is no evidence for a bone disease or skeletal dysplasia. She has had abnormal growth with no other clinical signs of pituitary disease for several years, and her thyroid tests are normal.

5. The answer is D. This child has been consistently in the fifth percentile, so his growth velocity is normal. He has genetic short stature, which is a normal variant. No testing or treatment is indicated. Genetic short stature is not an indication for treatment with GH at this time, although studies are being done to determine the efficacy of GH in increasing final height in such patients. No significant benefit of GH has been demonstrated thus far.

6. The answer is D. This child has classic symptoms of hypothyroidism (fatigue, constipation, cold intolerance) along with dramatic failure of linear growth. Congenital GH deficiency would have presented at an earlier age. She has no symptoms or signs of Cushing's disease, and her weight has remained in the 50th percentile. Her growth chart data are not consistent with constitutional delay. There is no evidence of psychosocial deprivation.

■ REFERENCES

Allen DB, Brook CGB, Bridges NA, et al: Therapeutic controversies: growth hormone treatment of non–growth hormone deficient subjects. *J Clin Endocrinol Metab* 79:1239–1248, 1994.

Frasier SD, Lippe BM: Clinical review. Rational use of growth hormone during childhood. *J Clin Endocrinol Metab* 71:269–273, 1990.

Greulich WW, Pyle SL. *Radiographic Atlas of Skeletal Development of the Hand and Wrist*, 2nd ed. Stanford, CA: Stanford University Press, 1959.

Goddard AD, Covello R, Shiuh-Ming L, et al: Mutations of the growth hormone receptor in children with idiopathic short stature. *N Engl J Med* 333(17):1093–1098, 1995.

LeRoith D, Clemmons D, Nissley P, et al: Insulin-like growth factors in health and disease. *Ann Intern Med* 116(110):854–862, 1992.

Moran A, Brown DM, Doherty L, et al: Diagnosis, monitoring and treatment of short stature in children: twin cities community standards. *Endocrinologist* 5:272–277, 1995.

Blethen SL (ed): National cooperative growth study: ten years of guidance in growth. In *Proceedings of the National Cooperative Growth Study Ninth Annual Investigators Meeting. J Pediatr* 128 (Suppl 1): 1996.

Walton A, Hammond J: The maternal effects on growth and confirmation in Shire horse–Shetland pony crosses. *Proc R Soc Lond B Biol Sci* 124:311–339, 1938.

Chapter 14
SEXUAL DETERMINATION, SEXUAL DIFFERENTIATION, AND PUBERTY

Erica A. Eugster, M.D., and Antoinette M. Moran, M.D.

■ CHAPTER OUTLINE

Case Study:
Introduction

Anna is a 5-year-old girl who came into the endocrinology clinic because of breast development that her mother noticed approximately a month ago. Anna's mother also reported that Anna has developed body odor and has had a recent growth spurt. Anna has needed larger shoes twice in the last 4 months. She has otherwise been healthy. On physical examination, her height, which had been at the twenty-fifth percentile, was now at the fiftieth percentile. Tanner stage-II breasts and Tanner stage-II pubic hair were noted, as well as mild acne. The vaginal mucosa appeared estrogenized. Bone age x-ray was 8 years (> 3 standard deviations [SD] above the mean).

■ INTRODUCTION

The sexual makeup of an individual is complex and is ultimately the result of a number of processes, including determination of genetic sex, development of the gonads, differentiation of internal and external sexual structures, establishment of gender role and gender identity, and postnatal pubertal development. Each of these processes takes place within a unique time frame during the evolution from fertilized ovum to complete sexual maturation. Successful completion of each stage is dependent on numerous factors, both endocrine and nonendocrine.

■ DETERMINATION OF GENETIC SEX

The chromosomal sex of the zygote is established with the fertilization of a normal ovum by an X or Y chromosome-bearing sperm at the moment of conception. Although conception usually takes place uneventfully, genetic accidents sometimes occur.

ABNORMALITIES OF SEX CHROMOSOMES

Abnormalities of the sex chromosomes occur at an approximate rate of 1:500 births. These abnormalities can occur in every cell or in a mosaic distribution. Sex chromosome abnormalities are usually sporadic events, and the phenotypes typically are milder than those observed with abnormalities of autosomal chromosomes. Either the number or the structure of the sex chromosomes may be affected.

Numerical abnormalities. Abnormalities in the number of chromosomes (either sex or autosomal chromosomes) is termed *aneuploidy*. Examples of sex chromosome aneuploidy include Klinefelter's syndrome (47,XXY karyotype) and Turner's syndrome (45,X).

Structural abnormalities. The most common structural abnormality of the sex chromosomes is duplication of the long arm of the X chromosome, with loss of all or part of the short arm. This type of chromosome is termed an isochromosome.

> **Mosaicism** refers to the presence of two or more different cell lines (such as 46,XX and 45,X) in the same individual.

■ DEVELOPMENT OF THE GONADS

Until approximately 6 weeks of fetal age the gonads of male and female fetuses are morphologically indistinguishable and can differentiate into either ovaries or testes. The primordial germ cells migrate from the yolk sac to the developing gonad in the urogenital ridge at approximately 4 weeks fetal age.

DEVELOPMENT OF THE TESTES

In the presence of a Y chromosome, the gonads differentiate into testes. This process is dependent on the existence of a gene known to be critical for male sexual differentiation, which has been given the name *SRY*, or sex-determining region of Y. The *SRY* gene is located on the short arm of the Y chromosome just distal to the pseudoautosomal region (Figure 14-1). The pseudoautosomal regions of the X and Y chromosomes are the portions of the sex chromosomes that pair with each other during male meiosis and, in this way, behave much like a pair of autosomes (thus the name pseudoautosomal). Genetic material may be exchanged between these portions of X and Y chromosomes during meiosis. In addition to *SRY*, several other autosomal or X-linked genes are involved in sexual differentiation.

> **46,XY females** may result from point mutations within *SRY*. **46,XX males** may result from the translocation of *SRY* onto an X chromosome during male meiosis.

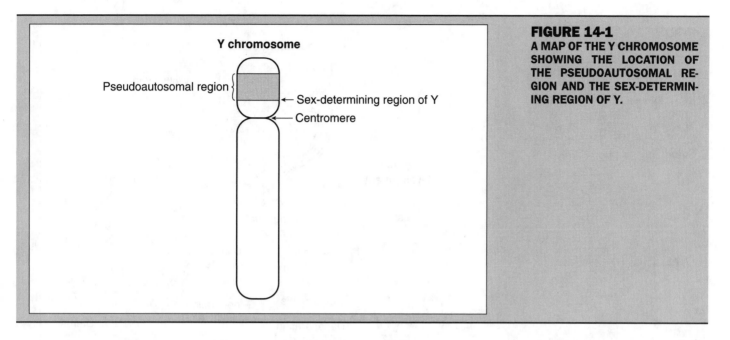

FIGURE 14-1
A MAP OF THE Y CHROMOSOME SHOWING THE LOCATION OF THE PSEUDOAUTOSOMAL REGION AND THE SEX-DETERMINING REGION OF Y.

Normal male sexual differentiation is also dependent on two hormones secreted by the testes, testosterone and müllerian-inhibiting hormone (MIH). Testosterone is secreted by the Leydig cells of the testes, and MIH is secreted by the Sertoli cells. Testosterone secretion, which begins at approximately 9 weeks of fetal life, results from stimulation of the testes by placental human chorionic gonadotropin (HCG) during the critical period of male sexual differentiation.

During later fetal and postnatal life the testes are stimulated primarily by pituitary luteinizing hormone (LH). However, LH levels are low during early fetal development. Because HCG is structurally similar to LH, it is able to bind to LH receptors and stimulate the testes.

Spermatogenesis. Primordial germ cells destined to become spermatogonia are found within the developing seminiferous tubules early in testicular development. After several mitoses, they become quiescent until the pubertal period when cell division again occurs, giving rise to primary spermatocytes.

DEVELOPMENT OF THE OVARIES

In the absence of *SRY*, the primordial gonad has the intrinsic tendency to develop into an ovary. Germ cells must be present for ovarian differentiation. Once ovarian differentiation has occurred, two normal X chromosomes are required to maintain the normal ovarian life span. Girls with Turner's syndrome have ovaries that appear histologically normal early in gestation. However, there is an accelerated rate of germ cell loss with subsequent fibrosis of ovarian stroma, leading to streak ovaries by the time the child is born or at a later point in postnatal life.

Oogenesis. During early development of the ovary, primary germ cells undergo many successive mitotic divisions to give rise to oogonia. The oogonia then enter meiotic division and become oocytes. Many oocytes degenerate during fetal life, but those that survive are arrested in the first meiotic division until ovulation occurs.

DEVELOPMENT OF THE GENITAL DUCTS AND EXTERNAL GENITALIA

GENITAL DUCTS

By the seventh week of fetal life, both male (wolffian) and female (müllerian) ducts are present, derived from the mesonephros. During the third fetal month, either the wolffian or the müllerian ducts become fully formed, while the opposite structures degenerate (Figure 14-2). The hormonal milieu plays the decisive role in determining which elements differentiate and which involute.

The classic concept of **female by default** has come under scrutiny because of the discovery of a gene on the short arm of the human X chromosome that, when duplicated, results in a male-to-female sex reversal, even in the presence of a functional *SRY* gene. Female sexual differentiation may be a more active process than was previously believed.

Karyotype 45,X
Turner's syndrome
Accelerated germ cell loss
Early ovarian fibrosis
Streak gonads
Short stature

FIGURE 14-2
DIFFERENTIATION OF THE MÜL-
LERIAN AND WOLFFIAN DUCTS
LEADING TO FORMATION OF IN-
TERNAL STRUCTURES. (*Source:*
Reprinted with permission from
Spence AP, Mason EB: *Human
Anatomy and Physiology*, 3rd
ed. Menlo Park, CA: Benjamin/
Cummings, 1987, p 810.)

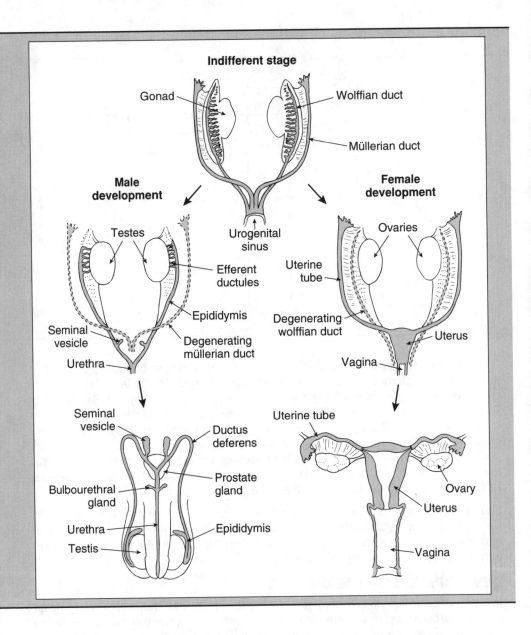

Development of the **wolffian structures** requires a high local concentration of testosterone. If only one functioning testis is present, male differentiation occurs only on one side, and female internal structures develop on the other side. MIH also acts locally and unilaterally.

Testosterone, produced by the fetal testes, causes the wolffian ducts to complete their development, leading to formation of the epididymis, vas deferens, and seminiferous tubules. MIH, also produced by the fetal testes, causes degeneration of the müllerian structures.

In the absence of functioning testes, the müllerian ducts differentiate, leading to the development of the uterus and fallopian tubes. This process is not dependent on the presence of an ovary. *Therefore, it is the presence or absence of functioning testes that determines whether male or female internal structures develop.*

EXTERNAL GENITALIA

At 8 weeks fetal life, the external genitalia of male and female fetuses are identical and can differentiate in the direction of either sex. Homologous structures are shown in Figure 14-3. Development of male external genitalia (and prostate) requires the presence of *dihydrotestosterone (DHT)* during weeks 8–12 of fetal life. DHT is formed from testosterone intracellularly by the action of the enzyme 5α-reductase.

During fetal life DHT binds to the androgen receptor with a greater affinity than testosterone. In the absence of DHT, female external genitalia develop.

In the female fetus, the vagina develops from the urogenital sinus. When normal müllerian structures are present, a septum develops that pushes the vaginal introitus

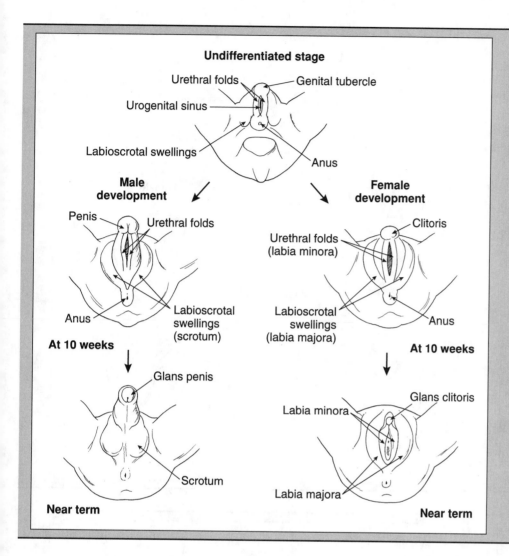

Undifferentiated stage

Urethral folds — Genital tubercle

Urogenital sinus

Labioscrotal swellings

Anus

Male development

Penis — Urethral folds

Anus

Labioscrotal swellings (scrotum)

At 10 weeks

Glans penis

Scrotum

Near term

Female development

Clitoris

Urethral folds (labia minora)

Labioscrotal swellings (labia majora)

Anus

At 10 weeks

Glans clitoris

Labia minora

Labia majora

Near term

FIGURE 14-3
DIFFERENTIATION OF THE EXTERNAL GENITALIA SHOWING HOMOLOGOUS MALE AND FEMALE STRUCTURES. (*Source:* Reprinted with permission from Spence AP, Mason EB: *Human Anatomy and Physiology,* 3rd ed. Menlo Park, CA: Benjamin/Cummings, 1987 p 811.)

posteriorly, creating a separate external opening. In the male, the prostate gland is derived from the urogenital sinus (Figure 14-4). After the twelfth fetal week, external genital formation is complete. Sexual determination and differentiation are summarized in Figure 14-5.

After the twelfth week of gestation, abnormalities in the hormonal environment can affect the size of the clitoris and phallus but not their morphologic structure.

FIGURE 14-4
DIFFERENTIATION OF THE URO-GENITAL SINUS. (*Source:* Reprinted with permission from Lifshitz F: *Pediatric Endocrinology*, 3rd ed. New York, NY: Marcel Dekker, 1996, p 285.)

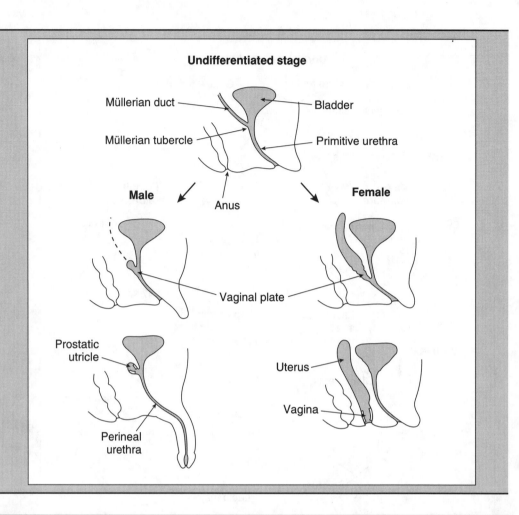

FIGURE 14-5
NORMAL SEXUAL DIFFERENTIATION FROM FERTILIZATION THROUGH FORMATION OF THE EXTERNAL GENITALIA. *SRY* = sex-determining region of Y.

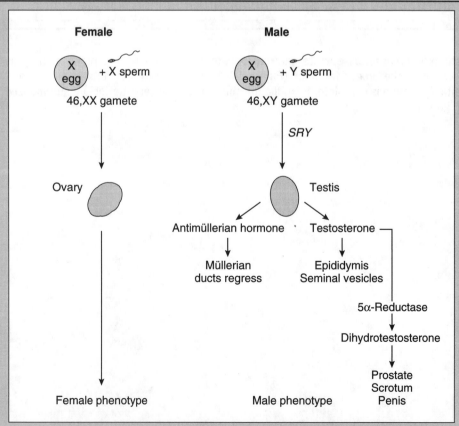

PSYCHOSEXUAL DIFFERENTIATION

In the area of psychosexual differentiation, the nature versus nurture debate is far from resolved. There are three main concepts that define psychosexual development: gender identity, gender role, and sexual orientation.

GENDER IDENTITY

Gender identity refers to the subjective sense of being "male" or "female," which is usually solidified between the ages of 2 and 2½. With time, gender identity becomes basic to all other aspects of personal identity. Factors influencing the formation of gender identity include parental attitudes, appearance of the genitalia, and sex assignment at birth.

GENDER ROLE

Gender role refers to objective behaviors within a given social group, which are assigned to either male or female members of the species. Differences in the behavior of boys and girls from early infancy have been observed, although such observations are influenced substantially by observer bias based on sexual stereotypes. There is evidence that gender role behaviors may be influenced by prenatal hormones, but these behaviors can also be learned. They are mediated initially by parents or other caregivers and later by same-sex peer groups.

Some researchers have found structural differences in certain areas of the brain in men and women. This has led to speculation about the role of the brain in human psychosexual differentiation.

SEXUAL ORIENTATION

Sexual orientation refers to an individual's sexual attraction to the opposite or same sex and usually develops after puberty.

AMBIGUOUS GENITALIA

The birth of an infant with ambiguous genitalia is considered both a medical emergency because potentially life-threatening conditions are part of the differential diagnosis and a psychologic emergency because of the need for an unequivocal sex assignment as soon as possible. This cannot be made before all the necessary information has been collected and analyzed. There are four general categories of ambiguous genitalia. These are virilization of the XX female infant, undervirilization of the XY male infant, intersex disorders, and anatomic or syndromic abnormalities.

VIRILIZATION OF THE XX FEMALE INFANT

Exposure of the female fetus to androgens prior to the twelfth fetal week results in labial fusion, clitoral hypertrophy, and sometimes even formation of a male urethra. After the twelfth fetal week, exposure to androgens causes only clitoral hypertrophy. There are three general categories of disorders that cause virilization of the XX female.

Congenital Adrenal Hyperplasia (CAH). CAH is the most common cause of ambiguous genitalia in female infants. This autosomal recessive disorder is caused by the deficiency of an enzyme involved in adrenal steroidogenesis.

The enzyme block is within the synthetic pathway of cortisol. If the defect is severe, synthesis of aldosterone also is affected. Low cortisol levels cause a rise in pituitary adrenocorticotropic hormone (ACTH) levels, producing hyperstimulation of the fetal adrenals. There is buildup of steroid precursors that are shunted into the androgen synthetic pathway, resulting in adrenal androgen excess (Figure 14-6). A defect in the enzyme 21-hydroxylase is the most common enzyme defect of CAH.

Approximately two-thirds of individuals with 21-hydroxylase deficiency have a defect in both cortisol and aldosterone synthesis, resulting in virilization and salt-wasting. The other one-third have only a defect in cortisol production, resulting in virilization.

Girls with CAH have a normal 46,XX karyotype and normal internal reproductive organs, but their external structures are virilized. In contrast, boys with a 21-hydroxylase deficiency appear normal at birth. This is due to the fact that androgens from the testes are very high in utero, so an extra contribution from the adrenals has no phenotypic

Fifty percent concordance for homosexuality among identical twins, as well as a higher than expected incidence of homosexuality in women with prenatal androgen exposure, indicates the contribution of both genetic and environmental factors in the development of sexual orientation.

Causes of Virilization of an XX Female
Congenital adrenal hyperplasia
Excess maternal or placental androgens
Idiopathic or teratogenic factors

The diagnosis of **21-hydroxylase deficiency** is made by finding an elevated level of plasma 17α-hydroxyprogesterone, the substrate for the defective enzyme in the synthetic pathway of cortisol.

If synthesis of **aldosterone** is blocked, patients with **CAH** are at risk for a "salt-wasting crisis," characterized by electrolyte abnormalities, dehydration, and shock. This usually occurs within the first 5–10 days of life. In many states, all newborns are screened for 21-hydroxylase deficiency.

FIGURE 14-6
PATHOPHYSIOLOGY OF CONGEN-ITAL ADRENAL HYPERPLASIA (CAH). This figure shows a block at the level of the 21-hydroxylase enzyme with accumulation of the cortisol precursor 17α-hydroxy-progesterone and increased production of adrenal androgens. The decreased production of cortisol leads to continued stimulation of the adrenals by pituitary adrenocorticotropic hormone (ACTH).

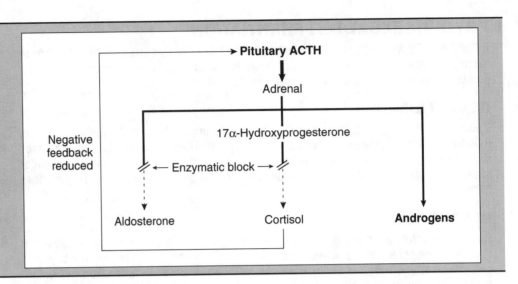

consequences. Boys may present in the newborn period if they are salt-wasters or later in life with precocious puberty (see Precocious Puberty).

Treatment of CAH involves glucocorticoid replacement and surgical correction of ambiguous genitalia. Mineralocorticoid replacement also may be required.

Maternal or Placental Androgens. Maternal or placental androgens may also cause virilization of a female fetus. Sources include maternal virilizing tumors (adrenal, ovarian), maternal CAH, ingestion of androgens or progestins, or abnormal placental enzyme activity (rare). In all of these cases, the mother is virilized.

Idiopathic or Teratogenic Virilization. Virilization of the XX female fetus can also be *idiopathic* or *teratogenic*. In idiopathic cases, the etiology of the virilization is not identified. Teratogenic implies a specific exposure.

UNDERVIRILIZATION OF THE XY MALE INFANT

Conditions giving rise to undervirilization of the male infant result in a spectrum of phenotypic findings, ranging from normal female genitalia to various degrees of ambiguous genitalia. The phenotype depends on the severity of the defect and the time of development during which the defect occurs. There are four general causes of undervirilization of the male infant.

Defect in the Pathway of Testosterone Synthesis. Deficiency of an enzyme needed for the synthesis of testosterone can be present in the adrenals and testes or in the testes alone. Patients with adrenal enzyme deficiencies may also be at risk for salt-wasting.

Patients with a 5α-reductase deficiency cannot convert testosterone to DHT. Since the development of normal male external genitalia is dependent on DHT, these patients have female or ambiguous external genitalia. Their internal reproductive structures develop normally since these structures are dependent only on the presence of testosterone. At puberty, receptor-affinity relationships change. The external structures become responsive to testosterone, leading to partial virilization of external genitalia. In some cultures, in which the incidence of 5α-reductase is quite high, complete reversal of sex assignment at puberty is an accepted and well-recognized phenomenon called "guevedoce," which means "penis at 12."

Androgen Resistance. Androgen resistance is another cause of undervirilization of male infants. End organ resistance to androgens, which can be complete or partial, is caused by abnormalities in the number or function of androgen receptors. These abnormalities are due to mutations in the genes coding for the androgen receptor on the X chromosome or other related molecules that cause postreceptor defects.

Complete androgen resistance due to a severe abnormality or absence of the androgen receptor results in *testicular feminization syndrome*. Testes are present and testosterone is produced, but tissues are unable to respond. The genotype is 46,XY, but the phenotype is unambiguously female. There are no wolffian structures because tissues

Causes of Undervirilization of an XY Male
Deficient enzyme for testosterone synthesis
Deficient 5α-reductase enzyme for DHT synthesis
Abnormal androgen receptors (androgen resistance)
    Complete (testicular feminization)
    Partial
Testicular regression
Maternal drug ingestion

cannot recognize testosterone. There are no müllerian structures because the testes produce MIH normally. The external genitalia are female.

At puberty, when testosterone increases, follicle-stimulating hormone (FSH) and LH levels remain high because the pituitary lacks testosterone receptors and cannot respond to negative feedback. Constant FSH and LH stimulation results in high levels of testosterone, which is converted to estrogen in peripheral tissues. Breast development occurs in response to estrogen stimulation. Patients present with primary amenorrhea, since the vagina ends in a blind pouch. They have little or no pubic hair and acne because both require effective androgens for development.

The testes are intra-abdominal and must be removed after puberty has been completed because intra-abdominal testes are at high risk for malignancy. Estrogen replacement therapy is given after the testes are removed.

Partial androgen resistance, resulting in variable degrees of genital ambiguity, accounts for most cases of ambiguous genitalia in boys. The pattern of inheritance in many kindreds is consistent with an X-linked recessive trait with variable penetrance. Wolffian duct structures are poorly developed.

Testicular Regression. Testicular regression, also known as "vanishing testes," refers to a 46,XY male infant with absence of identifiable gonads. The underlying defect is unknown but can result in varying degrees of genital ambiguity or micropenis, depending on the timing of the regression.

Maternal Drug Ingestion. Maternal drug ingestion can interfere with normal male sexual differentiation. Estrogens, progestins, and spironolactone are examples of drugs ingested by the mother that can result in undervirilization of a male fetus.

INTERSEX DISORDERS

Intersex disorders represent abnormalities of gonadal differentiation in which both male and female elements are present. Individuals with *true hermaphroditism* have ovarian and testicular tissue. The genitalia may be male, female, or ambiguous. The most common finding is an ovary on one side of the abdomen and a testis on the other, although both may be combined as an ovotestis. The most common karyotype is 46,XX.

In contrast, *mixed gonadal dysgenesis* is a disorder that is associated with mosaicism of two or more cell lines with different karyotypes, one of which includes a Y chromosome or portions of a Y chromosome. A wide range of phenotypes have been described. Various combinations of dysgenetic testes, ovotestis, or streak ovaries are present, as well as a rudimentary uterus and at least one oviduct. Approximately one-third of these patients have stigmata of Turner's syndrome (see Turner's Syndrome).

ANATOMIC AND SYNDROMIC CAUSES

Anatomic causes of ambiguous genitalia include morphologic defects, which often occur in association with other congenital anomalies of the hind gut such as imperforate anus or renal agenesis. In rare cases, ambiguous genitalia can be due to mechanical disruption such as that caused by a hemangioma or amniotic band. A number of *chromosomal abnormalities and syndromes*, including trisomy 13 and 18, CHARGE, Robinow's, Smith-Lemli-Opitz, and Vacterl's syndromes, are associated with ambiguous genitalia.

MANAGEMENT OF INFANTS WITH AMBIGUOUS GENITALIA

Sex assignment is based upon the potential for normal appearance and normal sexual function. Individuals with ambiguous genitalia usually are infertile. Virilized women in whom the internal reproductive organs are normal are exceptions. In male children, the most important factor is the potential size of the phallus in adulthood.

Once a sex assignment is made, the child should be raised unambiguously in that gender role. Throughout childhood and puberty, the appropriate hormonal and surgical interventions are instituted so that the phenotypic sex agrees with the assigned gender.

FSH, LH, testosterone, and estrogen levels are all high in **testicular feminization syndrome**. FSH and LH are high because the pituitary lacks receptors to recognize testosterone and cannot respond to negative feedback. Continual stimulation of the testes by high levels of LH results in high levels of testosterone, which are converted to estrogen in peripheral tissues.

MICROPENIS

Micropenis is defined as a phallic length that is 2.5 SD below the mean for age. In a term newborn, a phallus less than or equal to 2 cm is considered a micropenis.

Micropenis is the condition in which unambiguously male genitalia are abnormally small. The length of the phallus is at least 2.5 SD below the mean for age.

From the sixth to the twelfth fetal week, HCG from the placenta stimulates production of testosterone from the fetal testes. Testosterone is converted to DHT, which stimulates differentiation of the external genitalia. After the twelfth fetal week, LH from the fetal pituitary stimulates the testes to produce testosterone. A defect anywhere along the fetal hypothalamic-pituitary-gonadal axis or a defect in peripheral androgen action can result in failure of the phallus to grow.

Gonadotropin deficiency due to a pituitary defect is the most common cause of micropenis. LH deficiency can be isolated or can be associated with deficiencies in other pituitary hormones. Isolated gonadotropin deficiency also can be due to a hypothalamic defect resulting in failure of gonadotropin-releasing hormone (GnRH) secretion.

Primary hypogonadism can lead to micropenis if the testes cannot secrete enough testosterone for normal genital development. This can occur in boys with Klinefelter's syndrome (47,XXY) and with other causes of primary testicular failure such as "vanishing testes."

Mild *partial androgen resistance* can be the cause of micropenis. *Syndromes and chromosomal disorders* with micropenis as an associated feature include Noonan, Prader-Willi, and various trisomies. Some cases of micropenis are classified as *idiopathic*.

The newborn with a micropenis must be monitored closely for signs of other pituitary hormone deficiencies. Hypoglycemia may develop due to ACTH deficiency, GH deficiency, or both.

Newborn children with micropenis must be examined carefully for signs of multiple pituitary hormone deficiencies. If they are present, these infants are at risk for hypoglycemia due to growth hormone (GH) and ACTH deficiencies, hypothyroidism due to thyroid-stimulating hormone (TSH) deficiency, and adrenal insufficiency due to lack of ACTH. A karyotype may be necessary to rule out Klinefelter's syndrome. Children with micropenis due to inadequate testosterone production usually respond well to a trial of testosterone therapy. If the problem is due to resistance to androgen action and a 1–3 month course of testosterone fails to induce a significant increase in the size of the penis, gender reassignment may be necessary. As with infants with ambiguous genitalia, the major factor is the potential size of the phallus in adulthood.

Lack of response to exogenous androgens suggests that a male sex assignment is unrealistic.

Case Study:
Continued

Review of Anna's records confirmed that until recently she had been developing normally. Physical examination revealed that she had normal female genitalia. She had signs of estrogen action (breast development) and androgen action (body hair, acne), which would be expected at the time of puberty but were very inappropriate in a 5-year-old child. In addition, the acceleration in her growth velocity and advancement of skeletal maturation suggested a pathologic process. A GnRH stimulation test was performed.

PUBERTY

The onset of puberty marks the beginning of a complex process that results in complete sexual maturation. This process includes growth and development of primary sexual characteristics (genitalia and gonads), development of secondary sexual characteristics, psychologic changes, and the acquisition of fertility. These events are brought about by gonadal production of sex steroids resulting from the activation of the hypothalamic-pituitary-gonadal axis (Figure 14-7).

HYPOTHALAMIC-PITUITARY-GONADAL AXIS

Puberty can be thought of as part of a continuum of gonadal development. Hypothalamic-pituitary activity is very active during fetal life, becomes relatively quiescent during childhood, and then becomes active again at puberty.

Episodic release of GnRH from hypothalamic neurons known as the GnRH pulse generator stimulates intermittent release of the gonadotropins LH and FSH from the pituitary. Prior to puberty, infrequent, low-amplitude pulses of LH and FSH occur. Puberty

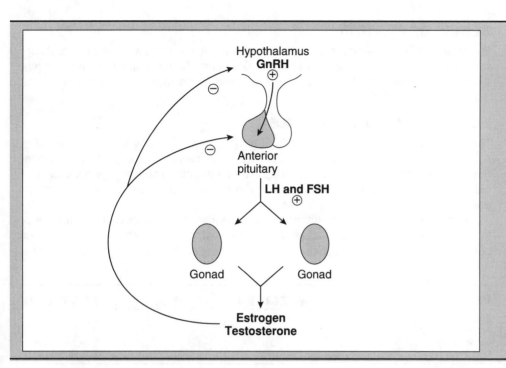

FIGURE 14-7

HYPOTHALAMIC-PITUITARY-GO-NADAL AXIS. This figure shows feedback relationships at the level of the pituitary and hypothalamus. GnRH = gonadotropin-releasing hormone; LH = luteinizing hormone; FSH = follicle-stimulating hormone.

is heralded by a dramatic increase in the amplitude and frequency of LH pulses. During the pubertal period, these pulses first occur during sleep and then later throughout the day. Patterns of gonadotropin secretion from infancy through puberty are shown in Figure 14-8.

SEX STEROIDS

The physical changes of puberty are caused by estrogens and androgens, both of which are present in male and female individuals. *Estrogen* is produced by the ovaries in females and by peripheral conversion of androgens in both sexes. Estrogen causes breast enlargement, maturation of the vaginal mucosa, growth acceleration, and advancement of skeletal maturation. *Androgens* are produced by the adrenals, by the testes (males), and by the ovaries (females). Androgens cause acne; axillary, pubic, and facial hair growth; body odor; voice changes; growth acceleration; and skeletal maturation.

Androgens and estrogens cause skeletal maturation, but estrogen is essential for complete epiphyseal fusion. This was demonstrated recently in a man with complete absence of estrogen receptors. At 28-years-old, he was 6'11" tall and still growing.

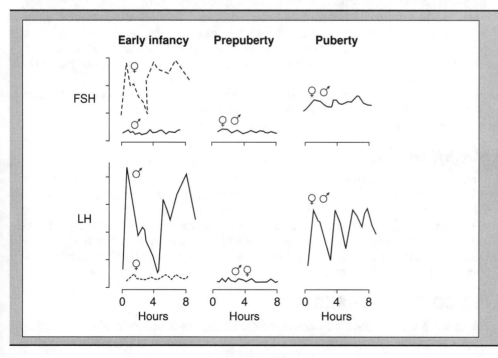

FIGURE 14-8

LEVELS OF LUTEINIZING HORMONE AND FOLLICLE-STIMULATING HORMONE IN AN 8-HOUR PERIOD IN MALES AND FEMALES DURING EARLY INFANCY, PREPUBERTY, AND PUBERTY. (*Source:* Reprinted with permission from Grumbach MM, Kaplan SL: The neuroendocrinology of human puberty: an ontogenetic perspective. In *Control of the Onset of Puberty.* Edited by Grumbach MM, Sizonenko PC, Aubert ML. Baltimore, MD: Williams & Wilkins, 1990, p 56.)

STAGES OF PUBERTY

Breast development, genital changes in boys, and pubic hair growth during puberty are staged according to the system derived by Dr. James Tanner (called Tanner staging). Tanner stage I represents the prepubertal stage, and Tanner stage V represents full sexual maturation.

PUBERTAL CHANGES IN GIRLS

The first visible sign of puberty in 70% of girls is breast budding known as *thelarche*. Appearance of pubic hair, known as *pubarche*, occurs first in 30% of girls. Whichever of these occurs first, the other usually follows within 6 months. The first physical change of puberty in girls is actually enlargement of the ovaries, but this is observable only by ultrasound.

Additional events during puberty include the pubertal growth spurt and *menarche*, or the first menstrual period. Menarche, the final milestone of puberty in girls, marks the point at which growth is almost complete. The timing of these events is shown in Table 14-1.

> The normal age range for the onset of puberty in girls is 8–13 years. There are ethnic variations, with this range being shifted downward approximately 6 months in girls of African-American or Hispanic descent.

> **Menarche** usually occurs 2–2.5 years after the onset of breast development. The average age of menarche in the United States is 12.8 years.

Table 14-1
Onset of the Events of Puberty

PUBERTY IN GIRLS[a]	AVERAGE AGE OF ONSET	AGE RANGE
Breast budding	11 years	8–13 years
Pubic hair appears	11 years	8–14 years
Growth spurt	11 years	9.5–14.5 years
Menarche	12.8 years	10–16.5 years

PUBERTY IN BOYS	AVERAGE AGE OF ONSET	AGE RANGE
Testes enlarge	12 years	9–14 years
Pubic hair appears	12.2 years	10–15 years
Penile enlargement	13 years	11–14.5 years
Growth spurt	13 years	10.5–16 years

[a] The first event of puberty in girls is ovarian enlargement, but this can only be detected on ultrasound.

PUBERTAL CHANGES IN BOYS

The first sign of puberty in boys is testicular enlargement. The timing and sequence of pubertal events in boys is shown in Table 14-1.

Pubertal Gynecomastia. Gynecomastia (excessive growth of male breast tissue) during puberty is due to an imbalance in the relative amounts of androgens and estrogens. Increased conversion of androgen to estrogen in fat cells during puberty temporarily lowers the testosterone:estrogen ratio expected in male individuals. Individual differences in sensitivity to normal levels of estrogen may also play a role. In most cases, gynecomastia resolves spontaneously within 1–2 years. However, if pubertal gynecomastia is persistent and cosmetically unacceptable, surgical removal of the breast tissue is possible.

Pathologic causes of gynecomastia include hypogonadism (another cause of a lower than normal testosterone:estrogen ratio), drug ingestion (marijuana, ketoconazole, estrogens), and very rare estrogen-producing tumors of the testes or adrenals.

> The age range of onset of puberty in boys is 9–14 years.

> The **pubertal growth spurt** is due to the combined effects of sex steroids and growth hormone. In boys, this begins later, lasts longer, and reaches a higher amplitude than the pubertal growth spurt in girls. As a result, men are taller on average than women.

> **Gynecomastia** occurs in nearly 90% of normal boys during puberty.

▌ADRENARCHE

Adrenarche refers to the rise in serum androgens resulting from the increased production of weak androgens (dehydroepiandrosterone [DHEA], dehydroepiandrosterone sulfate [DHEAS], androstenedione) from the adrenal glands. Adrenarche normally begins at the age of 6 or 7 years. This process is independent of *gonadarche*, which refers to the activation of the hypothalamic-pituitary-gonadal axis at the onset of "central" puberty. The levels of adrenal androgens continue to rise but usually are not high enough to cause physical changes until the age of puberty.

▌PRECOCIOUS PUBERTY

Precocious puberty is premature sexual development, which occurs at an age more than 2.5 SD below the mean age of puberty. Premature increases in estrogen and androgens cause acceleration of growth in the short term but ultimately compromise final adult height due to premature closure of the epiphyseal growth plates (see Chapter 13). Assessments of growth velocity and skeletal maturation are an important part of the evaluation of children with precocious puberty.

BENIGN VARIANTS

Premature Thelarche. Premature thelarche is a condition of isolated breast development in a girl with no other signs of puberty. Growth velocity and bone age are normal, and the onset of puberty occurs at a normal age. No treatment is needed, and there are no sequelae. The breast tissue may resolve, persist, or enlarge but does not usually surpass Tanner stage-III development. Asymmetric breast development is not a cause for concern; it is quite common for breasts to develop at different rates.

Premature Pubarche or Adrenarche. This refers to isolated pubic hair development in boys and girls. Body odor, axillary hair, and mild acne also may be present. Growth velocity is normal. Bone age often is mildly advanced but is usually within 2 SD of the mean. These children have mildly elevated levels of adrenal androgens, which do not interfere with the onset of normal puberty or with normal growth. This is a benign condition, although there is evidence that girls with premature pubarche may be at increased risk for developing polycystic ovarian syndrome as adults (see Chapter 12). The terms pubarche and adrenarche often are used interchangeably, but adrenarche refers to the biochemical changes in adrenal androgen levels; pubarche refers to the physical changes caused by these androgens.

CENTRAL PRECOCIOUS PUBERTY

This refers to puberty occurring via activation of the hypothalamic-pituitary-gonadal axis at a younger than normal age. In childhood, the pituitary is unresponsive to GnRH. Once central puberty has been activated, the pituitary responds to GnRH by secreting gonadotropins (Figure 14-9), and the gonads enlarge in response to LH and FSH stimulation.

Precocious puberty is defined as the onset of pubertal development in girls before age 8 and in boys before age 9.

Follow-up is essential for a child with premature thelarche. This could also represent the beginning of true precocious puberty.

Causes of Precocious Puberty

Benign Variants
   Premature thelarche
   Premature pubarche

Central Precocious Puberty
   Idiopathic
   Congenital CNS abnormality
   CNS trauma, infection, or ischemia
   CNS tumor
Peripheral Precocious Puberty
   CAH
   Androgen or estrogen ingestion
   Adrenal or gonadal tumor
   G-protein abnormality
   Ovarian cysts

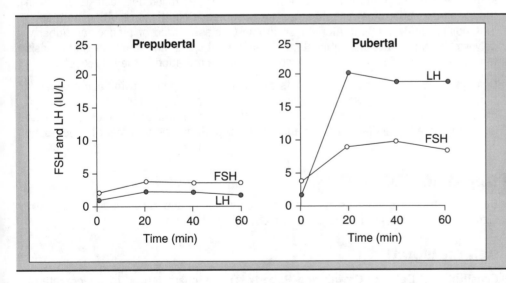

FIGURE 14-9
GONADOTROPIN-RELEASING HORMONE (GnRH) STIMULATION TEST. Luteinizing hormone (LH) and follicle-stimulating hormone (FSH) are measured sequentially after administration of intravenous GnRH. In the prepubertal child, there is no significant response to the GnRH analog. A pubertal response is characterized by a brisk rise in gonadotropins with a predominance of LH.

Random levels of LH and FSH are not helpful in making the diagnosis of central precocious puberty, since baseline values are indistinguishable in the prepubertal and pubertal state. The diagnosis of central precocious puberty can be made if administration of an exogenous GnRH analog results in a brisk rise in pituitary gonadotropins with LH predominance (a positive GnRH stimulation test).

Central precocious puberty can be caused by congenital central nervous system (CNS) abnormalities, such as septo-optic dysplasia, hypothalamic hamartoma, and neurofibromatosis, or by acquired CNS insults, such as infection, ischemia, trauma, and

Central precocious puberty is confirmed if a GnRH stimulation test elicits a brisk rise in pituitary gonadotropins with LH predominance.

Central precocious puberty is treated with long-acting GnRH analog therapy in the form of intramuscular or subcutaneous injections. Sustained high concentrations of GnRH lead to down-regulation of pituitary GnRH receptors and subsequent suppression of the pituitary-gonadal axis.

In **peripheral precocious puberty**, a GnRH stimulation test elicits no increase in FSH and LH, indicating that the hypothalamic-pituitary-gonadal axis is still immature.

CAH, which is due to **21-hydroxylase deficiency**, is the most common cause of postnatal virilization in boys and girls.

neoplasm. However, in 90% of cases of central precocious puberty in girls, the etiology of premature activation of the hypothalamic-pituitary-gonadal axis is unknown. In boys with central precocious puberty, approximately 50% of cases are idiopathic. Children with central precocious puberty are treated with a long-acting GnRH analog, which down-regulates GnRH receptors so that they no longer respond to GnRH pulses.

PERIPHERAL PRECOCIOUS PUBERTY

Peripheral precocious puberty is initiated by a process outside the central hypothalamic-pituitary-gonadal axis that results in either endogenous or exogenous androgen/estrogen exposure. Since the central axis is still immature, gonadotropin levels are low and do not respond to GnRH stimulation.

Congenital Adrenal Hyperplasia. CAH is an important cause of ambiguous genitalia, but CAH also can present as precocious puberty in girls and boys. The type of presentation depends on the severity of the enzyme block. Since the adrenals produce androgens but not estrogen, premature breast development does not occur in girls with peripheral precocious puberty due to CAH.

Exogenous Causes. Ingestion of androgens or estrogen found in birth control pills or contaminated meat also causes peripheral precocious puberty. Ingestion of estrogen results in breast development, whereas ingestion of androgens causes body hair and other signs of abnormal virilization.

Tumors. Adrenal, testicular, or ovarian *tumors* producing androgen or estrogen are very rare causes of peripheral precocious puberty in children. Tumors producing HCG can also cause precocious puberty because HCG is structurally similar to LH and stimulates the testes to produce testosterone.

G-Protein Abnormalities. G-protein abnormalities can cause peripheral precocious puberty. These are due to mutations in the gene coding for the G-protein stimulatory subunit (Gs_α) that result in constitutive activation of G-protein-driven formation of cyclic adenosine monophosphate (cAMP). Gonadal cells behave as though they are constantly stimulated with FSH and LH and continue to produce estrogen and testosterone even though the gonadotropin receptors are not occupied. Conditions resulting from such mutations include McCune-Albright syndrome (a classic triad of precocious puberty, polyostotic fibrous dysplasia of bone, and café au lait spots) and familial testotoxicosis (an autosomal dominant condition in which there is a mutation in the LH receptor).

Ovarian Cysts. Functional ovarian cysts can produce estrogen, causing acute onset of breast enlargement in girls. The cysts resolve spontaneously, often resulting in withdrawal bleeding from the estrogen-stimulated endometrium, after which the breast tissue regresses. The diagnosis is made by ultrasound, and no treatment is necessary.

▌DELAYED PUBERTY

Delayed puberty is defined as the failure of progression of puberty or the absence of any signs of puberty in a girl by age 13 or in a boy by age 14.

BENIGN VARIANT

Constitutional Delay of Growth and Puberty. This is characterized by a slow rate of growth during the first few years of life, delayed skeletal maturation (bone age is less than chronologic age), and delayed puberty. There is usually a family history of delayed growth. Puberty begins late, but because these children grow for a longer period of time than their peers, final adult height is normal (see Chapter 13).

PATHOLOGIC CAUSES OF DELAYED PUBERTY

Pathologic causes of delayed puberty include defects in the hypothalamic-pituitary-gonadal axis at any level and end organ resistance to gonadal hormones. Delayed puberty can also be seen in the context of *any* significant chronic disease or illness.

Gonadotropin Deficiency. This is the result of inadequate hypothalamic GnRH or inadequate pituitary LH and FSH. Hypothalamic causes of delayed puberty include Kallman's syndrome, which is due to a deletion of the gene coding for a protein involved in neuronal migration. This disorder is characterized by hypogonadotropic hypogonadism and a deficient or absent sense of smell (hyposmia or anosmia). Prader-Willi and Laurence-Moon-Biedl syndromes also are associated with hypogonadotropic hypogonadism. Patients with anorexia nervosa whose weight is markedly below normal have disturbances in the GnRH pulse generator. In some cases, gonadotropin deficiency is idiopathic.

Gonadal Failure. Gonadal failure in females most often is caused by Turner's syndrome (karyotype 45,X). The incidence of Turner's syndrome is approximately 1:2000 live female births. Approximately 30% of those affected are mosaics. This disorder is characterized by ovarian dysgenesis, short stature (see Chapter 13), and a spectrum of physical stigmata that include low posterior hairline, high-arched palate, webbed neck, shield-shaped chest, coarctation of the aorta, hyperconvex fingernails, cubitus valgus (increased carrying angle), and lymphedema. Most patients have normal intelligence but have difficulty with math, especially spatial relationships. Since many girls with Turner's syndrome lack some or most of the phenotypic features, the diagnosis must be made by chromosomal analysis.

Gonadal failure also occurs in boys with Klinefelter's syndrome (karyotype 47,XXY), which is characterized by seminiferous tubule dysplasia and varying degrees of testicular failure. The incidence of Klinefelter's syndrome is 1:400. Boys usually present at puberty with gynecomastia and small testes resulting from a lack of seminiferous tubules. Many are infertile from their first presentation; others become infertile in early adulthood due to premature testicular failure. Phenotypic features, which include decreased body hair, decreased muscle mass, and female-type subcutaneous fat distribution, vary widely, and a chromosomal analysis is required to make the diagnosis.

Causes of acquired gonadal failure include infection (tuberculosis), irradiation, trauma, and torsion.

End Organ Resistance. Delayed puberty due to end organ resistance to gonadal hormones occurs in patients with complete androgen resistance or testicular feminization syndrome (Chapter 13). These phenotypic females typically present at puberty with primary amenorrhea.

If **delayed puberty** is due to a **hypothalamic** or **pituitary disorder**, LH and FSH levels are low. Testosterone and estrogen levels also are low.

If **delayed puberty** is caused by **gonadal failure**, LH and FSH levels are high due to lack of pituitary suppression by testosterone or estrogen.

Case Study: *Resolution*

Anna had symptoms and signs of true (central) precocious puberty in which both estrogens and androgens are produced. If she had benign premature thelarche, she would have no other signs of puberty except breast enlargement, and her growth velocity would be normal. If she had benign premature pubarche due to adrenal androgens, she would not have breast development, and her growth velocity would have been normal.

To confirm central precocious puberty, a GnRH stimulation test was performed. Anna was given a bolus of an exogenous GnRH analog. This provoked a brisk rise in pituitary gonadotropins as shown in Figure 14-9. This rise was due to premature maturation of her hypothalamic-pituitary-ovarian axis. A magnetic resonance imaging scan of her head was normal, indicating that her central precocious puberty was not caused by a tumor or other CNS abnormality. Central precocious puberty in girls usually is idiopathic.

Anna was started on monthly injections of a potent, long-acting GnRH analog to down-regulate pituitary GnRH receptors. Within 6 months, the progression of her puberty had stabilized, her growth velocity had slowed, and the rapid increase in her bone age also decreased. She and her family were given counseling because children with precocious puberty may be teased by or feel uncomfortable with other children. Also, since these children do not have the social maturity to match their physical maturity, they may encounter unrealistic expectations from adults.

If Anna were left untreated, her growth chart would look very much like that shown in Chapter 13, Figure 13-15. She would be tall initially due to her early estrogen-induced growth spurt, but she would be short as an adult due to premature closure of her epiphyses.

▌REVIEW QUESTIONS

Directions: For each of the following questions, choose the **one best** answer.

1. An endocrinologist is called to evaluate a newborn with ambiguous genitalia. On examination, the gonads are palpable in the scrotum. The genitalia are ambiguous and include a phallic-like structure measuring approximately 1 cm. The parents are very concerned about the sex assignment. The endocrinologist should tell them that

    (A) it is up to them to decide what the sex assignment will be
    (B) since the infant has testes, the sex assignment will be male
    (C) the sex assignment will depend on what the chromosomes are
    (D) the sex assignment should be made on the basis of potential for normal function
    (E) the child should be allowed to choose his or her own sex at puberty

2. One week later, another child is born with ambiguous genitalia. The mother had an amniocentesis, so it is known that the infant's karyotype is 46,XX. No gonads are palpable. The external genitalia include a phallic-like structure measuring approximately 1 cm. An ultrasound done shortly after birth reveals a normal uterus, fallopian tubes, and ovaries. The most likely cause for this infant's ambiguous genitalia is

    (A) complete estrogen resistance
    (B) mixed gonadal dysgenesis
    (C) 21-hydroxylase deficiency
    (D) paternal androgen-secreting tumor
    (E) idiopathic

3. A mother is concerned because her 13-year-old daughter is only 4'9" tall. Her daughter is otherwise healthy and has been menstruating regularly for the last 1½ years. The mother wants to know if this child will grow taller. What is the most accurate response?

    (A) The child will grow but may need treatment with growth hormone
    (B) While *most* girls have their pubertal growth spurt before menarche, a few have it after menarche
    (C) The child will grow but only if she is given medication to stop her menses
    (D) During the 2 years after menarche the child should grow approximately the same amount as she grew in the 2 years before menarche
    (E) Menarche represents the end point of puberty in girls, and therefore, the child does not have any significant growth potential left

4. A 7-year-old boy comes to the clinic because he recently has developed pubic hair. The parents also report an adult body odor, which started about 1 month before the clinic visit. The child has otherwise been healthy. On examination, Tanner stage-II pubic hair and axillary odor are noted. The testes are 2 cc (normal prepubertal size: 1–3 cc), and the phallus is Tanner stage I. The examination is otherwise normal. Review of previous growth charts reveals that the child has been growing normally at about the seventy-fifth percentile. Bone age x-ray is normal (within 2 SD of the mean). Based on this information, the most likely diagnosis is

    (A) benign premature thelarche
    (B) congenital adrenal hyperplasia (CAH)
    (C) central precocious puberty
    (D) benign premature pubarche (adrenarche)
    (E) ingestion of anabolic steroids

5. A 17-year-old girl comes to see an endocrinologist because of primary amenorrhea. Breast development started several years ago, but she has had no menses. She has otherwise been well. On examination, height is above the ninety-fifth percentile. Breasts are a Tanner stage V, but there is no pubic or axillary hair. The endocrinologist attempts a pelvic examination but is unable to visualize the cervix. These findings are most consistent with which of the following syndromes?

(A) Turner's syndrome
(B) Kallman's syndrome
(C) Testicular feminization syndrome
(D) Klinefelter's syndrome
(E) Prader-Willi syndrome

6. A 3-year-old girl is brought to the endocrinologist's office because her mother noticed gradual enlargement of the right breast followed shortly by enlargement of the left breast during the last few months. The child has otherwise been healthy. No one in the home is taking birth control pills. Examination reveals height and weight to be at the fiftieth percentile (where they were 1 year ago), Tanner stage-II breast development with no axillary hair or odor, and Tanner stage-I pubic hair. Her records show that her growth velocity is normal. A bone age x-ray also is normal (i.e., equal to chronologic age). What is the most likely cause of this child's breast development?

(A) Premature thelarche
(B) Premature pubarche
(C) Congenital adrenal hyperplasia
(D) McCune-Albright syndrome
(E) Central precocious puberty

7. A 6-year-old boy is referred to the clinic for evaluation of pubic hair, which his father first noticed about 6 months ago. It has increased in amount since then. He also thinks that his child's penis has gotten bigger and states, "He is growing like a weed." His son has otherwise been healthy. Examination reveals height and weight above the ninety-fifth percentile and Tanner stage-III pubic hair and genital development. The testes are 3 cc (normal prepubertal size: 1–3 cc). A bone age is read as 12 years. Laboratory tests include a serum 17α-hydroxyprogesterone level of 3900 ng/dL (normal 3–90 ng/dL). This child has

(A) idiopathic central precocious puberty
(B) congenital adrenal hyperplasia (CAH)
(C) premature pubarche
(D) McCune-Albright syndrome
(E) familial testotoxicosis

8. A 14-year-old girl has not yet had menses. She developed pubic hair at approximately 12 years but has had no breast development. She has always been short but has otherwise been healthy. On examination, height and weight are below the fifth percentile. Other findings include Tanner stage-I breasts, Tanner stage-III pubic hair, low posterior hairline, a webbed neck, and cubitus valgus (increased carrying angle). Chromosome analysis reveals a 45,X karyotype. Her hormone profile is most likely to be

(A) low follicle-stimulating hormone (FSH), low luteinizing hormone (LH), and low estrogen
(B) normal FSH, normal LH, and low estrogen
(C) high FSH, high LH, and high estrogen
(D) high FSH, high LH, and low estrogen

■ ANSWERS AND EXPLANATIONS

1. The answer is D. While the genotypic sex *is* most likely male (ovaries do not descend), sex assignment must be made on the basis of the potential for normal function. In a boy, the most important determinant is the size of the phallus. This infant's phallus is very small and may or may not respond to exogenous androgens. Lack of growth of the phallus after a course of testosterone would indicate that a male sex assignment would be inappropriate.

2. The answer is C. The most common cause of ambiguous genitalia in a female infant is congenital adrenal hyperplasia (CAH) caused by 21-hydroxylase deficiency. Mixed gonadal dysgenesis is associated with mosaicism and the presence of male and female internal structures. Estrogen resistance and paternal tumor are not causes of ambiguous genitalia.

3. The answer is E. Menarche is the final milestone of puberty in girls. Most girls do not gain more than an additional 1–2 inches in height after menarche. By 1½ years postmenarche, linear growth is essentially complete. Once the epiphyseal growth plates are fused, there is no way to increase stature. Unfortunately, it is too late to do anything about this child's short stature.

4. The answer is D. Isolated pubic hair and body odor with prepubertal testes and phallus and a normal growth velocity and bone age are consistent with premature pubarche (adrenarche). However, this child needs to be followed to be sure that his condition remains stable.

5. The answer is C. Complete androgen resistance, or testicular feminization syndrome, is due to absence of functional testosterone receptors, resulting in a phenotypic female with normal breast development but a paucity of body hair (which requires androgen action). The testes are intra-abdominal. Müllerian structures are absent because the testes produce müllerian-inhibiting hormone. Wolffian structures do not develop because testosterone receptors are absent. The vagina ends in a blind pouch. The other syndromes listed can present with delayed puberty, but they are not consistent with the findings in this patient.

6. The answer is A. This child has isolated breast development. She has no pubic hair, no signs of virilization, and no other signs of puberty. Her growth velocity and her bone age are normal. She needs no treatment, but she does need follow-up to be sure that this is not the beginning of true precocious puberty.

7. The answer is B. The physical findings and advanced bone age indicate that puberty is underway. The testes are small, indicating that they are not the source of the androgen and that this is a type of peripheral precocious puberty. The high level of 17α-hydroxyprogesterone confirms a block in cortisol synthesis and the diagnosis of CAH.

8. The answer is D. This girl has classic features of Turner's syndrome, which is confirmed by the karyotype 45,X. Since her ovaries are fibrous streaks without follicle cells, she is unable to produce ovarian estrogen. Her pituitary gonadotropins are high due to lack of estrogen feedback. She has developed some pubic hair due to adrenal androgens.

■ REFERENCES

Bardoni B, Zanaria E, Floridia G, et al: A dosage sensitive locus at chromosome Xp21 is involved in male to female sex reversal. *Nat Genet* 7:497–501, 1994.

Bogan JS, Page DC: Ovary? Testes?—a mammalian dilemma. *Cell* 76:603–607, 1994.

Ferguson-Smith MA: Abnormalities of human sex determination. *J Inher Metab Dis* 15:518–525, 1992.

Kulin HE, Müller J: The biological aspects of puberty. *Pediatr Rev* 17:75–86, 1996.

Pescovitz OH: Precocious puberty. *Pediatr Rev* 11:229–237, 1990.

Rosen DS, Kletter GB, Kelch RP: Puberty—what to do when the clock doesn't ring. *J Pediatr Endocrinol* 5:129–140, 1992.

Smith EP, Boyd J, Frank GR, et al: Estrogen resistance caused by a mutation in the estrogen-receptor gene in a man. *N Engl J Med* 331:1056–1061, 1994.

Chapter 15

ENDOCRINOLOGY OF PREGNANCY AND LACTATION

Virginia R. Lupo, M.D.

■ CHAPTER OUTLINE

Case Study:
Introduction

A 28-year-old woman came to the company health service for a physical examination, as she had just started a new job as a computer programmer. She has had one normal pregnancy and was breastfeeding her 6-month-old infant. She has not yet had a recurrence of menses. She used oral contraceptives in the past, but since her child was born, she has used a diaphragm for contraception. Recently, she has experienced frequent nausea and increased fatigue, which she attributed to the stress of her new job. Her medical history was unremarkable except for an appendectomy at age 7. She has a sister with hypothyroidism and two grandmothers who have type II diabetes mellitus.

Physical examination revealed a modestly obese woman with mild acne. She has lost 5 lbs since her examination 3 months ago. Her blood pressure is within normal limits. Her resting heart rate (HR) is 88 beats/min (previous HR: 76 beats/min). Her eye examination was unremarkable. Her thyroid gland was slightly enlarged but not changed from her last examination. Her urine human chorionic gonadotropin (HCG) level was high.

■ HORMONAL EVENTS OF EARLY PREGNANCY

Fertilization of the egg by the sperm occurs in the fallopian tube within 48 hours of ovulation. Tubal peristalsis propels the zygote into the endometrial cavity. The endometrium is primed to receive a fertilized egg by the estrogen already secreted during the first half of the menstrual cycle (see Chapter 12). As soon as ovulation occurs, the

For most pregnancies, the date of conception is not known. By convention "week of gestation," or "gestational age," is dated from the first day of the last menstrual period.

remaining granulosa cells in the follicle that has released the egg begin producing progesterone in large quantities. Progesterone deposits appear yellow, and after ovulation, the follicle is called a corpus luteum ("yellow body"). Progesterone stabilizes the endometrium in preparation for implantation, which occurs 6–7 days after conception when the embryo is at the blastocyst stage.

If implantation does not occur, the corpus luteum makes progesterone for approximately 10 days after ovulation. Progesterone feedback inhibits luteinizing hormone (LH) production by the pituitary gland. This results in menses because without LH the corpus luteum fails. However, if implantation does occur, the developing embryo begins making HCG within 24 hours. HCG is a peptide hormone that mimics the effect of LH. HCG stimulates the corpus luteum to continue progesterone production, the endometrial lining is maintained, and menses do not occur. Ablation of the corpus luteum at this time causes loss of the pregnancy because there is no other adequate source of progesterone. By approximately 9 weeks after conception (approximately 11 weeks gestation), the rudimentary placenta is able to synthesize enough progesterone to support the pregnancy, and the corpus luteum involutes.

HORMONES OF THE PLACENTA

The placenta is an active metabolic factory, producing peptide hormones, steroid hormones, and many releasing and inhibiting factors for these hormones. The role of many of these hormones in pregnancy is not well understood.

POLYPEPTIDE HORMONES

Polypeptide hormones are made entirely within the placenta. They are too large to cross the placental barrier into the fetus, so they are found only in the maternal circulation. Their impact on maternal metabolism is uncertain. Several cytokines and growth factors also are produced by the placenta and may act locally. Polypeptide-releasing hormones synthesized by the placenta include gonadotropin-releasing hormone (GnRH), thyrotropin-releasing hormone (TRH), and corticotropin-releasing hormone (CRH). Pituitary-like products from the placenta include placental lactogen (similar to prolactin [PRL]), HCG (similar to LH), chorionic thyrotropin (similar to thyroid-stimulating hormone [TSH]), and chorionic adrenocorticotropin (similar to adrenocorticotropic hormone [ACTH]).

HUMAN CHORIONIC GONADOTROPIN (HCG)

Specific biochemical identification of the pregnant state requires measurement of HCG, which is present only during pregnancy.

HCG is produced by placental tissue and rare germ-cell tumors and is virtually undetectable in the maternal circulation before pregnancy. HCG is a glycoprotein with two subunits. The α-chain is common to HCG, LH, follicle-stimulating hormone (FSH), and TSH; the β-chain has some homology to the LH β-chain but is unique to HCG. In the past, pregnancy tests identified the entire HCG molecule. When other hormones with the common α-subunit were present in high concentrations, cross-reactivity occurred and resulted in false-positive pregnancy tests. Now pregnancy tests measure only the β-subunit of HCG, eliminating false-positive results. Home urine pregnancy tests use a monoclonal antibody specific for the β-subunit of HCG and give highly accurate results within a few minutes. Quantitative measurement of serum HCG is used primarily to distinguish between a viable pregnancy and an ectopic pregnancy or a miscarriage. Serum and urine tests can be positive 9 days after conception unless the urine is very dilute.

Pregnancy tests measure HCG, a placental hormone, which is detectable in serum and urine as early as 9 days after ovulation.

The HCG level doubles every 48 hours during the first few weeks of pregnancy, rising to a peak at 10 weeks gestation (Figure 15-1). After 10 weeks gestation, the HCG level decreases but remains above the nonpregnant level until delivery. Pregnancy tests can remain positive for several weeks after delivery because the half-life of HCG is 24 hours.

An abnormal rise in HCG early in gestation indicates a nonviable pregnancy. A very high HCG level indicates a trophoblastic tumor such as a hydatidiform mole or a choriocarcinoma.

HUMAN PLACENTAL LACTOGEN (HPL)

As pregnancy progresses, exponential growth of the placenta results in an exponential increase in the placental polypeptide hormone HPL. HPL is a single polypeptide chain of 191 amino acids, sometimes referred to as human chorionic somatomammotropin (HCS), which has some structural homology to pituitary growth hormone. Placental growth, fetal growth, and HPL levels all increase exponentially in the third trimester of pregnancy. The role of HPL during pregnancy is uncertain, but HPL stimulates maternal lipolysis, making more fatty acids available for fuel during periods of fasting. HPL is thought to contribute to the increase in maternal insulin resistance that occurs as pregnancy progresses.

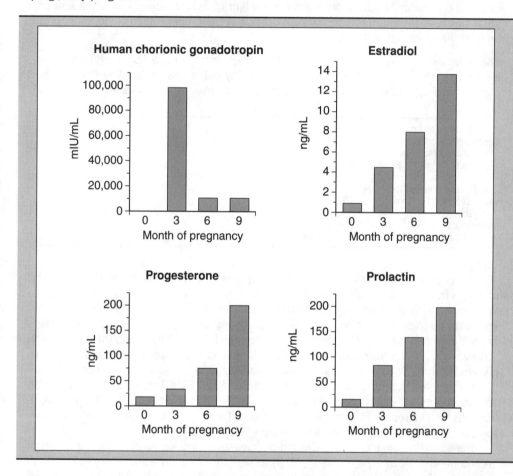

FIGURE 15-1
PLASMA LEVELS OF HUMAN CHORIONIC GONADOTROPIN, ESTROGEN, PROGESTERONE, AND PROLACTIN BEFORE AND DURING PREGNANCY. Since prepregnancy levels of estrogen and progesterone fluctuate throughout the menstrual cycle, values shown are at the upper limits of the normal ranges in nonpregnant women.

Case Study:
Continued

The patient's high urine HCG level indicated that she was pregnant again. Her nausea, fatigue, and mild tachycardia might be due to pregnancy, but because of her family history of thyroid disease, thyroid function tests were obtained. She had an elevated total thyroxine (T_4) level, with a normal free T_4. Her TSH level was within normal limits. Her fasting plasma glucose level was lower than a previous nonpregnant level.

As her pregnancy progressed the patient's acne resolved, but she complained of chronic sinus drainage and constipation. During her second trimester, her fasting plasma glucose was higher than expected, and an oral glucose tolerance test revealed a blood glucose level more than 2 standard deviations (SD) above the mean for her stage of pregnancy.

STEROID HORMONES

The placenta is unable to synthesize steroid hormones de novo. Cholesterol precursors from the maternal compartment are required for placental synthesis of progesterone. Placental estrogen synthesis requires cholesterol precursors from the maternal com-

Placental steroid synthesis requires cholesterol precursors from the maternal compartment. Placental estrogen synthesis also requires processing by the fetal adrenal and fetal liver.

partment, but these precursors must be further metabolized by the fetal adrenal and fetal liver. Most estrogens are actually metabolites of androgens, which require fetal and placental steps in their synthesis. When the precursors do become available, the syncytiotrophoblast has an extraordinary ability to complete estrogen and progesterone synthesis and to secrete the hormones into the maternal and fetal circulations.

Maternal estradiol levels increase markedly during pregnancy (see Figure 15-1), as do the levels of estrone and estriol. Since estrogen synthesis requires synergy between the fetus and the placenta, estrogen levels were once thought to reflect the metabolic integrity of the placenta, and serial estrogen levels were used to assess fetal well-being. Now more direct measures of fetal well-being are used. Maternal progesterone levels also increase dramatically during pregnancy (see Figure 15-1). Placental estrogen and progesterone have profound effects on the mother, but their roles in the development of the fetus still are not well defined.

Estrogen. Major physiologic effects of increased estrogen are listed in Table 15-1. Hepatic synthesis of most proteins, including thyroid hormone–binding globulin and cortisol-binding globulin, is increased, but serum transaminase levels are not elevated.

Table 15-1
Effects of Increased Estrogen during Pregnancy

Increased hepatic protein synthesis
Peripheral vasodilatation
   Increased heart rate
   Increased stroke volume
   Increased cardiac output
   Increased uterine blood flow
Increased blood volume
   Physiologic anemia
Increased coagulation factors
Increased renal perfusion and creatinine clearance

Estrogen-induced vasodilation is responsible for the following:
Increased sinus congestion
Increased epistaxis (nosebleeds)
Bleeding gums
Better healing of acne and chronic ulcerations
Sensation of warmth

Estrogen is a profound vasodilator. Blood flow to the uterus increases due to the estrogen-induced decrease in uteroplacental resistance. Peripheral vasodilation requires an increase in cardiac output. Both stroke volume and heart rate rise, and cardiac output increases up to 50%. Women with lesions restricting cardiac output may suffer worsening of their heart disease. Peripheral blood pressure falls initially due to the vasodilation but eventually returns to prepregnancy levels. Blood vessels are less sensitive to angiotensin during pregnancy, probably due to a change at the angiotensin receptor level.

Plasma volume increases more than red blood cell (RBC) mass, and a physiologic anemia occurs routinely in pregnant women. Coagulation factors and venous thromboembolic disease increase. This problem persists until estrogen levels fall postpartum. One-third of thromboses occur in the early postpartum period.

The increase in venous thromboembolic disease during pregnancy is due to the following:
Increased coagulation factors
Stasis
Vessel wall damage

Renal perfusion increases. Creatinine clearance increases by 50%, and serum creatinine and blood urea nitrogen (BUN) levels fall. The glomeruli cannot reabsorb all the glucose filtered, so many pregnant women have glucosuria even with normal plasma glucose levels.

Progesterone. Major physiologic effects of increased progesterone are listed in Table 15-2. Progesterone acts on the central respiratory centers to produce a sense of air hunger and a compensated respiratory alkalosis. Tidal volume and minute ventilation increase, but the respiratory rate does not.

Table 15-2
Effects of Increased Progesterone during Pregnancy

Increased minute ventilation
Compensated respiratory alkalosis
Smooth muscle relaxation
   Lower esophageal sphincter relaxation
   Decreased intestinal motility
   Urinary collecting system stasis
   Decreased uterine contractions
Stasis of ureters and urethra

Progesterone is responsible for smooth muscle relaxation during pregnancy. Relaxation of the lower esophageal sphincter can result in reflux esophagitis. Gastric emptying is delayed. Decreased intestinal motility causes constipation in many women. Increased stasis in the ureters and urethra contributes to the increase in urinary tract infections during pregnancy.

ADDITIONAL HORMONAL AND METABOLIC ALTERATIONS OF PREGNANCY

The metabolic and hormonal adaptations to pregnancy are extensive (Table 15-3). Pituitary production of LH and FSH remains suppressed by the high circulating levels of estrogen and progesterone until delivery. Pituitary size increases, primarily due to the estrogen-induced stimulation of lactotrophs, which synthesize PRL.

Progesterone-induced smooth muscle relaxation causes:
Increased esophageal reflux and
  esophagitis
Delayed gastric emptying
Constipation
Urinary tract stasis and infections

Higher estrogen
Higher progesterone
Low LH and FSH
Increasing prolactin
High total T_4; normal free T_4 and TSH
Increased total and free cortisol
Increased calcium absorption; normal ionized calcium
Lower fasting glucose; increased postprandial glucose
Higher postprandial insulin; increased insulin resistance

Table 15-3
Major Maternal Hormonal and Metabolic Changes during Pregnancy

Note. LH = luteinizing hormone; FSH = follicle-stimulating hormone; T_4 = thyroxine; TSH = thyroid-stimulating hormone.

Renal clearance of iodide is increased during pregnancy. Mild thyroid enlargement is common during pregnancy, especially in areas of iodine deficiency. The concentrations of total T_4 and total T_3 levels increase as a result of the estrogen-induced increase in thyroxine-binding globulin (TBG) [see Chapter 4], but free thyroid hormone concentrations and TSH are normal. Maternal TSH does not cross the placenta. Only minute amounts of maternal T_4 and T_3 cross the placenta, but they are sufficient for a fetus without a thyroid gland to develop normally until after delivery.

The concentration of total cortisol increases. This is due in part to the estrogen-induced increase in cortisol-binding globulin, but it also is due to an increase in free cortisol. The diurnal variation of cortisol levels is maintained.

Calcium (Ca^{2+}) is needed for the fetal skeleton, especially in the third trimester. Maternal parathyroid glands become hyperplastic, and Ca^{2+} absorption efficiency increases. Ionized Ca^{2+} remains normal.

Fetal nutritional requirements alter maternal fuel metabolism. Fasting glucose levels decrease because glucose is transported across the placenta to the fetus by facilitated diffusion, and amino acids actively transported to the fetus are not available for maternal gluconeogenesis. Lipolysis and ketogenesis increase, and fasting ketone and free fatty acid levels are higher. Fatty acids do not cross the placenta. Maternal insulin is bound and degraded by the placenta and does not cross into the fetal compartment. The fetus depends on its own insulin for glucose disposal; fetal insulin is produced by 12 weeks gestation.

There is a shift in maternal carbohydrate metabolism after meals, especially as pregnancy advances from the second to the third trimester. Postprandial glucose levels are higher than in nonpregnant women, even though postprandial insulin secretion increases. This insulin resistance has been attributed to higher maternal levels of HPL, progesterone, and cortisol. Lipolysis is suppressed after meals despite the insulin resistance. Triglyceride synthesis increases due to the high estrogen levels.

ENDOCRINE CHANGES AT PARTURITION

Levels of placental hormones fall precipitously after the placenta is delivered. The plasma half-lives of the placental hormones determine how quickly they disappear from the maternal circulation. Some women are sufficiently sensitive to the rapid fall in estrogen levels that they perceive hot flashes similar to those that occur after menopause. The decrease in circulating estrogen quickly returns peripheral vascular resistance to nonpregnant levels. The diminished smooth muscle tone of pregnancy resolves as progesterone levels fall. In the nonlactating woman, estrogen and progesterone are back to prepregnancy levels by 6 weeks postpartum. At this time the increased risk of thromboembolism from estrogen-induced hepatic synthesis of coagulation factors is over, the renal collecting system is back to normal, and the risk of urinary tract infections is back to the prepregnancy level.

In lactating women, estrogen levels are suppressed for months by the increased PRL secretion (see below). Bone loss occurs as a result of this hypoestrogenism, but this is promptly reversed after lactation ceases.

The insulin resistance induced by pregnancy resolves very rapidly after delivery.

■ DIABETES MELLITUS AND PREGNANCY

In women who have diabetes *before* pregnancy, control of blood glucose at conception and during the first few weeks of gestation influences the occurrence of congenital malformations in the fetus.

In women who have diabetes *before* pregnancy, control of blood glucose early in gestation influences the occurrence of congenital malformations. Glucose is transported across the placenta by means of facilitated diffusion, so maternal hyperglycemia exposes the fetus to hyperglycemia. Poor diabetes control at the time of conception is highly correlated with increases in fetal heart and neural tube defects, spontaneous abortion, and premature deliveries. Infants of mothers with poorly controlled diabetes are at risk for death at term. The mechanisms are not known.

Gestational diabetes develops in the second half of pregnancy. Because it occurs after organogenesis, the risk for congenital malformations is not increased.

Some women develop diabetes *during* pregnancy because they cannot increase insulin secretion enough to counteract the physiologic increase in insulin resistance. Prospective screening with an oral glucose challenge test in mid pregnancy reveals maternal glucose levels several standard deviations higher than expected. This is called *gestational* diabetes. Because gestational diabetes develops after organogenesis already has occurred, the risk of congenital malformations is not increased.

Fetuses of diabetic mothers often are larger than those of non-diabetic mothers (**macrosomia**). Macrosomia is due to the excessive fuel (glucose) supplied to the fetus and to fetal hyperinsulinemia.

When maternal hyperglycemia results in fetal hyperglycemia, the fetus secretes more insulin. Insulin is a major growth hormone for the fetus, and fetuses of diabetic mothers are more likely to be large (*macrosomia*) as a result of the hyperinsulinemia and the increased fuel supply. Macrosomia increases the risk for birth trauma, especially shoulder dystocia, and the need for cesarean section.

Most women with gestational diabetes are treated with changes in diet alone, but sometimes insulin therapy is necessary. If so, large doses of insulin may be required to overcome the insulin resistance. All pregnant women with diabetes need careful blood glucose monitoring to avoid fasting hypoglycemia as well as hyperglycemia. Ketosis increases the fetal death rate.

Newborns of diabetic mothers are at risk for hypoglycemia.

After delivery of the infant, maternal insulin requirements plummet because the factors produced by the placenta that cause insulin resistance are no longer present. Gestational diabetes resolves as the insulin resistance resolves unless pregnancy has unmasked underlying diabetes that was unrecognized previously. Approximately 40% of women with gestational diabetes will develop diabetes within 10–15 years. The risk of subsequent diabetes increases if women are obese or have a family history of diabetes.

Women with diabetes need very careful glucose monitoring during pregnancy to avoid the complications of hyperglycemia, hypoglycemia, and ketosis.

Exposure of the infant to hyperglycemia stops abruptly at delivery, but fetal hyperinsulinemia still is present. Therefore, newborns of diabetic mothers must be watched for the development of hypoglycemia. Infants of diabetic mothers also are more likely to have polycythemia, hyperbilirubinemia, and hypocalcemia, the causes of which are uncertain. Lactation is not contraindicated for women with diabetes.

■ THYROID DISORDERS AND PREGNANCY

Some of the symptoms of pregnancy mimic those of hyperthyroidism: nausea, a sensation of warmth due to vasodilation, tachycardia, and increased cardiac output. Thyroid function testing and pregnancy testing are required to make the correct diagnosis.

Hyperthyroidism causes menstrual irregularity and infertility, but this is not universal, and hyperthyroid women can become pregnant. Maternal hyperthyroidism most often is due to Graves' disease, with thyroid-stimulating immunoglobulins (TSI) causing stimulation of the thyroid gland (see Chapter 4). TSI can cross the placenta into the fetal compartment and stimulate the fetal thyroid gland. This results in fetal tachycardia, hypermetabolism, and fetal growth restriction. Since hyperthyroidism can be life-threatening for both the mother and fetus, hyperthyroidism must be treated during pregnancy. However, the antithyroid medications used to treat maternal hyperthyroidism do cross the placenta and can cause fetal hypothyroidism. The minimum dose required to bring the mother's thyroid function tests into the upper limit of the normal range should be given. Inadvertent administration of radioactive iodine to a pregnant woman can result in destruction of the fetal thyroid gland. Since untreated hypothyroidism in the newborn period causes irreversible brain damage, many states perform routine heel-stick capillary screening for hypothyroidism after birth.

Maternal hypothyroidism has no impact on the fetal thyroid axis unless the hypothyroidism is due to previously treated Graves' disease, and antibodies still remain in the maternal circulation. Thyroid hormone replacement for the mother crosses the placenta in such small amounts that fetal thyroid hormone levels are not increased. Several studies have shown that requirements for thyroid hormone replacement increase during pregnancy, so thyroid function tests should be followed carefully.

Case Study:
Continued

The patient's thyroid function tests were typical for a pregnant woman. The high total T_4 level reflected the estrogen-induced increase in TBG (see Chapter 4). Her normal free T_4 and TSH indicated that she is euthyroid. The improvement in her acne and her increased sinus drainage were consequences of estrogen-induced vasodilation, and the constipation was caused by progesterone-induced smooth muscle relaxation.

Initially her fasting plasma glucose level was lower than before her pregnancy, an expected adaptation to the nutritional requirements of the fetus. However, by mid pregnancy she had developed gestational diabetes. After this diagnosis was made, she watched her caloric intake carefully, and her glucose control was excellent. She delivered a 9-lb girl 2 weeks before her due date. Within a week of delivery, her plasma glucose levels were similar to those prior to her pregnancy. Her constipation and excessive sinus drainage resolved after delivery. She decided to breastfeed this infant also.

■ THE BREAST AND LACTATION

ANATOMY OF THE BREAST

The breast is composed of alveoli, which empty into ducts. These ducts empty into large collecting ducts that converge under the nipple (Figure 15-2). The alveoli proliferate during pregnancy. They are lined by cuboidal epithelial cells, which produce milk under the influence of PRL. The alveoli are surrounded by myoepithelial cells, and the contraction of these muscle cells causes ejection of the milk in the alveoli into the ducts. A symphony of hormones is necessary for breast enlargement and for priming of lactation during pregnancy. Estrogen, progesterone, insulin, growth hormone, adrenal steroids, PRL, TSH, and ACTH are required for breast development. Each breast enlarges by approximately 0.5 kg during pregnancy.

ROLE OF PROLACTIN (PRL)

PRL is the main hormonal support of lactation. It is a polypeptide consisting of 198 amino acids held together by three disulfide bonds. It is made in the lactotroph cells of the anterior pituitary. In nonpregnant women PRL secretion is kept tonically suppressed by dopamine from the hypothalamus.

The rise in PRL production during pregnancy probably is due to the inhibition of dopamine by estrogen. Unlike many other peptide hormones, PRL does not use the cyclic adenosine monophosphate (cAMP) pathway. It binds to a membrane receptor on breast alveolar cells and passes directly into nuclear and cytoplasmic sites where it stimulates production of the milk protein casein.

Although PRL levels rise early and dramatically under the influence of estrogen, milk production does not occur during pregnancy because estrogen and progesterone block the interaction of PRL with its receptors on alveolar cell membranes (Figure 15-1). The fluid produced and stored in the breast during pregnancy is colostrum, a thick mixture composed of desquamated epithelial cells, lymphocytes, and transudate.

At term, with delivery of the placenta, estrogen and progesterone levels fall dramatically, and lactation can begin. Usually milk production begins within 3 days of delivery.

In the nonpregnant state, the lactotrophs make up 10%–25% of the pituitary, and PRL production is tonically suppressed by dopamine. During pregnancy, PRL levels rise as much as 20–40-fold, and up to 70% of the pituitary gland is involved in synthesis of PRL.

During pregnancy, milk production is suppressed by estrogen and progesterone.

FIGURE 15-2
ANATOMY OF THE BREAST. A cluster of alveoli showing alveolar and myoepithelial cells.

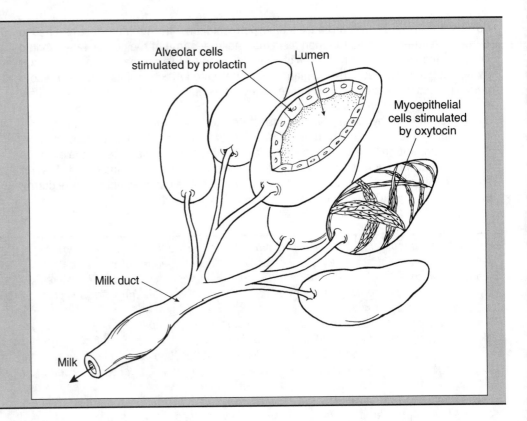

Suckling on the breast activates sensory receptors and transmission of impulses via thoracic nerves (usually T_4, T_5, and T_6) to the spinal cord and to the hypothalamus. Dopamine secretion is suppressed. This results in release of stored PRL from the anterior pituitary (Figure 15-3). The PRL level can increase 10–20 fold. PRL released during suckling stimulates milk production in the breast for 3–4 hours, allowing alveolar cells to replenish the milk supply.

Over time, PRL levels fall even in women who continue to breastfeed. Nevertheless, a rise in PRL still occurs with each episode of breastfeeding. Even at 6 months after delivery PRL levels are higher than nonpregnant levels and increase two-fold with suck-

FIGURE 15-3
NEURAL RESPONSES TO SUCKLING RESULTING IN PROLACTIN SECRETION FROM THE PITUITARY GLAND.

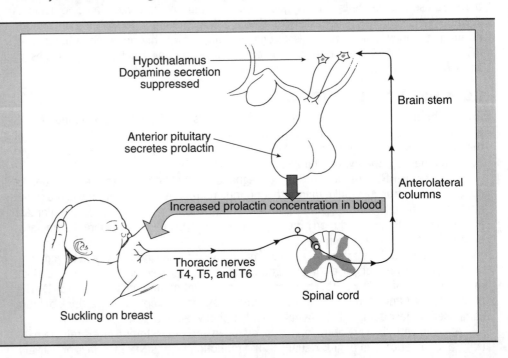

ling. If a woman does not breastfeed, PRL levels fall immediately after delivery and within approximately 1 month are back to nonpregnant levels.

PRL is found in ovarian follicle fluid, in the lining of the pregnant uterus, and in amniotic fluid. In other species, PRL plays a role in osmotic regulation. Some studies suggest that the very high PRL concentrations in amniotic fluid help to maintain fetal water balance until squamous epithelium develops, and fetal skin becomes impermeable to water.

ROLE OF OXYTOCIN

Suckling on the areola stimulates afferent nerves running with thoracic nerves T4, T5, and T6, and impulses are transmitted to the spinal cord and the hypothalamus. Oxytocin, a peptide produced in the supraoptic and paraventricular nuclei of the hypothalamus, is then released into the circulation from the posterior pituitary (see Chapter 3). Oxytocin stimulates contraction of the myoepithelial cells surrounding breast alveoli, causing milk to be expressed into the nipple. The infant's tongue strokes the nipple from back to front, stripping the milk out of the nipple. Initially, the oxytocin level is elevated only during the time of actual breastfeeding. However, after women have been breastfeeding for a time, central nervous system (CNS) effects also can cause oxytocin secretion. Hearing an infant cry can be sufficient stimulation for oxytocin release.

Oxytocin receptors also are found in the uterus. Oxytocin increases the frequency and strength of uterine contractions. Estrogen potentiates the action of oxytocin by altering membrane potentials of uterine smooth muscle cells. The uterus is especially sensitive to oxytocin at the end of pregnancy when the estrogen levels are very high. Dilation of the lower uterus, cervix and vagina during delivery also stimulates oxytocin secretion. In the postpartum period, a woman who is breastfeeding may experience uterine contractions. Oxytocin-induced muscle contraction helps the uterus return to its normal size and reduces postpartum bleeding.

> Milk release from the breast is due primarily to suckling-induced release of the hormone oxytocin.

COMPOSITION OF BREAST MILK

Breast milk is the ideal energy source for the growing newborn. It is digestible, sterile, always the correct temperature, and contains immunoglobulins that provide protection against many illnesses in the first few months of life. It provides 20 kcal/oz, which is the caloric equivalent of whole cow's milk. Breast milk has a high fat content, with approximately 1.3 g/oz (30 cc). The fat content gradually increases for up to 3 months after delivery. The milk from the breast at the end of a breastfeeding session has a higher fat content than the earlier milk. This may trigger satiety in the infant when most of the milk has been extracted from that feeding. Preterm milk contains more protein, lower lactose, and more essential long-chain fatty acids than term milk, making it ideal for preterm infants needing more brain growth than term infants.

The main proteins of human milk are very easily absorbed by the newborn. The main sugar of milk is lactose, a combination of glucose and galactose. IgA is present in colostrum and breast milk and helps to protect the infant's mucosal surfaces from infection. Immunocompetent cells are also present in breast milk and help boost neonatal immunologic defenses. Iron is available in very small amounts in breast milk, but its bioavailability is so great that levels are as high in breastfed infants as in infants fed iron-fortified formula.

> Breastfed infants have fewer gastrointestinal illnesses, food allergies, and ear infections in the first year of life.

Maternal nutrition during lactation should include 1500 mg calcium daily from dairy products or other foods or supplements. Maternal iron supplementation often is required during breastfeeding, although adequate dietary intake is possible with attention to iron-rich foods. Drugs taken by the mother are transported into breast milk mainly by passive diffusion, but lipid solubility, ionization, and protein binding affect the concentration in breast milk. Lactic acid, which accumulates after heavy exercise, and alcohol also are transported into breast milk. Many women note aversion of the newborn to breastfeeding after maternal alcohol ingestion or vigorous exercise. Nicotine decreases milk production.

SUSTAINING LACTATION

There is a synergism between breastfeeding and milk production that allows increased milk production as the infant grows. The more an infant suckles, the more milk a woman produces. Supplementation of breastfeeding with formula or food can decrease the infant's suckling frequency and intensity very quickly. This diminishes milk supply and results in greater hunger for exogenous nutritional sources by the infant. Only with long-standing breastfeeding can milk production be maintained if feedings are decreased to only once or twice a day.

Breastfeeding can be maintained for several years after birth. Occasionally women breastfeed through a subsequent pregnancy, although this is uncommon in the United States. Only 50% of women in the United States are breastfeeding when they are discharged from the hospital, and by 6 months after delivery only 5% of all women are still breastfeeding.

Motivation to breastfeed is culturally influenced to a large extent. Maternal infections and medications also may limit lactation. Other barriers to lactation are listed in Table 15-4.

Table 15-4
Barriers to Lactation
	Maternal
	  Cultural
	  Infection
	  Medications
	Neonatal
	  Marked prematurity
	  Hypotonia
	  Ventilator support
	  Congenital malformations

Human immunodeficiency virus (HIV) is transmitted in breast milk, and in the United States, breastfeeding is not recommended for HIV-positive women. The World Health Organization does not discourage breastfeeding among HIV-positive women internationally, since infants in Third World countries are more likely to die of diarrheal disease if they are not breastfeeding, than of HIV infection if they are breastfeeding. Maternal hepatitis B virus (HBV) infection is not a contraindication to lactation, as long as the newborn receives passive prophylaxis for HBV shortly after delivery and begins the primary immunization series against the virus while in the hospital.

Breastfeeding is contraindicated in women taking cocaine or methadone, which are transferred into breast milk. Tetracyclines can cause staining of baby teeth and permanent teeth. Quinoline antibiotics can cause disordered growth of the cartilaginous epiphyses during the first year of life.

Infant barriers to suckling include marked prematurity, hypotonia, congenital malformations such as facial clefts, and need for ventilator support.

Pharmacologic suppression of lactation with bromocriptine, a dopamine agonist that blocks PRL release, is no longer approved by the Food and Drug Administration because of the side effects (hypertension, seizures, strokes, nausea). Failure to complete a full 2-week course of the drug can result in rebound breast engorgement. When women do not wish to breastfeed, firm support of the breasts and ice packs are used for the discomfort of breast engorgement. Breast stimulation should be avoided. The pressure stasis of not breastfeeding causes prompt cessation of new milk production.

Estrogen can be used to suppress lactation. Estrogen releases dopamine inhibition, causing PRL levels to rise, but at the breast alveolar cell level, estrogen antagonizes PRL action.

LACTATION AND CONTRACEPTION

Breastfeeding is a low estrogen state. The high PRL level suppresses pulsatile GnRH secretion, and FSH and LH levels are tonically reduced to the low-normal range. Estrogen production is decreased, and ovulation is suppressed. Lactation is an effective contraceptive from the standpoint of large populations where breastfeeding is common. However, in a given individual, return of ovulatory function is unpredictable, and lactation is not a dependable method of contraception. As breastfeeding frequency wanes, baseline

PRL levels fall. Eventually only a small peak is seen with each breastfeeding episode. Ovulation may occur and will precede the return of menses. In general, the period of anovulation during breastfeeding lasts longer when maternal nutrition is poor.

Hormonal contraception during lactation is highly effective, but estrogen-containing pills can decrease milk production and should not be prescribed until several months after breastfeeding is well established. A progesterone-only contraceptive is a good choice while breastfeeding. Progesterone does antagonize PRL binding to its receptors on breast alveolar cells, but the doses used in these contraceptives are too low to have much effect. Barrier methods of contraception such as diaphragms or condoms do not interfere with breastfeeding, but they are less effective than hormonal contraception.

The patient breastfed her daughter for 6 months and experienced amenorrhea during that time. Since she became pregnant while breastfeeding her first child and using a barrier method of contraception, she decided to use a progesterone-only contraceptive while breastfeeding her second child. Her risk for developing diabetes in the future is increased because she is moderately obese and she has a family history of diabetes. After she finished breastfeeding her daughter, the patient was given a modest weight reduction diet. Her exercise level increased as she coped with the demands of her job and two small children.

Case Study:
Resolution

■ REVIEW QUESTIONS

Directions: For each of the following questions, choose the **one best** answer.

1. A 34-year-old woman's last menstrual period began 9 weeks ago. She is fatigued and nauseated, and she has lost 3 lbs in the past few weeks. Primary evaluation should consist of

   (A) urine human chorionic gonadotropin test
   (B) thyroid-stimulating hormone and total thyroxine tests
   (C) oral glucose tolerance test
   (D) follicle-stimulating hormone (FSH) test

2. The early pregnancy is maintained by

   (A) maternal gonadotropin-releasing hormone (GnRH)
   (B) human chorionic gonadotropin (HCG) from the endometrium
   (C) progesterone from the corpus luteum
   (D) luteinizing hormone (LH) from the developing fetal pituitary

3. Which of the following conditions is due to the effects of progesterone during pregnancy?

   (A) Increased reflux esophagitis
   (B) Peripheral vasodilation
   (C) Increased cardiac output
   (D) Decreased facial acne

4. A 22-year-old woman volunteers for a study of hormonal adaptation during the third trimester of pregnancy. She previously has been well except for mild hypothyroidism, which was treated with thyroid hormone replacement. If her pregnancy is progressing normally, the physician would be most likely to expect which of the following?

   (A) Increased fasting plasma glucose and decreased postprandial glucose and insulin levels
   (B) Decreased thyroid size and a decreased requirement for thyroid hormone replacement
   (C) Increasing prolactin (PRL) levels and post-peak levels of human chorionic gonadotropin (HCG)
   (D) Decreasing levels of estrogen and progesterone

5. A woman wishes to breastfeed her infant. Forty-eight hours after delivery she still has no milk production. Her infant has lost 5% of his initial birthweight. She is reassured when told that it usually takes 3 days for prolactin (PRL) to stimulate milk production in breast alveolar cells and that infants often lose up to 10% of their body weight before milk production begins. If she continues to be unable to lactate, the cause is most likely to be

   (A) a low estrogen level after delivery of the placenta
   (B) a low RRL level due to postpartum pituitary infarction
   (C) a low progesterone level after delivery of the placenta
   (D) a low oxytocin level due to excessive suckling

■ ANSWERS AND EXPLANATIONS

1. The answer is A. Pregnancy testing is mandatory in a premenopausal woman who presents with amenorrhea. Her complaints of fatigue, nausea, and weight loss are compatible with hyperthyroidism, but even if she had more compelling signs of hyperthyroidism such as tachycardia, proptosis, and lid lag, pregnancy must be excluded. Fatigue and nausea also can be presenting signs of diabetes, but in the absence of polyuria and polydipsia or ketosis, a pregnancy test should be done first. An oral glucose tolerance test would not be the first step in an evaluation for diabetes in any case (see Chapter 8). Evaluation for ovarian failure with measurement of FSH is not indicated unless pregnancy has been excluded and there are other symptoms or signs of premature ovarian failure.

2. The answer is C. Early pregnancy is maintained by progesterone. Withdrawal of progesterone from the estrogen-primed endometrium results in bleeding and loss of the newly implanted blastocyst. HCG is made in the *trophoblast* not the endometrium. HCG stimulates progesterone production, but it is the progesterone from the corpus luteum that maintains the early pregnancy until the placenta can make enough progesterone to take over this function. Maternal GnRH pulses are suppressed by negative feedback from the high progesterone levels during pregnancy. Maternal LH and FSH also are suppressed to the low-normal range during pregnancy. The fetal pituitary has not developed into a hormone-secreting gland early in pregnancy.

3. The answer is A. Estrogen causes marked systemic peripheral vasodilation during pregnancy. A compensatory increase in cardiac output then occurs as a response to decreased afterload. Facial acne is often ameliorated in pregnancy because estrogen-induced peripheral vasodilatation increases blood supply to the skin. Progesterone has generalized effects on smooth muscle, decreasing its tone. Progesterone-induced relaxation of the lower esophageal sphincter is most likely responsible for the frequent complaints of heartburn during pregnancy.

4. The answer is C. Fasting plasma glucose is lower during pregnancy, and postprandial glucose levels are higher due to postprandial insulin resistance. Hypothyroidism often worsens and requirements for thyroxine replacement are higher during pregnancy. The thyroid gland often is mildly enlarged during pregnancy. PRL levels increase throughout pregnancy, but HCG levels peak during the first trimester. After the placenta matures, HCG no longer is required to sustain progesterone production. Estrogen and progesterone levels are high until delivery of the placenta.

5. The answer is B. Postpartum pituitary infarction (Sheehan's syndrome) is likely to present as failure of lactation because the pituitary gland is unable to secrete PRL. During pregnancy, high levels of estrogen and progesterone inhibit PRL action on the breast. Estrogen and progesterone levels must drop, as they do after delivery, for milk production to occur. Newborn suckling stimulates milk production and letdown by stimulating both PRL and oxytocin secretion.

■ REFERENCES

Baird DT, Glasier AF: Hormonal contraception. *N Engl J Med* 328:1543–1549, 1993.

Buchanan TA: Glucose metabolism during pregnancy: normal physiology and implications for diabetes mellitus. *Israel J Med Sci* 27:432–444, 1991.

Burrow GN: The management of thyrotoxicosis in pregnancy. *N Engl J Med* 313:5762–5765, 1985.

Burrow GN, Fisher DA, Larsen PR: Maternal and fetal thyroid function. *N Engl J Med* 331:1072–1078, 1994.

Freed GL, Clark SJ, Sorenson J, et al: National assessment of physicians' breastfeeding knowledge, attitudes, training, and experience. *JAMA* 273:472–476, 1995.

Garner P: Type I diabetes and pregnancy. *Lancet* 346:157–161, 1995.

Hyman BT, Tanzi R: Management of gestational diabetes mellitus. *N Engl J Med* 333:1281–1283, 1995.

Larsen RP: Maternal thyroxine and congenital hypothyroidism. *N Engl J Med* 321:44–46, 1989.

INDEX

NOTE: An f after a page number denotes a figure; a t after a page number denotes a table.